SPEECH SOUNDS

A Pictorial Guide to Typical and Atypical Speech

SPEECH SOUNDS

A Pictorial Guide to Typical and Atypical Speech

Sharynne McLeod, Ph.D.
Sadanand Singh, Ph.D.

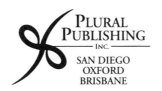

PLURAL
PUBLISHING
INC.

SAN DIEGO
OXFORD
BRISBANE

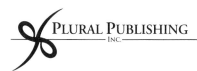

5521 Ruffin Road
San Diego, CA 92123

e-mail: info@pluralpublishing.com
Web site: http://www.pluralpublishing.com

49 Bath Street
Abingdon, Oxfordshire OX14 1EA
United Kingdom

Library of Congress Cataloging-in-Publication Data:
McLeod, Sharynne.
  Speech sounds : a pictorial guide to typical and atypical speech / Sharynne McLeod and Sadanand Singh.
       p. ; cm.
  Includes bibliographical references and index.
  ISBN-13: 978-1-59756-106-8 (alk. paper)
  ISBN-10: 1-59756-106-1 (alk. paper)
 1. Speech—Atlases. 2. English language—Phonetics—Atlases. 3. Mouth—Atlases. 4. Speech disorders—Atlases.
  [DNLM: 1. Phonetics—Pictorial Works. 2. Speech—physiology—Pictorial Works. 3. Speech Disorders—physiopathology—Pictorial Works. WV 17 M478s 2007] I. Singh, Sadanand. II. Title.
  QP306.M353 2007
  612.7'80223—dc22
                                                                    2007052273

Contents

Foreword

Speech sounds have intrigued me since I first read about phonetics while I was a high school student. I did not expect then that I would pursue a career in which the sounds of speech would have a central and continuing place. I still marvel over the way in which thoughts and emotions are sent from one person to another through the invisible channel of sound. Having taught phonetics and speech science, I am familiar with the challenge of cataloging and describing the sounds of speech. Although we call them "speech sounds" they are not only sounds (auditory events), because they also can be described as articulatory actions that correlate with a certain auditory impression. Speech movements, like auditory events, are largely invisible without the aid of specialized technology. To understand phonetics, we must make visible those things that are usually invisible. We want to visualize the acoustic pattern that underlies the perception of speech along with the articulatory pattern that underlies the acoustic one. Only in this way do we come to a reasonably complete understanding of phonetics. So we come to rely on the tools of the speech scientist or phonetician, because these tools enable us to visualize the acoustic and articulatory domains of phonetics.

However, the array of available tools has not been brought to bear on the subject of speech sounds, at least not until the appearance of McLeod and Singh's ambitious and painstaking text, which documents speech sounds with the methods of cinematography, ultrasound, electropalatography, and spectrography. The rich descriptions afforded by these tools enable the student of phonetics or speech science to grasp the essence of speech sounds—how they are molded in the vocal tract and how they are expressed as acoustic patterns. The success of this text is proof of the adage that the whole is greater than the sum of its parts. Certainly, the sum of the parts is important enough, but a synthesis of the parts gives us the whole, in this case, the manifold nature of a speech sound. McLeod and Singh have marshaled phonetic tools and knowledge to create an authoritative yet friendly text that guides the reader through the phonetic landscape of the sounds of English. *Speech Sounds: A Pictorial Guide to Typical and Atypical Speech* offers a comprehensive and lucid examination of the elements of speech.

With this book, speech sounds come into view (literally) as articulatory and acoustic images. This new text is a resource that is unrivaled among phonetics or speech science books, and it sets a standard for the use of technology to reveal the essential nature of the sounds that are the substance of speech communication.

Ray D. Kent, Ph.D.
Professor Emeritus
University of Wisconsin-Madison

Preface

Speech Sounds: A Pictorial Guide to Typical and Atypical Speech contains maps of the mouth. Literally, an atlas is a collection of maps in book form; so this book contains a collection of images or maps that have captured different aspects of the production of the consonants and vowels of English. As an atlas highlights topographies and landmarks, this book highlights relevant articulatory and acoustic aspects for the production for each English speech sound.

Each chapter profiles a different English consonant or vowel. There are 24 chapters to describe each English consonant and 11 chapters to describe most English vowels and diphthongs. Analytic comments are presented for each. These comments focus on key dimensions of speech production and speech acoustics that differentiate one speech sound from another. Within each chapter there are different representations for the profiled speech sound organized according to static and dynamic representations. The static representations include:

- a photograph of the lower portion of the face,
- a schematic drawing of tongue position (created by superimposing ultrasound images onto a midsagittal image of the face),
- an ultrasound image of the tongue, and
- electropalatographic images of tongue/palate contact.

Dynamic representations profile words containing each speech sound and include:

- a filmstrip,
- sound spectrogram, and
- continuous electropalatographic frames of tongue/palate contact.

For each of the lingual consonants, multiple images demonstrating inter- and intraspeaker variability also are included. These images have been compiled from a comprehensive research project (McLeod, 2003) of eight typical English adults' productions of lingual speech sounds in word-initial and word-final contexts within five vowel environments.

An important feature of *Speech Sounds: A Pictorial Guide to Typical and Atypical Speech* is that data from an extensive range of research papers have been assembled to demonstrate similarities and differences between productions of speech sounds by adults and children, speakers of different English dialects, speakers of languages other than English, and people with impaired speech. Images from research papers have been redrawn using the same template so that extensive comparisons can be made. EPG Images from an extensive range of characteristics of people are found within *Speech Sounds: A Pictorial Guide to Typical and Atypical Speech*:

- English dialects: Australian, Canadian, English, Scottish, United States
- Languages other than English: Catalan, German, Greek, Japanese, Norwegian, Polish, Putonghua (Modern Standard Chinese)
- Impairments: cerebral palsy, cleft palate, Down syndrome, articulation and phonological delay and disorder ("speech impairment"), lateral lisp, hearing impairment, Parkinson's disease.

As many images as possible are included in each chapter. As discussed in Chapter 1, researchers have focused more on some speech sounds than on others. Consequently, the diversity of images in each chapter reflects the focus of the world's speech researchers. Chapters that contain numerous comparative images include Chapter 4, which focuses on /t/, and Chapter 15, which focuses on /s/.

Readers (viewers) are advised to examine each chapter in detail, first one at a time and then comparatively. Chapter 37 has been designed to facilitate comparison of images of consonants and vowels by presenting the same representation type for every consonant or every vowel highlighted in this book.

For example, there is one table of all the ultrasound images and other tables of all the electropalatography images. Additionally a companion flip chart enables ready comparison of key images for each consonant and vowel. This flip chart will be of particular importance for speech-language pathologists working with adults and children to change their articulation of sounds and for students of phonetics as they develop an understanding of the similarities and differences between sounds. The flip chart is McLeod and Singh's *Seeing Speech: A Quick Guide to Speech Sounds*.

Chapter 1 provides explanatory material for the interpretation of each image or map, whereas Chapter 38 provides extensive detail regarding the creation of the images included in the *Speech Sounds: A Pictorial Guide to Typical and Atypical Speech*. Finally, Chapter 39 provides exercises to assist students' understanding of the content.

This book will be of interest to speech-language pathologists, phoneticians, linguists, teachers, people who have a non-English speaking background, and students of these disciplines. For those who require further explanatory detail, a companion book that elucidates the theory underpinning *Speech Sounds: A Pictorial Guide to Typical and Atypical Speech* is S. Singh and K. Singh (2006) *Phonetics: Principles and Practice* (3rd ed., San Diego, CA: Plural). Additional complementary texts are listed in References at the end of the text.

Acknowledgments

First, thank you to Dr. Sadanand Singh who created and analyzed the excellent filmstrips, line drawings, and spectrographs of speech sounds. It has been a great pleasure to work with such a renowned person in our profession.

Preparation of this book was supported by a British Academy Visiting Fellowship that enabled the first author to spend time at Queen Margaret University, Edinburgh (QMU). Thanks are extended to everyone in Speech and Hearing Sciences at QMU, who were extremely supportive, provided excellent advice, and facilitated the creation of the single electropalatographic (EPG) and ultrasound images for this book. Dr. Alan Wrench from Articulate Instruments and Professors Fiona E. Gibbon, William J. Hardcastle, and Dr. Jim Scobbie from QMU deserve special mention.

Support for the recording of the single and cumulative electropalatographic images of the eight Australian adults was provided by a Charles Sturt University competitive grant. Special thanks to the eight volunteers who, prior to the recordings, had no contact with speech-language pathology. Each participant agreed to go to the dentist to have a dental impression made, and then wore an electropalatographic palate while making the speech recordings for an extended period of time, all in the name of science. The comprehensiveness of the data these eight volunteers provided is an important feature of this book. Thanks also to Amber Roberts who painstakingly analyzed these electropalatographic images.

Thanks are extended to all the speech scientists, phoneticians, and speech-language pathologists who undertook extensive research in order to demonstrate typical and impaired speech production. The richness of their data has been redrawn so that EPG images can be compared across speakers and languages.

Finally, my family has constantly supported and accompanied me throughout the meticulous process of compiling this book. Thank you David, Brendon, and Jessica.

Sharynne McLeod
Bathurst, Australia

About the Authors

Sharynne McLeod, Ph.D. /ʃæɹən məklaʊd/

Dr. McLeod is Professor in speech and language acquisition at Charles Sturt University, Australia. She is the Vice President of the International Clinical Linguistics and Phonetics Association and a Fellow of both the American Speech-Language-Hearing Association and Speech Pathology Australia. Professor McLeod is editor of the *International Journal of Speech-Language Pathology* (informa) (www.informaworld.com/ijslp) and on the editorial board of *Clinical Linguistics and Phonetics* (informa). She has edited a landmark book titled *The International Guide to Speech Acquisition* (Thomson Delmar) and has been invited as a speaker at a number of American Speech-Language-Hearing Association and other international conventions.

Sadanand Singh, Ph.D. /sədanænd sɪŋ/

Dr. Singh is a Fellow of the American Speech-Hearing-Language Association (ASHA) and an active member and contributor to the direction of that organization. Currently Chairman of Plural Publishing, Inc., which specializes in the communication sciences, he has been a Professor at Ohio State University, Professor and Department Chair at Howard University, Professor and Director at the University of Texas Health Science program, and Professor and Chairman of the Communicative Disorders Department at San Diego State University. He also has served on advisory boards with leading scientists, clinicians, and professors in several areas of key academic and clinical concentration. Dr. Singh has authored undergraduate and graduate texts in phonetics, phonology, measurements, and clinical procedures.

THE INTERNATIONAL PHONETIC ALPHABET (revised to 2005)

CONSONANTS (PULMONIC)

	Bilabial	Labiodental	Dental	Alveolar	Postalveolar	Retroflex	Palatal	Velar	Uvular	Pharyngeal	Glottal
Plosive	p b			t d		ʈ ɖ	c ɟ	k ɡ	q ɢ		ʔ
Nasal	m	ɱ		n		ɳ	ɲ	ŋ	N		
Trill	B			r					R		
Tap or Flap		ⱱ		ɾ		ɽ					
Fricative	ɸ β	f v	θ ð	s z	ʃ ʒ	ʂ ʐ	ç ʝ	x ɣ	χ ʁ	ħ ʕ	h ɦ
Lateral fricative				ɬ ɮ							
Approximant		ʋ		ɹ		ɻ	j	ɰ			
Lateral approximant				l		ɭ	ʎ	L			

Where symbols appear in pairs, the one to the right represents a voiced consonant. Shaded areas denote articulations judged impossible.

CONSONANTS (NON-PULMONIC)

Clicks		Voiced implosives		Ejectives	
ʘ	Bilabial	ɓ	Bilabial	ʼ	Examples:
ǀ	Dental	ɗ	Dental/alveolar	pʼ	Bilabial
ǃ	(Post)alveolar	ʄ	Palatal	tʼ	Dental/alveolar
ǂ	Palatoalveolar	ɠ	Velar	kʼ	Velar
ǁ	Alveolar lateral	ʛ	Uvular	sʼ	Alveolar fricative

OTHER SYMBOLS

ʍ	Voiceless labial-velar fricative	ɕ ʑ	Alveolo-palatal fricatives
w	Voiced labial-velar approximant	ɺ	Voiced alveolar lateral flap
ɥ	Voiced labial-palatal approximant	ɧ	Simultaneous ʃ and x
ʜ	Voiceless epiglottal fricative		
ʢ	Voiced epiglottal fricative	Affricates and double articulations can be represented by two symbols joined by a tie bar if necessary.	k͡p t͡s
ʡ	Epiglottal plosive		

VOWELS

Where symbols appear in pairs, the one to the right represents a rounded vowel.

SUPRASEGMENTALS

ˈ	Primary stress	ˌfoʊnəˈtɪʃən
ˌ	Secondary stress	
ː	Long	eː
ˑ	Half-long	eˑ
̆	Extra-short	ĕ
ǀ	Minor (foot) group	
ǁ	Major (intonation) group	
.	Syllable break	ɹi.ækt
‿	Linking (absence of a break)	

DIACRITICS

Diacritics may be placed above a symbol with a descender, e.g. ŋ̊

̥	Voiceless	n̥ d̥	̤	Breathy voiced	b̤ a̤	̪ Dental	t̪ d̪
̬	Voiced	s̬ t̬	̰	Creaky voiced	b̰ a̰	̺ Apical	t̺ d̺
ʰ	Aspirated	tʰ dʰ	̼	Linguolabial	t̼ d̼	̻ Laminal	t̻ d̻
̹	More rounded	ɔ̹	ʷ	Labialized	tʷ dʷ	̃ Nasalized	ẽ
̜	Less rounded	ɔ̜	ʲ	Palatalized	tʲ dʲ	ⁿ Nasal release	dⁿ
̟	Advanced	u̟	ˠ	Velarized	tˠ dˠ	ˡ Lateral release	dˡ
̠	Retracted	e̠	ˤ	Pharyngealized	tˤ dˤ	̚ No audible release	d̚
̈	Centralized	ë	̴	Velarized or pharyngealized	ɫ		
̽	Mid-centralized	e̽	̝	Raised	e̝ (ɹ̝ = voiced alveolar fricative)		
̩	Syllabic	n̩	̞	Lowered	e̞ (β̞ = voiced bilabial approximant)		
̯	Non-syllabic	e̯	̘	Advanced Tongue Root	e̘		
˞	Rhoticity	ɚ a˞	̙	Retracted Tongue Root	e̙		

TONES AND WORD ACCENTS

LEVEL			CONTOUR		
e̋ or ˥	Extra high		ě or ˩˥	Rising	
é ˦	High		ê ˥˩	Falling	
ē ˧	Mid		e᷄ ˦˥	High rising	
è ˨	Low		e᷅ ˩˨	Low rising	
ȅ ˩	Extra low		e᷈ ˧˩˧	Rising-falling	
↓	Downstep		↗	Global rise	
↑	Upstep		↘	Global fall	

Courtesy of the International Phonetic Association (c/o Department of Theoretical and Applied Linguistics, School of English, Aristotle University of Thessaloniki, Thessaloniki 54124, GREECE)

Chapter 1

Visualizing Speech Sounds

OVERVIEW

As an atlas provides maps of the world demonstrating topography and landmarks, *Speech Sounds: A Pictorial Guide to Typical and Atypical Speech* provides images (or maps) of the mouth for the production of speech sounds. These maps have been created using cinematography, ultrasound, electropalatography, and spectrography. Interpretation of each of the types of maps is described in depth in Part 1 of this chapter. An understanding of phonetic transcription and the International Phonetic Alphabet will assist users' understanding of the nomenclature used to describe vowels and consonants in this book. The International Phonetic Alphabet is provided in the front material of *Speech Sounds: A Pictorial Guide to Typical and Atypical Speech*.

The production of speech sounds occurs by movement of air through the human respiratory and speech apparatus (Figure 1–1). The major anatomic structures involved in speech production are the tongue, lips, teeth, hard palate, velum (soft palate), larynx (vocal folds), nasal cavity, mandible (jaw), and lungs. Different configurations of these structures result in the production of discrete consonants and vowels. In the English language there are 24 consonants and at least 19 vowels and diphthongs. Each consonant can be differentiated according to their place of production, manner of production, and whether they are voiced or voiceless. Each vowel can be differentiated according to the advancement and height of the tongue, and tenseness and roundedness of the lips. Part 2 of this chapter describes these features of consonants and vowels in depth. Readers who have prior knowledge of phonetics may wish to skip Part 2 and continue to Chapter 2. Each subsequent chapter profiles a different English consonant or vowel.

Speech-language pathologists (SLPs) frequently assess and provide intervention to "correct" the production of speech sounds. Inaccurate productions of speech sounds often are difficult to alter in therapy. This may be due to an absence of objective knowledge regarding the tongue positioning involved in the production of speech sounds (Gibbon, 1999b). Much of the information used within speech-language pathology clinics regarding typical production of speech sounds is based on perceptual analysis techniques such as impressionistic phonetic transcription. Weismer (1980, p. 50) indicates "if we are committed to a phonological analysis of speech sound errors; however, an analysis that relies solely on auditory skills is unacceptable." The description of speech can be enhanced using instrumental techniques such as photographs, filmstrips, spectrography, electropalatography (EPG), ultrasound, electromagnetic articulography (EMA), x-ray, and medical resonance imaging (MRI) (Ball et al., 2001; Hardcastle & Gibbon, 1997; Stone, 2005). These instrumental measures provide objective and detailed, real-time information about speech production. The next part of this chapter enables the interpretation of images created by the different instrumental techniques.

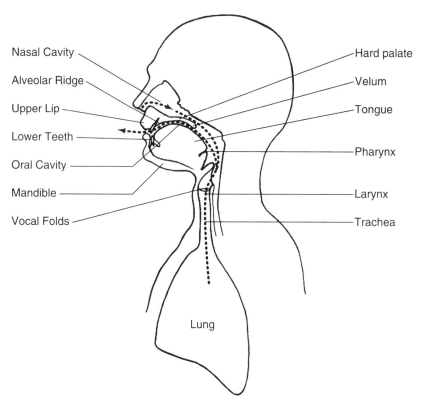

Nasal Cavity

Alveolar Ridge

Upper Lip

Lower Teeth

Oral Cavity

Mandible

Vocal Folds

Hard palate

Velum

Tongue

Pharynx

Larynx

Trachea

Lung

Figure 1–1. Human respiratory and speech apparatus (*Source:* Singh, S. and Singh, K. [2006]. *Phonetics: Principles and Practice* 9 [3rd ed.]. San Diego, CA: Plural. Figure 4–3c, p. 48).

PART 1: INTERPRETATION OF IMAGES OF CONSONANTS AND VOWELS

Each instrumental technique provides different insights into the production of consonants and vowels (see Table 1-1 for an overview). It can be seen from Table 1-1 that in order to comprehensively map speech sounds, a variety of imaging techniques are necessary. Images of speech sounds can either be static or dynamic. A static image is one distinctive image that is frozen in time and captures the most significant aspects of the consonant or vowel being studied. However, speech is a continuous stream of sound created by continuous movement of the oromusculature. As a result, it is not enough to segment speech into discrete units. Dynamic images, which demonstrate continuous production, are essential for understanding the contextual coarticulatory influences of consonants and vowels on one another. Thus, dynamic images typically consist of a series of frames extending over the production of an entire sound, word, or phrase. The purpose of *Speech Sounds: A Pictorial Guide to Typical and Atypical Speech* is to make available the direct viewing of the phenomenon of speech production to facilitate a thorough understanding of the differences and similarities in the articulation of consonants and vowels produced under varying contextual influences.

The presentation of the total picture of phoneme production in context is contained within Chapters 2 through 36. With certain limitations, each chapter is a self-contained, complete story of a sound of speech as it is being produced. There are 24 chapters depicting the English consonants, 10 chapters depicting vowels, and one chapter for the diphthongs. Analytic comments are presented in each chapter. These comments focus on dimensions of speech production and speech acoustics that the authors consider important. The readers (viewers) are advised to examine them in detail, first one at a time and then comparatively. Chapter 37

Table 1–1. Features of Consonants and Vowels Viewed Using Different Technologies

	Feature	Photograph	Filmstrip	Schematic diagram	Ultrasound	Electropalatograph (EPG)	Spectrogram	Waveform	X-ray	Magnetic Resonance Imaging (MRI)
Consonants	Voicing			*			*	*		
	Advancement				*	*			*	*
	Labiality	*	*	*						
	Sonorancy						*	*		
	Continuancy						*	(*)		
	Sibilancy						*			
	Nasality			*			*			
Vowels	Advancement				*	*			*	*
	Height				*				*	*
	Tenseness	*	*							
	Rounding	*	*							
	Voicing						*	*		

assists in comparing images by placing similar imaging techniques side-by-side in tables of consonants and vowels. Chapter 38 provides detailed information about the creation of the static and dynamic images of speech production in this book.

INTERPRETING STATIC IMAGES OF CONSONANTS AND VOWELS

In Chapters 2 through 36, static images are presented to depict speech sounds in isolation. Each chapter contains at least 4 different static representations of a given speech sound: (1) photograph, (2) schematic drawing of tongue position, (3) ultrasound, and (4) electropalatography frame(s). Interpretation of each of these image types is described in turn.

Photographs

The photographs emphasize the front, or outside, of the mouth. They provide detail regarding the placement of the lips, teeth, jaw, and in some cases, the tongue at a single moment during the production of a consonant or vowel.

Schematic Line Drawings

Schematic line drawings are provided to visualize the overall function of the tongue—its elasticity, its flexibility, and its limits—all of which contribute to its systematic movements in the oral cavity. The line drawing accompanying each chapter emphasizes the position of the tongue during the production of a particular consonant or vowel. The voicing of a phoneme is indicated by the use of a plus or minus sign at the approximate point of the larynx. In most images, the velopharyngeal port is closed, indicating oral airflow. However, in the line drawings for /m, n, ŋ/ the velopharyngeal port is open.

The schematic diagrams are extremely simplified. The tongue shapes are based on ultrasound images of the tongue during the production of each sound in connected speech. The schematic diagrams were created by superimposing these ultrasound images of the tongue onto a template of the nasooropharynx (see Chapter 38).

It is also important to note that the schematic diagrams represent only the midsagittal plane, that is, the midline of the body. Consequently, detail regarding the lateral margins of tongue movement is not included. This can lead to the misconception that the sides of the tongue are in similar configuration to the midline. This is particularly relevant in the production of alveolar sounds. For example, during the production of the following alveolar sounds, the midpoint of the tongue is raised to the alveolar ridge: /t, d, n, s, z, l/; However, comparison between the schematic line drawings and the electropalatography (EPG) images reveals that it is only the /l/ sound that has a similar shape along the lateral margins of the palate. For the other five sounds, the sides of the tongue are raised to rest near the teeth in order to provide lateral bracing.

Ultrasound

Ultrasound enables us to view the surface of the tongue during speech. To create an ultrasound a transducer is held below the chin and a wedge-shaped scan of sound waves emanates from the transducer. The sound waves travel through the body of the tongue until they reach the upper tongue surface. The white line on the ultrasound image is a reflection of the air above the surface of the tongue, or the tongue on the palatal surface. The thickness of this line is not relevant. Typically, approximately 1 cm of the tongue tip is not visible in the production of alveolar sounds due to the acoustic shadow of the jaw. Similarly, the tongue root may be obscured due to the acoustic shadow of the hyoid bone. Stone (2005) provides an extensive tutorial regarding recording and interpretation of ultrasound images.

Ultrasound images of the midsagittal plane of the tongue were taken during production of speech sounds and words. Figure 1–2 shows the tongue at rest, which can be used as a comparison with the other ultrasound images in *Speech Sounds: A Pictorial Guide to Typical and Atypical Speech*. The bright white line is the surface of the tongue. The air shadow can be seen above this bright white line and the muscles and fatty tissue of the tongue can be seen below the white line. Chapter 38 describes the creation of the ultrasound

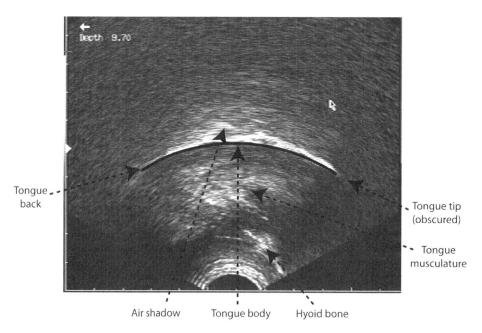

Figure 1–2. Ultrasound image of the tongue at rest.

images and the use of a purpose-built helmet to ensure stability of the ultrasound probe so that each image within this book can be compared with one another. In each image an arrow cursor has been included at approximately the level of the nose (top right quadrant), so that comparisons can be made.

The tongue tip is on the right for the ultrasound images. As for the schematic line drawings, it is also important to note that the ultrasound images only represent the midsagittal plane. It is important to compare the ultrasound images with the EPG images to determine the location and movement of the lateral margins of the tongue. Again, this is particularly important for the production of the alveolar sounds: /t, d, n, s, z, l/.

Figure 1–3 illustrates the relationship of the tongue to the palate in the ultrasound image of the production

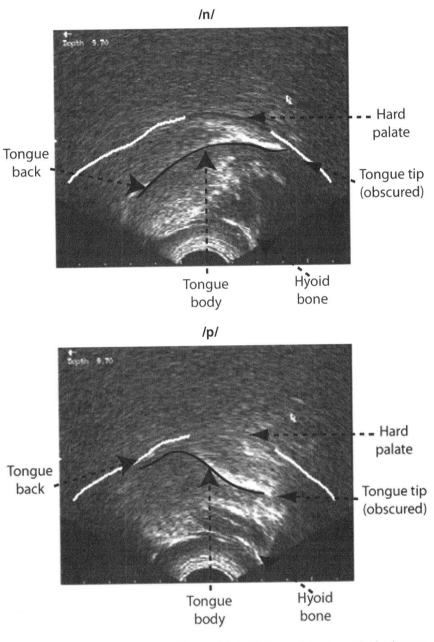

Figure 1–3. Ultrasound image of /n/ and /p/ with the palate drawn in the image. Note the bright white line representing the tongue. The tip of the tongue is at the right of the image. The tongue tip is up for /n/ and down for /p/.

of /n/ and /p/. At the beginning of the simultaneous ultrasound and electropalatograph recording, the speaker swallowed so that the imprint of the palate could be drawn; this was then superimposed on the subsequent image of the productions of /n/ and /p/. Below the bright white line of the tongue, there are diagonal lines reflecting muscles and fat within the tongue. There is also an air shadow above the tongue in this image.

Figure 1–4 compares simultaneous productions of ultrasound and electropalatographic images of the sentence "I see pop again." Readers can observe the difference in tongue position on the midsagittal ultrasound images and the coronal electropalatographic images. Readers also can compare the difference in tongue position for each sound within the sentence. For example, the tongue tip is up for production of

/s/ and /n/, but down for production of the vowels, /p/ and /g/.

Researchers of typical speech production have used the ultrasound to study aspects such as:

◆ tongue surface of English consonants and vowels (Stone, Faber, Raphael, & Shwaker, 1992; Stone & Lundberg, 1996)
◆ protrusion, grooving, and symmetry of the tongue during speech (Bressmann, Thind, Uy, Bollig, Gilbert, & Irish, 2005)
◆ production of schwa in /z/+ consonant sequences (Davidson, 2005)
◆ trough effect in coarticulatory sequences (Vazquez Alvarez, Hewlett, & Zharkova, 2004)
◆ swallowing (Chi-Fishman, 2005).

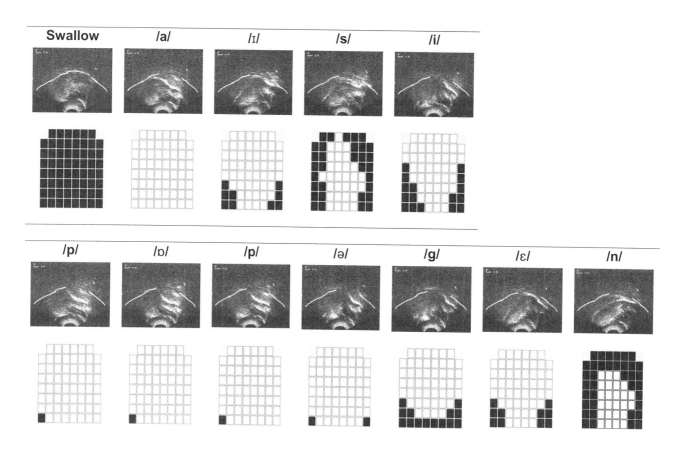

Figure 1–4. Simultaneous ultrasound and electropalatographic images of the sounds in "I see pop again." *Note*: The right of the ultrasound image corresponds with the tip of the tongue. The palate trace has been drawn on the ultrasound images based on the swallow image to demonstrate the range of tongue movement. The top of the EPG image corresponds with the palate immediately behind the front teeth.

Researchers of people with speech impairment have used the ultrasound to study aspects such as:

- vowel production of adolescents with hearing impairment (Bacsfalvi, Bernhardt, & Gick, 2007)
- consonant production (/s, z, l, r/) of adolescents with hearing impairment (Bernhardt, Gick, Bacsfalvi, & Ashdown, 2003).

Electropalatography: Single Frames

The electropalatograph (EPG) records tongue contact with the palate during speech production, providing a printout of activated electrodes every 10 milliseconds.

The EPG has an artificial palate (Figure 1–5) that is individually molded to fit the roof of the mouth. The Reading/WINEPG used to create the images in this book has 62 electrodes that record tongue contact with the surface of the palate. The Reading/WIN palate is usually around 1.5 millimeters thick. The EPG provides a printout of the electrodes that are activated during speech. These are taken every 10 milliseconds. Figure 1–5 shows one frame. The black squares represent the activated electrodes where tongue to palate contact has occurred. The white squares indicate that no contact has occurred. The areas of the palate can be separated into three zones: alveolar, palatal, and velar (Hardcastle & Gibbon, 1997). These are also presented in Figure 1–5. It can be seen that the top of the EPG frame corresponds with the alveolar region immediately behind the front teeth. The final row of squares corresponds with the juncture between the hard and soft palates. The maximum point of contact is often selected for analyzing the place of articulation for individual speech sounds as it provides a point of comparison (Hardcastle & Gibbon, 1997). This is selected by identifying the frame that has the highest number of contacted electrodes. An example of the maximum contact frame for /s/ is shown in Figure 1–5.

Electropalatography: Cumulative Frames

A cumulative EPG display is created by accumulating data from maximum contact frames for each consonant. Chapter 38 describes the study of eight speakers' productions of speech sounds that have been used in this book (McLeod, 2003). Figure 1–6 presents the

Row	EPG frame of the maximum point of contact for /s/	Region of palate	Hypothesized area of tongue	EPG palate	Dental cast with junction between hard and soft palate drawn
1 2 3 4 5 6 7 8	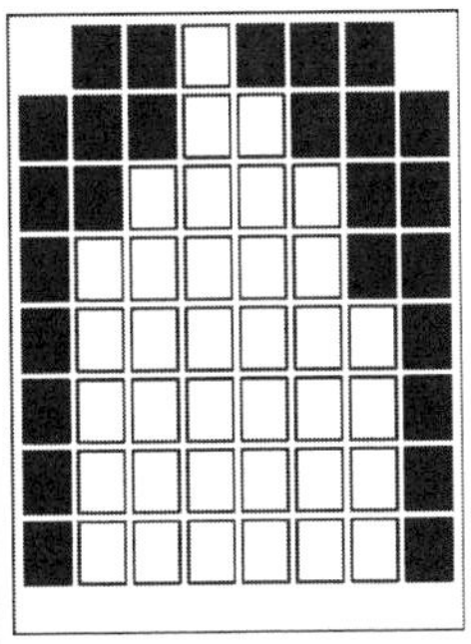	Alveolar (2 rows) Palatal (3 rows) Velar (3 rows)	Anterior (tip) Blade Posterior (body)	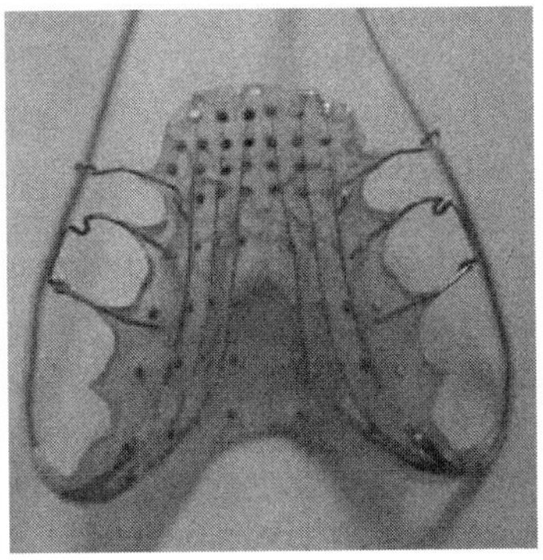	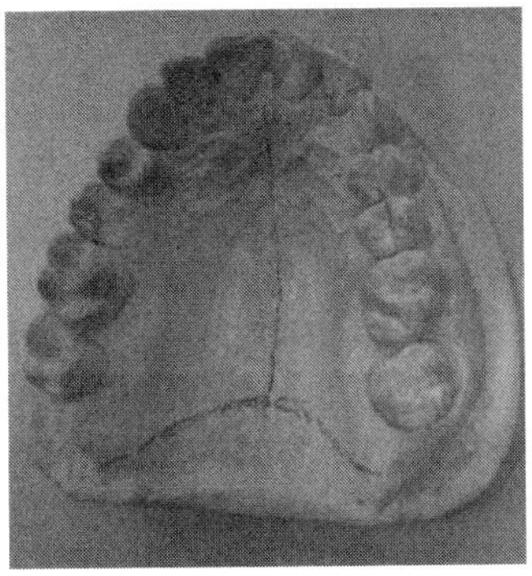

Figure 1–5. An example of an EPG frame for the production of /s/ juxtaposed with an EPG palate. The black squares represent the contacted electrodes. The zoning scheme is adapted from Gibbon (1999b). The EPG frame, EPG palate, and dental cast are from the speaker who produced the EPG images for *Speech Sounds: A Pictorial Guide to Typical and Atypical Speech.*

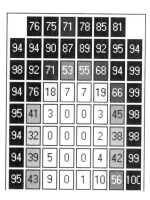

Figure 1–6. Cumulative EPG display for eight English adults' productions of /t/.

cumulative display for /t/ for eight typical adults as shown in Chapter 4. The darker the shading on rectangle (representing the electrode) the greater proportion of tongue/palate contact. The number in each box indicates the percentage of occasions each electrode was activated by all the participants during their productions of /t/. For example, the bottom left-hand electrode was contacted 95% of the time by the participants during their productions of /t/.

Electropalatography: Single Frames Demonstrating Intra- and Interspeaker Variability

A range of EPG studies have been published that describe typical and impaired productions of vowels and consonants. A summary is provided in Tables 1–2 and 1–3. As can be seen, some sounds have received a large amount of attention. Others have received none. Gibbon and Paterson (2006) indicated that the most commonly treated sounds using the EPG were /s, z, t, d/ and this is evident in Table 1–3.

It was considered important to demonstrate variability in the images presented in research. Many of the following chapters include additional EPG images from others' research in order to demonstrate variability in the production of speech sounds across English accents, languages other than English, children, and people with speech impairment. Specifically, *Speech Sounds: A Pictorial Guide to Typical and Atypical*

Speech includes images of differences between studies of:

◆ adults speaking English,
◆ children speaking English,
◆ adults speaking languages other than English, and
◆ people with speech impairment.

The selected images have been redrawn with permission to simplify the complexity and individuality of the published images. A simplified EPG template was created. A black rectangle indicates that that electrode was contacted at least 67% of the time in the originally published EPG image. A gray rectangle indicates that that electrode was contacted less than 67% of the time. There are a few exceptions to this where the published studies have used different criteria (for example, Guizik and Harrington (2007) used a criterion of 50%); however, any departure from the 67% is mentioned in the text.

INTERPRETING DYNAMIC IMAGES OF CONSONANTS AND VOWELS

In Chapters 2 through 36, dynamic images are presented to depict speech sounds while they are being produced contextually. Each English consonant is presented in one or more contexts in a meaningful word (initial, within word, and/or final positions). Each of the vowels and diphthongs is presented within meaningful words to show the influence of consonants on vowel formants. For example, Chapter 2 depicts the English phoneme /p/ at the word-initial and word-final positions in the word "pop" as well as /p/ at the word-initial and within-word positions in the word "puppy." A careful study of these two words independently and simultaneously provides a better understanding of the phoneme /p/.

Each chapter contains at least 3 different dynamic representations of a given speech sound: (1) filmstrip, (2) sound spectrogram, and (3) a series of electropalatography frames. By carefully studying these three segments, the reader can develop an understanding of the correlation between articulation and acoustics.

Table 1–2. Selected EPG Studies of Typical Production of Consonants and Vowels

Study	Language/ Dialect	Population	p	b	t	d	k	g	m	n	ŋ	f	v	θ	ð	s	z	ʃ	ʒ	tʃ	dʒ	w	l	ɹ	j	Vowels	Non-English
Cheng, Murdoch, Goozée, & Scott (2007)	Australian English	12 adults; 36 children			t		k									s								l				
McAuliffe, Ward, & Murdoch (2003)	Australian English	10 adults			t											s								l				
McAuliffe, Ward, & Murdoch (2006a & 2006b)	Australian English	15 adults#			t											s								l				
McAuliffe, Ward, & Murdoch (2007)	Australian English	15 adults#			t											s								l				
McLeod (2006)	Australian English	7 adults								n																		
McLeod & Gibbon (2007)	Australian English	8 adults			t	d	k	g		n	ŋ					s	z	ʃ	ʒ					l	ɹ	j		
McLeod & Roberts (2005)	Australian English	8 adults			t	d	k	g		n	ŋ					s	z	ʃ	ʒ					l	ɹ	j		
Liker, Gibbon, Wrench, & Horga (2007)	English	7 adults			t															tʃ								
Gibbon, Lee, & Yuen (2007)	Scottish English	8 adults	p	b					m																			
Gibbon, McNeill, Wood, & Watson (2003)	Scottish English	1 child			t		k																					
Gibbon, Smeaton-Ewins, & Crampin (2005)	Scottish English	5 adults#																									i, ʉ, ɪ, o, ɔ	

continues

Table 1–2. continued

Study	Language/Dialect	Population	p	b	t	d	k	g	m	n	ŋ	f	v	θ	ð	s	z	ʃ	ʒ	tʃ	dʒ	w	l	ɹ	j	Vowels	Non-English
Shannon (2001) in Gibbon (2004)	Scottish English	1 adult; 1 child																ʃ									
Stone & Lundberg (1996)	US English	1 adult								n	ŋ			θ		s		ʃ					–			i, ɪ, e, ɛ, æ, ɑ, ɔ, o, u, ʌ, ɝ	
Stone, Faber, Raphael, & Shawker (1992)	US English	1 adult														s		ʃ					–			i, ɛ, o, ɑ	
McLeod, Roberts, & Sita (2006)	US, Canadian, UK, Australian English	10 adults														s	z										
Recasens (2004)	Catalan	15 adults																					–				
Fuchs, Brunner, & Busler (2007)	German	7 adults														s	z	ʃ	ʒ								
Recasens (2004)	German	5 adults																					–				
Nicolaidis (2004)	Greek	1 adult#			t		k			n						s							–				x, r
Fujiwara (2007)	Japanese	5 adults#			t																						
Moen & Simonsen (2007)	Norwegian	4 adults			t	d																					ʈ, ɖ
Simonsen & Moen (2004)	Norwegian	7 adults																ʃ									ʂ
Guzik & Harrington (2007)	Polish	3 adults														s		ʃ									ʑ, x
Stokes & Zhen (1998)	Putonghua	1 adult														s											ʂ, ɕ, ʐ, ts, tsʰ, tʂʰ, tɕ, tɕʰ

Primary purpose of the study was to examine people with speech impairment.

Table 1–3. Selected EPG Studies of Impaired Production of Consonants and Vowels

Study	Language/Dialect	Population	p	b	t	d	k	g	m	n	ŋ	f	v	θ	ð	s	z	ʃ	ʒ	tʃ	dʒ	w	l	ɹ	j	Vowels	Non-English/Other
McAuliffe, Ward, & Murdoch (2006a & 2006b)	Australian English	9 adults: Parkinson's disease (+15 typical)			t											s							–				
McAuliffe, Ward, & Murdoch (2007)	Australian English	8 adults: Parkinson's disease (+15 typical)			t											s							–				
Martin, Hirson, Herman, Thomas, & Pring (2007)	British English	1 adolescent: hearing impaired			t	d																					
Bernhardt, Gick, Bacsfalvi, & Ashdown (2003)*	Canadian English	4 adolescents: hearing impaired														s		ʃ					–	ɹ			
Bacsfalvi, Bernhardt & Gick (2007)*	Canadian English	4 adolescents: hearing impaired																								i, ɪ, u, ʊ, ɛ	
Howard (2003)	English	3 adolescents: cleft palate	p	b	t	d	k	g	m	n	ŋ	f	v	θ	ð	s	z	ʃ	ʒ	tʃ	dʒ	w	l	ɹ	j		
Howard (2004)	English	5 children: speech impaired	p	b	t	d	k	g		n	ŋ					s	z	ʃ	ʒ								
Howard (2007)	English	6 children: speech impaired																									connected speech + prosody

continues

Table 1–3. *continued*

Study	Language/Dialect	Population	p	b	t	d	k	g	m	n	ŋ	f	v	θ	ð	s	z	ʃ	ʒ	tʃ	dʒ	w	l	ɹ	j	Vowels	Non-English/Other
Pantelemidou, Herman, Thomas (2003)	English	1 child: hearing impaired					k	g																			
Scobbie, Wood, & Wrench (2004)	Scottish English	1 child: cleft palate			t		k																				
Gibbon & Crampin (2002)	Scottish English	27 adults & children: cleft palate	p	b					m																		
Gibbon, Ellis, & Crampin (2004)	Scottish English	15 children: cleft palate			t	d	k	g																			
Gibbon, Smeaton-Ewins, & Crampin (2005)	Scottish English	18 children: repaired cleft lip and palate			t	d																				i, ʉ, ɪ, o, ɔ	
Gibbon, Stewart, Hardcastle, & Crampin (1999)	Scottish English	1 child: speech impaired																									
Gibbon & Wood (2003)	Scottish English	1 child: cerebral palsy					k	g			ŋ																
Gibbon, McNeill, Wood, & Watson (2003)	Scottish English and Hungarian	1 child: Down syndrome					k	g			ŋ																

Study	Language/Dialect	Population	p	b	t	d	k	g	m	n	ŋ	f	v	θ	ð	s	z	ʃ	ʒ	tʃ	dʒ	w	l	ɹ	j	Vowels	Non-English/Other
Lee, Gibbon, Crampin, Yuen, & McLennan (2007)	Scottish English	1 child: cleft lip and palate			t	d				n						s	z			tʃ	dʒ		l				
Shannon (2001) cited in Gibbon (2004)	Scottish English	1 child: cleft palate																ʃ									
Schmidt (2007)	US English	13 children: speech impaired					k	g			ŋ					s	z	ʃ		tʃ	dʒ			ɹ			
Nicolaidis (2004)	Greek	4 adults: hearing impaired (+ 1 typical)			t		k			n						s							l				x, ɾ
Fujiwara (2007)	Japanese	5 children: cleft palate			t																						

*Also included ultrasound.

Filmstrips

The high-speed motion picture presentations provide important information regarding the articulatory gestures involved in the production of speech sounds. These pictures primarily emphasize the front portion of the mouth and provide detail regarding the movement of the lips, teeth, jaw, and the tongue (in some cases). The filmstrips were made from negatives of 35-mm high-speed motion picture film. The filmstrips are in absolute continuation; the bottom of the first strip continues at the top of the second strip. The approximate midpoint of the speech sounds are indicated using phonetic transcription (see the International Phonetic Alphabet). Arrows have been added to the left-hand margin to indicate the general area of transition between phonemes, not to the discrete phoneme boundary. The corresponding acoustic waveform is shown along the left-hand sides of the filmstrips.

Spectrogram

The spectrogram, also called "sound spectrogram," and less commonly known as "sonography," is the plotting of frequency, time, and intensity—three important physical attributes of speech sounds. Time is plotted along the horizontal axis, frequency is plotted along the vertical axis, and the intensity is contained in the relative darkness of the bandwidth. The beauty of this representation lies in the fact that intensity is shown as the property of both time and frequency, thus indicating what is critical in speech production, and what is not.

Formants are marked by concentration of energy in a relatively narrow area of frequency across the continuum of time. Formants are more applicable to describing vowels than consonants, simply because the energy concentration in the relative frequency areas for vowels are clearly discernable. Intensity is the energy denoted by the density of the darkness on the axis of time and frequency. The higher the darkness, the greater the intensity. Nasality, deflected in the acoustic terms, is best described as a phenomenon of antiresonance which is shown by a reverse frequency-intensity relationship to the oral counterparts. The first formant is relatively weaker. There is a bandwidth showing the presence of nasality, and second formant is relatively stronger.

Silence is the property of stop consonants reflecting the complete closure of the airstream, thereby having no noticeable acoustic energy present at the sound spectrogram. This silence is indicated by stoppage of any noticeable acoustic energy at the medial word position and voice onset time (VOT) at the initial position. Voice onset time is the time elapsed from the release of the oral occlusion of the stop gestures and the onset of voicing.

Burst is the presence of abrupt release of energy, as in stop consonants at the initial position of a word. Plusive burst is known to show the aspiration of the noise for consonants /p/, /t/, /k/, at the beginning of a word.

Frication is the continuous presence of energy in the high-frequency region of speech without any appreciable formation of either stop or formant-like features. Examples for fricatives are such sounds as /s/ and /z/.

Spectrograms reflect the dialect and sex differences of speakers. Because the speaker in this book is female, the overall frequency components are elevated.

The spectrogram has been used to assist in the understanding of typical speech, as well as to understand speech impairment. There are hundreds of documented studies by phoneticians, linguists, SLPs, and others. The following serve to provide an example of the range. Researchers of typical speech have used the spectrograph to study:

- intonation contours of children (Snow, 2001)
- typical /s/ production in children (Flipsen, Shriberg, Weismer, Karlsson, & McSweeny, 1999)
- acoustic properties of stops (Hewlett, 1988)
- speaking rate for different dialects of English (Robb, Maclagan, & Chen, 2004)
- voice onset time in French speakers (Ryalls et al., 1997).

Researchers of people with speech impairment have used the spectrograph to study:

- intonation of children with hearing impairment (O'Halpin, 2001)
- tonal accents in Swedish children with language impairment (Samuelsson & Löfqvist, 2006)
- dysprosody in people with Parkinson's disease (Penner, Miller, Hertirch, Ackermann, & Schumm, 2001)

◆ diadochokinesis in people with traumatic brain injury (Wang, Kent, Duffy, Thomas, & Weismer, 2004)

◆ speech segment timing in children who stutter (Onslow, Stocker, Packman, & McLeod, 2002)

◆ fundamental frequency patterns in people with cerebral palsy (van Doorn & Sheard, 2001)

◆ differentiation between liquids in a child with speech impairment (McLeod & Isaac, 1995)

◆ distortions of rhotics in children with speech impairment (Flipsen, Shriberg, Weismer, Karlsson, & McSweeny, 2001).

A number of researchers have compared the correlation between acoustic and electropalatographic measures. Tabain (2001) indicated that there is high correlation between articulatory (EPG) and acoustic (spectral) data for the production of fricatives. Hoole, Ziegler, Hartmann, and Hardcastle (1989, p. 59) indicated that electropalatographic and acoustic measures of fricatives "appeared comparable in sensitivity."

Electropalatography: Dynamic Frames

Interpretation of electropalatographic images were described earlier under the heading of Electropalatography: Static Images. To represent tongue palate contact dynamically, sequential EPG frames are presented in Chapters 2 through 35. Using the Reading/WINEPG 10 frames are sampled every millisecond, providing extensive information on minute differences in tongue/palate contact during speech. In the sequential EPG frames, viewers will note that each individual palate has a number above it. This corresponds to the numbers of EPG frames that were recorded in that entire speech sample. Although the specific number is not relevant; the frame numbers are very useful as a label for identifying relevant segments of speech. Additional information about selection of the frames for each word can be found in Chapter 38. Dynamic EPG images have been included in *Speech Sounds: A Pictorial Guide to Typical and Atypical Speech* as it is important to examine the coarticulatory influence of the surrounding vowels and consonants on the focus sound. There is a large body of data that indicates the effect of the vowel context on the tongue placement of consonants (e.g., Gibbon, Lee, & Yuen, 2007; Tabain, 2001).

Summary

Speech Sounds: A Pictorial Guide to Typical and Atypical Speech presents multiple static and dynamic images of each consonant and vowel using a range of imaging techniques. Comparison of these images provides a comprehensive overview of important articulatory and acoustic features of each consonant and vowel and provides clues to the coarticulatory influences each consonant and vowel has on the others.

PART 2: CONSONANTS AND VOWELS

The second part of Chapter 1 describes key features of the production of consonants and vowels. Those who are familiar with phonetics may wish to skip this section and move forward to the next chapter.

CONSONANTS: PLACE, MANNER, AND VOICING

All consonants can be described according to their place of articulation (where in the oral cavity the sound is formed), *manner* of articulation (how the airstream is passed through the oral cavity), and *voicing* (whether the vocal folds vibrate during sound production). Consonants differ from one another because they have different combinations of the following binary principles (see box):

Advancement (information about place)

Voicing (information about voice)

Labiality (information about place)

Sonorancy (information about manner)

Continuancy (information about manner)

Sibilancy (information about manner)

Nasality (information about manner)

Consonants can be distinguished using the following concepts:

Place of articulation: bilabial/labiodental/ linguodental/alveolar/palatal/velar/glottal

Advancement: front/back

Voicing: voiced/voiceless

Labiality: labial/nonlabial

Sonorancy: sonorant/nonsonorant (obstruent)

Continuancy: continuant/noncontinuant

Sibilancy: sibilant/nonsibilant

Nasality: nasal/nonnasal (oral)

Place of Articulation

For the sake of simplification, let us examine the oral cavity along its horizontal axis. The horizontal axis starts at the front of the mouth and terminates at its back. The front of the mouth includes the lips, the teeth, and the alveolar ridge. The middle and back of the mouth includes the hard palate, the soft palate, and the pharynx. The horizontal axis determines the place of articulation of the consonants. The contact of the tongue with the different points of articulation causes an alteration in the shape of the resonating cavities in front of and behind the point of contact. Figure 1–7 shows the changes in the shapes and sizes of the resonating cavities during the production of the various consonant sounds.

Bilabial

Sounds produced at the lips are known as labial sounds. The English phonemes /p/, /b/, /m/, and /w/ are produced at the lips and are referred to as *labials*. In the articulation of these sounds, the resonating cavity size is almost null in front of the point of contact and is large behind it, as shown in Figure 1–7. The upper and lower lips act as *articulators*, which are movable speech organs involved in the shaping of speech sounds.

Specifically, because the production of /p/, /b/, /m/, and /w/ involves both lips, these sounds are called *bilabial* sounds. It should be noted that /w/ is a labiovelar sound. The back of the tongue is raised in addition to the lip closure.

Labiodental

The production of /f/ and /v/ involves the contact of the lower lip and the upper teeth. The resonating cavity size is altered a bit, in the sense that there is a slight shortening of the resonation chamber behind the point of contact. This oral cavity configuration is shown in Figure 1–7, in the view labeled labiodental.

Linguadental

The two sounds called "theta" and "thorne" are represented phonemically by /θ/ and /ð/, respectively. These sounds are produced when the tip of the tongue is between the upper and lower teeth. The cavity size resulting from this contact is further reduced behind the point of constriction and is slightly enlarged in front of the point of constriction. Shown in Figure 1–7, the oral cavity configuration labeled *linguadental* uniquely relates to the nature and quality of phonemes /ð/ and /θ/. These two phonemes are described as linguadentals because the tongue and teeth are involved in their production. Some phoneticians refer to them as interdentals because they cannot be produced effectively without the tongue tip being securely placed between the upper and lower teeth.

Alveolar

When the tongue contacts the alveolar ridge, the cavity in front of the constriction is the largest of all the cavity configurations described so far. The portion of the cavity behind the constriction, although further reduced, is still slightly larger than that in front. In Figure 1–7, this configuration is labeled alveolar. The alveolar ridge is a very prominent point of tongue contact in many languages of the world, including English. Many sounds are produced when the tongue tip touches it, and it seems to be the most natural point of contact for the tongue tip. In order to enunciate the sound /t/, one merely has to lift the tongue tip and touch the alveolar ridge, thus stopping the airflow,

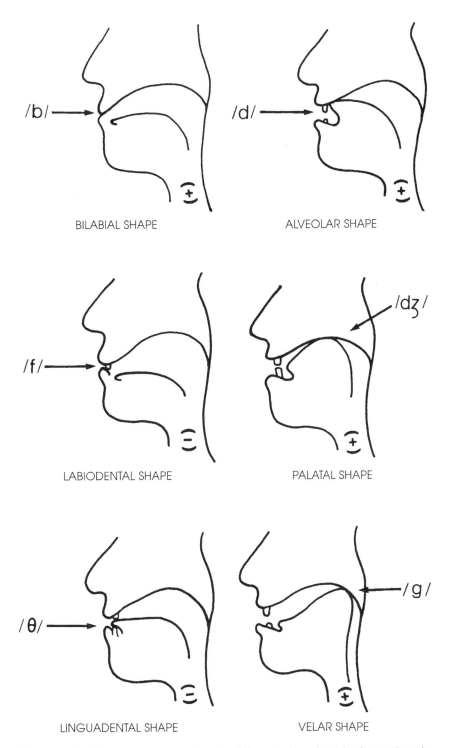

Figure 1–7. Diagram showing the six different alterations in the oral cavity shape controlled by lip and tongue contacts at the six different places along the horizontal line of the oral cavity. (*Source*: Singh, S. and Singh, K. [2006]. *Phonetics: Principles and Practice* [3rd ed.]. San Diego, CA: Plural. Figure 3–6).

and then release it to produce /t/. English sounds such as /t/, /d/, and /n/ are produced at the alveolar ridge and are called lingua-alveolar sounds. In addition, the consonants /s/, /z/, /l/, and /ɹ/ are also produced with the tongue tip in the general vicinity of the alveolar ridge.

In the production of the labial, labiodental, linguadental, and alveolar sounds, the size of the resonating cavity is larger behind the point of constriction than in front of it; therefore, these consonants are referred to as front consonants.

Palatal

The consonants /ʃ/, /ʒ/, /tʃ/, /dʒ/, and /j/ are produced by the body of the tongue contacting or approximating the postalveolar region of the hard palate. In Figure 1-7 this configuration is labelled *palatal*. The size of the resonating cavity in front of the constriction is enlarged, whereas the size of the cavity behind the constriction is reduced. Because the cavity is now larger in front of the constriction point than behind it, these consonants are referred to as *back consonants*.

Velar

Velar sounds are produced when the point of tongue contact is farthest back in the oral cavity. The back of the tongue touches or approximates the soft palate to form the constriction necessary for the production of the velar sounds /k/, /g/, /ŋ/, and /h/. Some phoneticians classify /h/ as a glottal fricative.

Summary

We have now mapped in the oral cavity each of six important locations involved in the pronunciation of English consonants: (1) lips, (2) lip and teeth, (3) tip of the tongue and teeth, (4) tip of the tongue and alveolar ridge, (5) body of the tongue and hard palate, and (6) back of the tongue and soft palate (velum). The different sizes of the resonating cavities in front and behind the constriction have been utilized as the criterion for determining the front and back sounds in English. Front sounds are those in which the cavity size is larger behind the point of constriction. Back sounds are those in which the cavity size is larger in front of the point of constriction.

The number of English consonant sounds associated with the different place categories is as follows: four sounds are bilabial, two are labiodental, two are linguadental, seven are alveolar, five are palatal, and three are velar. Thus, the different points of articulation have an unequal number of consonants associated with them. The consonant sounds associated with each place category are presented in Table 1-4.

Table 1–4. Distribution of English Consonant Phonemes According to Place of Articulation and Resonating Cavity

Place of Articulation	Consonant	Point of Articulation in Oral Cavity	Resonating Cavity (front/back sound)
Bilabial	/p/, /b/, /m/, /w/	Lips	Front
Labiodental	/f/, /v/	Lower lip and upper teeth	Front
Linguadental	/θ/, /ð/	Tip of tongue and teeth	Front
Alveolar	/t/, /d/, /n/, /s/, /z/, /l/, /ɹ/	Tip of tongue and alveolar ridge	Front
Palatal	/ʃ/, /ʒ/, /tʃ/, /dʒ/, /j/	Body of tongue and hard palate	Back
Velar	/k/, /g/, /ŋ/	Back of tongue and soft palate	Back
Glottal	/h/		Back

So far, we have examined the vocal tract subdivisions of an English speaker from the point of view of tongue contact at the various locations of the oral cavity. It must be noted here that the six categorizations or the six places of articulation are specifically related to English speakers. In the analysis of other languages of the world, certain details of this classification system may be altered. For example, Arabic languages include one additional point of contact further beyond the velum to account for the voiceless and voiced uvular fricative consonants /χ/, /ʁ/. The International Phonetic Alphabet provides a description of the speech sounds for all of the worlds' languages.

Manner of Articulation

As you have just read in the previous section, the exact point in the vocal tract where the airstream is modified, subdivides consonants into six discrete categories. Consonants also can be divided by their manner of articulation. "Manner" means the way in which an act is performed. Manner of articulation refers to the way in which speech sounds are produced. This section explains and differentiates between the different manners of articulation, so that students will be able to visualize the strategy that people utilize in speech production.

According to the manner of articulation, English consonants may be divided and subdivided into many binary classifications. Figure 1–8 illustrates these classifications, and this section explains them in detail. To provide an overview, English consonants may be classified as either sonorant or obstruent. The sonorant consonants may be divided into oral and nasal categories, and the obstruent consonants may be divided into stop and continuant categories. In addition, stops and continuants may be subdivided into sibilant and nonsibilant categories.

Figure 1–8 displays the division of the consonants of English into a system of manner, place, and voicing categories. The place categories of front or back and labial or nonlabial have been integrated with the voicing category and with the manner categories of sonorant or obstruent, nasal or oral, stop or continuant, and sibilant or nonsibilant. Each of the categories is denoted by two specifications only. This description is not unlike the description of the two sides of a coin, where one side is directly opposite to the other and where each side is considered independent of the other. Such a description is also called a binary function. For example, sonorant is opposite obstruent, nasal is opposite oral, stop is opposite continuant, voiced is opposite voiceless, and front is opposite back. These opposite specifications are important in developing an elegant system for describing the sounds of a language. Although this binary designation is useful for learning the classification of English consonants, it sacrifices a great deal of articulatory detail. It must be understood that a student of phonetics cannot afford to sacrifice the details of phonetic descriptions when pursuing a comprehensive study of speech sounds. It is important to note that within the field of speech-language pathology, tradition has prevailed to describe manner of articulation using the necessary and additional phonetic details such as plosive, fricative, liquid, nasal, and glide. These categories are explained later in this chapter.

Figure 1–8 can be used to identify the features of each consonant phoneme in the English language. The utility of this figure lies in its ability to illustrate how elegant the sound system is. Selecting any node at the bottom, you can see the meaningful distinctions between two phonemes by traveling toward the top. In subsequent chapters, a box containing distinguishing binary features is provided for each consonant and vowel.

Sonorant/Obstruent

The sonorant/obstruent classification distinguishes all consonants according to the amount of vocal tract obstruction necessary for their production. The *obstruent* consonants are produced by a considerable amount of obstruction of the laryngeal airstream in the vocal tract. The sonorant consonants, on the other hand, require only a negligible amount of obstruction in the vocal tract.

The phonetic description of sonorants includes a relatively unobstructed flow of air between the articulator and the point of articulation. These consonants contain vowel-like qualities, although their predominant function in English is consonantal. The sonorants in English are /m/, /n/, /ŋ/, /l/, /ɹ/, /j/, and /w/. Three of these seven sonorants /m/, /n/, and /ŋ/ are nasal and the remaining four, /l/, /ɹ/, /j/, and /w/ are classified as oral. Sonorants are the most open of all the conso-

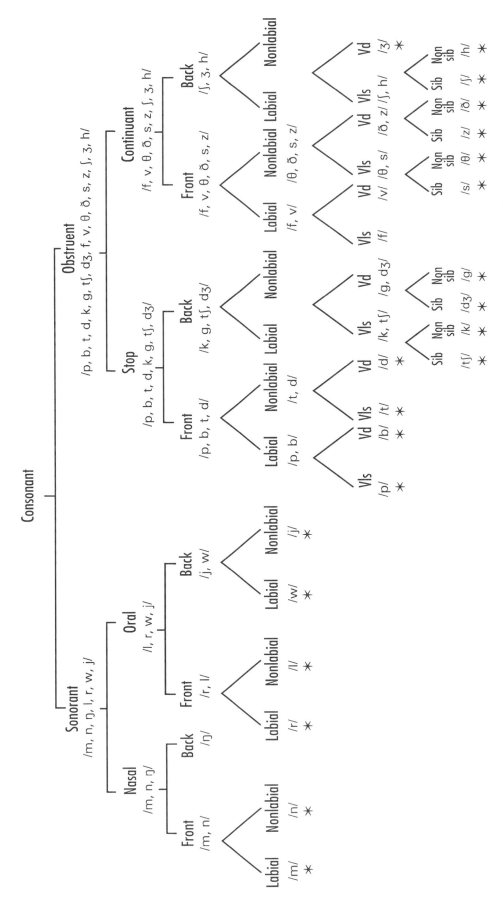

Figure 1–8. Division of consonants, on binary principles, into sonorant/obstruent, nasal/oral, stop/continuant, front/back, labial/nonlabial, voiceless/voiced (Vls/Vd), and sibilant/nonsiblinant (Sib/Non-Sib) groups. (*Source:* Singh, S. and Singh, K. [2006]. *Phonetics: Principles and Practice* [3rd ed.]. San Diego, CA: Plural. Figure 3–7).

nant categories. Only vowels show greater open quality than the sonorant consonants.

Nasal/Oral

Nasal/oral is also considered a manner category. It distinguishes speech sounds primarily according to the difference in the resonating cavities. For oral consonants, the resonating cavity is the entire portion of the vocal tract excluding the nasal cavity and the nasopharynx. For nasal consonants, however, the resonating cavity is the entire vocal tract, including the nasal cavity and the nasopharynx. Because the airstream is passed through the nose and the point of constriction is in the mouth, there is an added complexity to the nature of the resonator for the nasal consonants. Nasal consonants are considered nasal stops because during the production of each, /m/, /n/, and /ŋ/, airflow is completely interrupted in the oral cavity prior to their releases.

Stop/Continuant

The stop/continuant category of obstruents is an important manner category. In English, the stop category includes the consonants /p/, /b/, /t/, /d/, /tʃ/, /dʒ/, /k/, and /g/; the continuant category includes the consonants /f/, /v/, /θ/, /ð/, /s/, /z/, /ʃ/, /ʒ/, and /h/. *Stops* are produced with maximal closure at the point of constriction and maximal or total obstruction of the laryngeal airstream. *Continuants* are produced with relatively less closure and relatively less airstream obstruction. Because all stops and continuants require obstruction in the vocal tract, they are labeled as obstruents.

One major difference between stops and their opposite class, continuants, is the amount of time involved in their production. As a class, stops are relatively shorter in duration than continuants. In addition, stops involve a complete closure at a given point in the vocal tract, whereas the continuants do not. This closure is caused by contact of the lips or of the different portions of the tongue with the various points of articulation described above. At the lips, for example, there is a complete closure for the stop consonants /p/ and /b/. There is, however, some opening for the continuant consonants /f/ and /v/. At the alveolar ridge, there is a complete closure for the stops /t/ and /d/ but the continuants /s/ and /z/ involve some degree of opening.

Table 1–5 shows that the manner of articulation helps to make systematic distinctions within the different phoneme groupings at the six places of articulation described earlier. In this table, the six discrete places of articulation are on a horizontal axis, and the three manners of articulation (stop, continuant, and sonorant) are on a vertical axis. The clearly discernable distribution of the stop-continuant-sonorant continuum in relation to the six places of articulation can be seen in Table 1–5.

Plosives Versus Stops. The phonetic category stop is also called plosive, mainly because of phoneticians' differences in viewpoints. Although the term "stop" denotes the complete stoppage of the airflow at the point of constriction in the vocal tract, the term

Table 1–5. Description of English Consonants According to the Six Places of Articulation and Three Manners of Articulation[1]

Manner	Place						
	Bilabial	**Labiodental**	**Linguadental**	**Alveolar**	**Palatal**	**Velar**	**Oral Cavity**
Stop	/p/, /b/			/t/, /d/	/tʃ/, /dʒ/	/k/, /g/	Closed
Continuant		/f/, /v/	/θ/, /ð/	/s/, /z/	/ʃ/, /ʒ/	/h/	Slight opening
Sonorant	/m/, /w/			/n/, /ɹ/, /l/	/j/	/ŋ/	Opening

[1]Similar to the place of articulation, the manner of articulation has been treated on a continuum: stops are closed, continuants are slightly open, and most sonorants have greater opening in the oral cavity.

"plosive" implies the release of, or explosion of, the airflow following that closure. The explosion of stops is mainly realized when the stops are produced at the initial place of a word or syllable. Functionally, then, the term "plosive" is only relevant to initial stop consonants. However, the production of the six consonants /p/, /t/, /k/, /b/, /d/, and /g/ involves a total stoppage, irrespective of their position in a word. Thus, functionally the term "stop" is more inclusive of the overall nature of English stops than the term "plosive." Stop consonants belong to a universal phonetic inventory, implying that all languages of the world include this category of sounds. Stop consonants appear uniformly at prominent places of articulation with consistent contrast of voicing (in English), voicing and aspiration (in Indic languages), and aspiration and release (in some Southeast Asian languages).

Continuants. Phonetically, although stops and continuants are descriptions of independent articulatory gestures, phonologically they can be defined by utilizing the presence (+) or the absence (−) of one and only one feature. The term "continuancy" may be used to describe the complete stop/continuant dichotomy. Thus, all continuants are labeled as plus continuant and all stops are labeled as minus continuant. In this kind of notation system, those sounds that are neither stops nor continuants are not considered for either the plus or minus specifications. For example, the /l/ consonant is neither a stop nor a continuant, and therefore /l/ will not be marked by either the plus (+) or minus (−) specification of the feature continuancy. In other words, the feature of continuancy is redundant for /l/ and other sonorant consonants.

Groove and Slit Fricatives. Molding the opening of the vocal tract by shaping the tongue to create either a slit or a groove opening at the alveolar ridge may create continuants. In both instances (slit or grove), the airstream is allowed to pass through the opening in the vocal tract. A slit implies a small, flat opening, whereas a groove refers to a larger and valley-shaped opening, both of which create some friction during the passage of the airstream through the constriction in the vocal tract. The slit continuants include /f/, /v/, /θ/, and /ð/ while the groove continuants include /s/, /z/, /ʃ/, /ʒ/. The phoneme /h/ is neither a slit nor a groove continuant because it does not require much restriction in the vocal tract.

Voiced and Voiceless Consonants

The feature of *voicing* relates to the presence or absence of vibration of the vocal folds in the production of consonants. Therefore, the term voicing applies to all place and manner categories of consonants. Voiced consonants are produced with the vibration of the vocal folds, whereas voiceless consonants are produced without such vibration. In English, voicing is used to distinguish among the consonants within the obstruent group. Only the consonants /p/, /t/, /k/, /f/, /θ/, /s/, /ʃ/, /tʃ/, and /h/ do not involve the vibration of the vocal folds. To the contrary, all sonorant consonants are voiced and, thus, like vowels, the voicing feature is not necessary for their description. In other words, what is sonorant is automatically voiced and, therefore, it is unnecessary and uneconomic to apply voicing to characterize sonorants.

In English, voicing distinguishes eight pairs of consonants: /p/-/b/, /t/-/d/, /k/-/g/, /f/-/v/, /θ/-/ð/, /s/-/z/, /ʃ/-/ʒ/, /tʃ/-/dʒ/. Consider the pair /p/-/b/: /p/ is identical to /b/ in terms of its place (bilabial) and manner (oral stop) of articulation. The single difference between them is voicing. Thus, /p/ is the voiceless cognate of the /b/ phoneme, and /b/ is the voiced cognate of the /p/ phoneme.

VOWELS

All English vowels are voiced. Vowel production involves a smooth vibration of the vocal folds. The wave motion is rhythmic; the form of each wave cycle is similar if not identical to the previous one. This type of rhythmic wave motion is called *periodic*. Wave motions that involve interruptions in the wave form to make them irregular in shape are called *aperiodic*. Waves of this type are found in noise, for example, static from a radio. In contrast, voiced consonants have both a periodic component (voicing) and an aperiodic component (for example, friction). In addition, consonant production requires a closure in the oral cavity, but vowel production does not. Those students who have a background in music will understand why singers always prolong the periodic waveforms of vowels which are quite pleasant to the ear rather than prolonging the aperiodic wave forms of voiced consonants.

Vowels can be distinguished using the following concepts

Advancement: front/central/back

Height: high/mid/low

Tenseness: tense/lax/neutral

Rounded: rounded/unrounded

Advancement

English vowel production is accomplished by the positioning of the tongue in three general locations along the horizontal axis of the oral cavity. The tongue body either protrudes forward toward the *front* of the mouth to produce the front vowels, remains in a relatively neutral or central location for the production of the central vowels, or retracts toward the *back* of the mouth for the production of the back vowels. The forward movement of the tongue along the horizontal axis is also referred to as tongue *advancement*. Front vowels have the most resonating cavity in the back of the mouth, central vowels have about half of the resonating cavity in the front and half in the back of the mouth, and back vowels have most of the resonating cavity in the front of the mouth.

Height

Besides the positioning of the tongue along the horizontal dimension of the oral cavity, the tongue also moves simultaneously along the vertical axis. The tongue is either at its highest position to produce *high* vowels, at its mid-position to produce *mid* vowels, or at its lowest position to produce *low* vowels. The movement of the tongue along the vertical axis is also referred to as *tongue height*. Reserve the term *central* when describing tongue advancement and the term *mid* as you think about the vertical dimension of the tongue movement pattern.

Because the tongue assumes three positions along the horizontal axis and three positions along the vertical axis, a simultaneous movement along these two axes allows the tongue to assume a total of nine positions. As a result, the tongue can be high-front, mid-

front, low-front, high-central, mid-central, low-central, high-back, mid-back, or low-back.

Tenseness

Describing vowels by placement alone creates difficulty, as two vowels would have identical specifications: /i/ and /ɪ/ would be labeled as high-front and /u/ and /ʊ/ would be labeled as high-back. Two additional articulatory features: *tenseness* and *placement* provide additional nomenclature for differentiating vowels.

Tense vowels are produced with added muscle tension, whereas lax vowels are produced without as much tension. The following English vowels are usually tense: /i, e, ɝ, u, o, ɚ/. Five vowels are usually lax: /ɪ, ə, ɜ, ʊ, ɔ/. Three vowels are neutral for the feature of tenseness: /æ, a, ɑ/, because each has a unique tongue position, and so does not need to be differentiated using tenseness.

In English, the feature tenseness is functional in the formation of open and closed syllables. An *open syllable* is one that is terminated by a vowel. A *closed syllable* ends with a consonant. Tense vowels may appear in open or closed syllables, whereas lax vowels generally appear in closed syllables only.

Roundedness

Of the English vowels, some vowels are accompanied by *lip rounding*, others are not, and still others are neutral for the feature of rounding. The round vowels are produced with added lip rounding and the unround vowels are produced without lip rounding. In English, the four round vowels are, in order of degree of roundedness, /u, ʊ, o, ɔ/. The five unround vowels are: /i, ɪ, e, ɛ, æ/. Generally, rounding corresponds with advancement, the front vowels are unrounded, the back vowels are rounded, and the central vowels are neutral for rounding.

Dilectal differences

Table 1–6 provides a comparison of phonemic symbols for the pronunciation of vowels across seven English dialects based on information from McLeod (2007). It can be observed that whereas some vowels (such as /i/ appear across these dialects, others (such as the r-colored vowels) do not.

Table 1–6. A Comparison of Phonemic Symbols for the Pronunciation of Vowels Across Seven English Dialects

American English Location	American English Vowels (Smit, 2004)	English Received Pronunciation (RP) (Wells, 1982)	Scottish English (Scobbie, Mennen, & Matthews, 2007)	Northern Irish English (Rahilly, 2007)	Southern Irish English (Rahilly, 2007)	Australian English (Mitchell, 1946)	Australian English (Harrington et al., 1997)	New Zealand English (Maclagan & Gillon, 2007)
High-front	i	i	i/iː	i	i	i	iː	i
	ɪ	ɪ		ɪ	ɪ	ɪ	ɪ	ɪ
	e			ɛi/ei/ɛɪ/e	ei/ei		e	e
Mid-low front	ɛ	ɛ	ɛ	eə/ɛ	ɛ	ɛ		
	æ	æ				æ	æ	æ
High-back, rounded	u	u	ʉ↔ʉː	ʉ	ɔe/ʊ/u	ʊ	ʉː	ʉ
	ʊ	ʊ	ʉ↔uː	ʉ/ʊ/ʌ	ʊ/ʌ	ʊ	ʊ	ʊ
Mid-back, rounded	o			eo/oː	ov/eo/oː		oː	
	ɔ	ɔ	ɔ	ɔ	ɔ/ɒ	ɔ	ɔ	ɔ
		ɒ	ɔ	a/ɑ	a/ɒ	ɒ		ɒ
Low-back	ɑ	ɑ	a↔ɑ	ɑ	ɑ	a	ɐː	a
[r]-colored	ɝ	ɜ	ɹe↔ɹʌ	ɝ	ə̆	ɜ	ɜː	ɜ
	ɚ			ə̆				
	ɪr		ɹi	ɹɪ/ɜ/ɹʌ	ɹɪ			
	ɛr		ɹɛ	ɹɜ/ɹɜ	ɹə/ɹɜ			
	ʊr		ɹɐf	ɹeɐ/ɹʌ	ɹɔe/ɹʊ			
	ɔr		ɹɔ	ɹɛɔ/ɹɔ	ɹɔe/ɹɔ			
	ɑr		ɹɒ	ɹɑ	ɹɑ/ɹɒ			
				ɹʌ	ɹʌ			

American English Location	American English Vowels (Smit, 2004)	English Received Pronunciation (RP) (Wells, 1982)	Scottish English (Scobbie, Mennen, & Matthews, 2007)	Northern Irish English (Rahilly, 2007)	Southern Irish English (Rahilly, 2007)	Australian English (Mitchell, 1946)	Australian English (Harrington et al., 1997)	New Zealand English (Maclagan & Gillon, 2007)
Central	ə	ə		ə	ə	ə	ə	ə
	ʌ	ʌ	ʌ	ʌ	ʌ	ʌ	ɐ	ʌ
Diphthongs	aɪ	aɪ	ʌi/ɑːe	ai/ɛi	ʌi	aɪ	ɑe	ai
	aʊ	aʊ	ʌʉ	ɐʉ	ʌʊ	aʊ	æɔ	aʊ
	ɔɪ	ɔɪ	ɔe	ɔi	ʌi	ɔɪ	ɔɪ	ɔɪ
		eɪ	e ↔ eː	ei/e	ɛi	ɛɪ	æɪ	eɪ
		əʊ				oʊ	ɐe	oʊ
		eɪ		ei	ei	eɪ	eɪ	eɪ
		eɜ	ɔ ↔ o	ɜː/eɜ	ɜː/eɜ	eɜ	iː	eɪ
		eʊ		eʊ	eʊ	eʊ	eʊ	eʊ
				iɜ/ei	iɜ			
			ɑe					

25

Summary

The basic features of consonants and vowels have been described in Part 2 of this chapter. Interested readers are directed to References at the end of the text for recommended readings to continue exploration of these topics. The following chapters describe each consonant and vowel in turn.

Chapter 2

/p/

The consonant /p/ is a voiceless bilabial stop.

Place of articulation: bilabial

Advancement: front

Voicing: voiceless

Labiality: labial

Sonorancy: nonsonorant (obstruent)

Continuancy: noncontinuant (stop)

Sibilancy: nonsibilant

Nasality: nonnasal (oral)

STATIC IMAGES OF THE ARTICULATORY CHARACTERISTICS OF /p/

The static images of /p/ are presented via a photograph, schematic diagram, ultrasound, and electropalatograph images (Figure 2–1).

Photograph

In this photograph (Figure 2–1A), the upper and lower lips are approximated to create closure of the airstream to produce /p/. The front view of the lip approximation can be compared with the lateral (side) view of lip approximation in the schematic diagram.

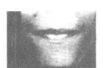

A. Photograph

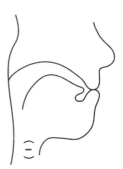

B. Schematic diagram

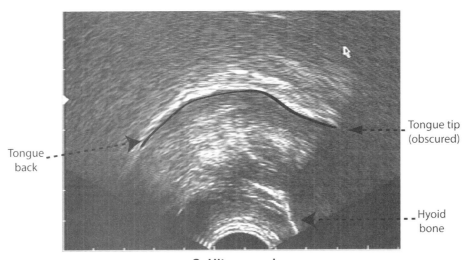

Tongue back

Tongue tip (obscured)

Hyoid bone

C. Ultrasound

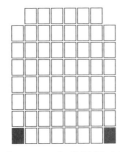

D. Electropalatograph (EPG) (single frame)

Figure 2–1. Static images of the articulatory characteristics of /p/.

Schematic Diagram

The involvement of both the upper and lower lips in the production of /p/ is shown by the drawing of lip approximation in Figure 2–1B. The tongue is not involved in the production of this labial consonant as shown by its location at a rest position. The symbol (–) has been chosen to indicate that the vocal folds do not vibrate systematically in the production of this speech sound.

Ultrasound

The bright white line on the ultrasound image of /p/ in Figure 2–1C shows the air above the tongue surface. The tongue tip is on the right and is toward the floor of the mouth. The back of the tongue is somewhat raised in the oral cavity. An air shadow can be seen above the tongue and diagonal muscle fibers can be seen below the surface of the tongue.

Electropalatograph (EPG)

The primary oral mechanisms involved in shaping the oromusculature to produce a /p/ are the lips and the soft palate (see Figures 2–1A and 2–1B). There is extremely limited tongue/palate contact for the EPG image of /p/ in Figure 2–1D. In this image the tongue touches the most posterior corners of the palate, as shown by the dark boxes. There is no contact with the central regions of the palate. In other productions of /p/, it is possible that there could be no tongue contact with the palate during production of /p/. Gibbon and Crampin (2002) stated that "simultaneous valving [that is, complete constriction] in the linguapalatal region throughout the period of lip closure is not a feature of normal speakers' productions of bilabials" (p. 41). Gibbon, Lee, and Yuen (2007) found that the extent of tongue/palate contact for the production of /p/ was significantly correlated with the extent of contact for the surrounding vowels.

DYNAMIC IMAGES OF THE ARTICULATORY AND ACOUSTIC CHARACTERISTICS OF /p/

In order to obtain a comprehensive view of the production of this consonant, the dynamic aspects of the production of /p/ are shown in a filmstrip, spectrogram, and EPG images in two words containing /p/ in different word positions (Figures 2–2 and 2–3).

/p/ in Word-Initial and Word-Final Contexts: "pop"

Filmstrip: /pɑp/ "pop"

The phoneme /p/ is at the initial and final positions of the word /pɑp/ (Figure 2–2A). The complete closure of the lips can be seen in the first frame, a slight opening in the second frame, and a full opening pertaining to the target vowel /ɑ/ in the sixth frame. The subsequent 9 frames (7 through 15) sustain the lip position exclusively attributable to the vowel /ɑ/. The next 7 frames (16 through 22) gradually show the accomplishment of the final target /p/. Because final stops in English are sometimes unaspirated as in this case, no lip opening can be seen in the final frame. The arrows along the sides of these strips indicate the general location of the transition between adjacent phonemes. The first arrow marks the transition between the initial /p/ and the vowel /ɑ/. The second arrow marks the transition between /ɑ/ and the acoustic energy for the final /p/. The vowel /ɑ/ is clearly marked in the sound track by waveforms characterized by high amplitude and a repetitive pattern.

Sound Spectrogram: /pɑp/ "pop"

The phoneme /p/ is presented in both the initial and final positions in the word "pop" (Figure 2–2B). Lip involvement for /p/ is associated with energy mainly in the low-frequency region of the sound spectrogram.

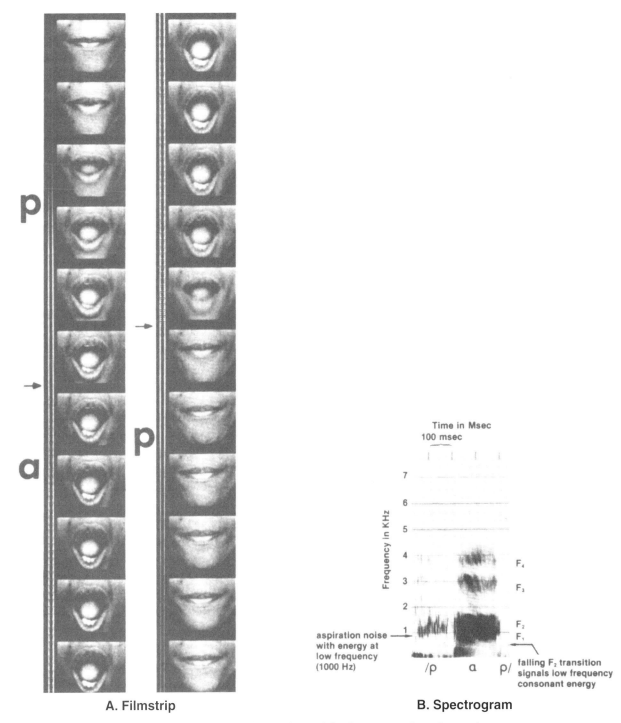

A. Filmstrip   B. Spectrogram

Figure 2–2. Dynamic images of /p/ in word-initial and word-final contexts: "pop." *continues*

Most of the energy for the phoneme /p/ in the initial position is concentrated around 1000 Hz, which is relatively low for a consonant. The first and second formants for the vowel /ɑ/ are somewhat indistinguishable, whereas there is an appreciable distance between the second and third formants. The final consonant /p/ is denoted by the transitional elements of the first two formants of the vowel /ɑ/. Both the F1 and F2 show a downward slant accommodating the final consonant /p/, which has energy in the low-

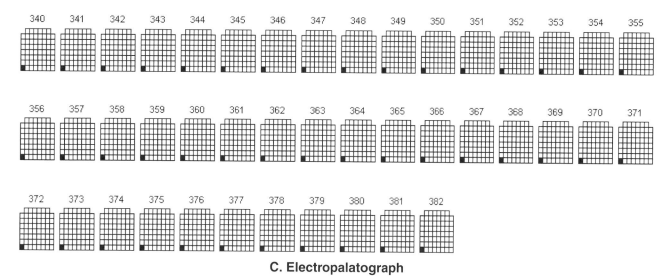

C. Electropalatograph

Figure 2–2. *continued*

frequency areas. Although the articulatory gesture of lip closure is denoted by these formant transitions, there is an absence of any noticeable consonant energy at the final position. This is permissible in English, because stops in the final position in a word may or may not be released. It is clear from this sound spectrogram that, once the information regarding place of articulation (labiality) is conveyed by the downward slope of these formants, it is not necessary for the acoustic information signifying a plosive burst to appear. Although there is a significant amount of aspiration noise present for the initial voiceless-labial-plosive consonant, it is absent in the final position.

Electropalatograph: /pɒp/ "pop"

The dynamic series of EPG palates for the production of the word /pɒp/[1] "pop" is presented in Figure 2–2C. The word "pop" was extracted from the sentence "I see a pop again." Within this sentence context, the word "pop" took 0.209 seconds to produce. Each EPG palate in the dynamic series shows minimal tongue contact palate throughout the whole word, with only one electrode being contacted at the bottom left of the palate. Tongue contact with the palate is not a feature of the production of the consonant /p/, nor the vowel /ɒ/.

/p/ in Within-Word Context: "puppy"

Filmstrip: /ˈpʌpɪ/ "puppy"

The criterion phoneme /p/ is at the initial and medial positions of the word /ˈpʌpɪ/. The first three frames of the filmstrip in Figure 2-3A show the complete lip closure for the initial /p/, and the middle four frames (11 through 14) show the complete lip closure for the medial /p/. Because the vowel /ʌ/ following the initial /p/ is more open than the vowel /ɪ/ following the medial /p/, the lip opening following the initial /p/ is relatively greater and more round (see frame 4) than the flat and small lip opening following the medial /p/ (see frame 15). At both the initial and medial positions, the acoustic tracing of /p/ starts after the lips have opened into the vowel.

Sound Spectrogram: /ˈpʌpɪ/ "puppy"

The phoneme /p/ is presented in both the initial and medial positions in the spectrogram of the word "puppy" (Figure 2-3B). The plosive nature of this consonant is marked by the presence of a plosive burst of energy in both the initial and medial positions. At the initial position, the energy starts at the very base of the sound spectrogram and terminates at over 4000 Hz.

---

[1]/pɒp/ is the Australian English pronunciation of "pop."

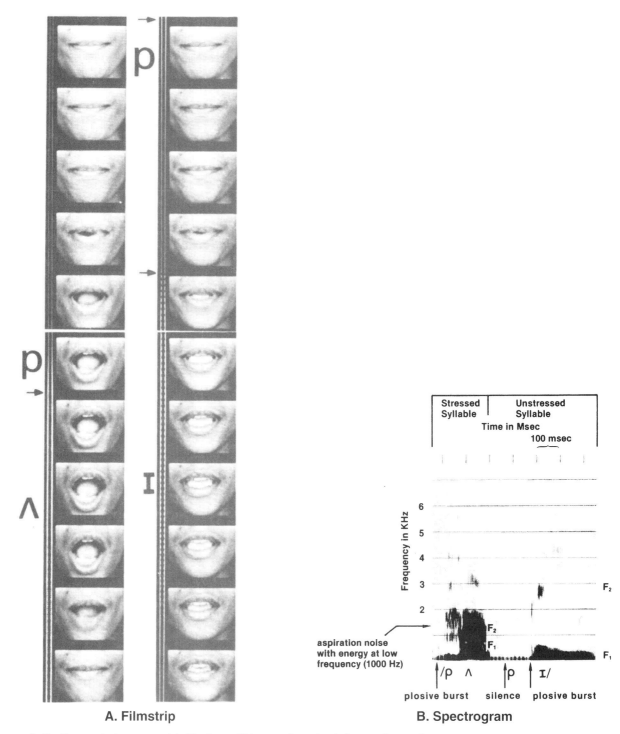

A. Filmstrip   B. Spectrogram

Figure 2–3. Dynamic images of /p/ in the within-word context: "puppy." *continues*

At the medial position, it again starts at the base and terminates at over 4000 Hz. The difference between the initial position and medial position /p/ is most apparent in the presence of an aspiration noise, which follows the initial plosive burst for approximately 80 msec. This aspiration noise is absent for the medial

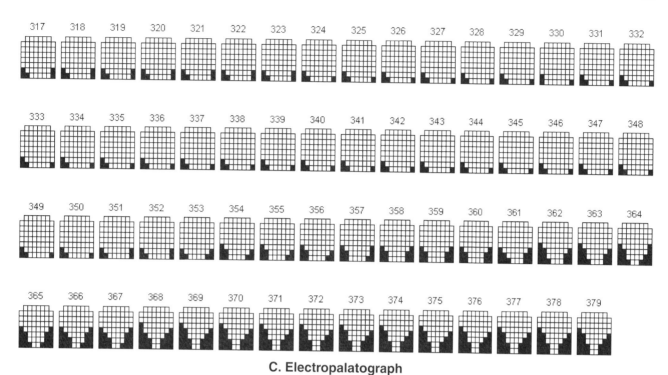

C. Electropalatograph

Figure 2–3. *continued*

/p/ and is replaced by a silence. It may be noted that the phoneme /p/ maintains allophonic variations in the English language—one of aspiration at the initial position of a word and one of lack of aspiration at the medial position. This spectrogram clearly provides an acoustic verification of this linguistic rule. Because of the labial nature of the phoneme /p/, most of the energy for the plosive burst at the initial and medial positions is concentrated below 2000 Hz. In addition, most of the aspiration energy of the initial stop is also below 2000 Hz. The coarticulatory influence of this stop can be seen in the mid-central vowel /ʌ/ and the high-front vowel /ɪ/. The second formant of the vowel /ɪ/ shows a sharp rising transition. Its energy connects with the medial plosive burst at 2000 Hz and rises to a steady state portion at about 2600 Hz.

Electropalatograph: /ˈpʌpi/ "puppy"

The dynamic series of EPG palates for the production of the word /ˈpʌpi/[2] "puppy" is presented in Figure 2–3C.

The word "puppy" was extracted from the sentence "I see a puppy again." Within this sentence context, the word "puppy" took 0.313 seconds to produce. There was limited lingualpalatal contact for the production of /p/ (frames 317–338), /ʌ/ (frames 339–346), and the second /p/ (frames 346–361). However, an increase in tongue palate contact was evident, commencing with frame 354, signaling the beginning of the coarticulatory phase for the vowel /i/ (frames 362–379). This vowel has more tongue/palate contact than for most other vowels (see Chapter 26).

INTRA- AND INTERSPEAKER VARIABILITY FOR /p/

Electropalatographic images enable consideration of intra- and interspeaker variability. First, production of /p/ by adult speakers of English is considered. Then

---

[2]/ˈpʌpi/ is the Australian English pronunciation of "puppy."

EPG images of productions of /p/ by children with cleft palate are displayed.

Inter- and Intraspeaker Variability in the Production of /p/ by English-Speaking Adults

Scottish English-Speaking Adults

Gibbon, Lee, and Yuen (2007) studied eight typical Scottish English-speaking adults' productions of bilabials. They found that the extent of tongue/palate contact for the production for /p/, /b/, and /m/ was significantly correlated with the contact for the surrounding vowels. They also found that under experimental conditions there was significantly more tongue/palate contact for /m/ than for /b/ or /p/. Figure 2–4 provides two EPG images from one adult's production of /p/ in two vowel contexts /ipi/ and /apa/. The black squares correspond to the contacted electrodes at the temporal midpoint of closure each of these nonsense words.

Interspeaker Variability for /p/ in Speakers with Impaired Speech

Children with Cleft Palate

Gibbon and Crampin (2002) described the production of /p, b, m/ for 27 Scottish-English speaking adults and children aged 5 to 62 years who had a history of cleft

palate and produced compensatory speech errors. Fifteen productions of words containing the bilabial consonants were produced by each speaker. Three speakers were described as frequently producing "labial-lingual double articulations (LLDAs)" (p. 40): speaker P (aged 9;07), speaker L (aged 9;10), and speaker J (aged 12;6). Speaker P produced LLDAs for all words containing /p/; speakers L and J inconsistently produced LLDAs during words containing /p/. Figure 2–5 illustrates the cumulative maximum contact EPG frames for the production of /p/ by these three Scottish English-speaking children (P, L, J). Black

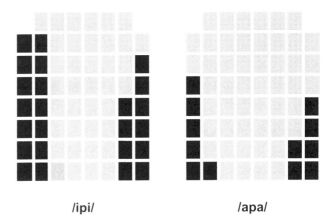

/ipi/   /apa/

Figure 2–4. EPG frames at the temporal midpoint of closure for the production of /p/ in the contexts /ipi/ and /apa/ by a typical Scottish English-speaking adult (adapted from Gibbon, Lee, & Yuen, 2007, Figure 4, p. 90).

P   L   J

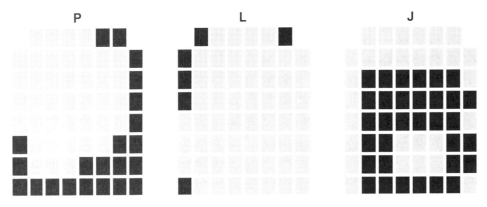

Figure 2–5. Cumulative maximum contact EPG frames for the production of /p/ by three Scottish English-speaking children (P, L, J) with cleft palate (adapted from Gibbon & Crampin, 2002, Figure 4, p. 45).

shading indicates that the electrode was contacted at least 80% of the time over five productions of words containing /p/. Evidence of production at both alveolar and velar edges of the palate is apparent for each of these three speakers. The importance of these images is that Gibbon and Crampin (2002, p. 46) suggest that LLDAs may "have been misclassified as correct productions in studies that have used transcription to identify articulation errors in cleft palate speech."

Chapter 3

/b/

The consonant /b/ is a voiced bilabial stop.

Place of articulation: bilabial

Advancement: front

Voicing: voiced

Labiality: labial

Sonorancy: nonsonorant (obstruent)

Continuancy: noncontinuant (stop)

Sibilancy: nonsibilant

Nasality: nonnasal (oral)

STATIC IMAGES OF THE ARTICULATORY CHARACTERISTICS OF /b/

The static representations of /b/ are presented via a photograph, schematic diagram, ultrasound, and electropalatograph images (Figure 3–1).

Photograph

As for the phoneme /p/, the upper and lower lips are approximated to create closure of the airstream to produce /b/ (Figure 3–1A).

A. Photograph

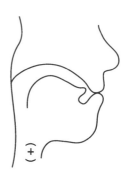

B. Schematic diagram

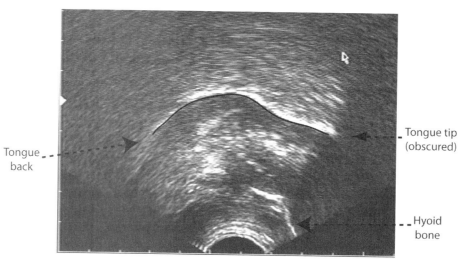

Tongue back

Tongue tip (obscured)

Hyoid bone

C. Ultrasound

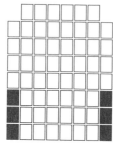

D. Electropalatograph (EPG) (single frame)

Figure 3–1. Static images of the articulatory characteristics of /b/.

Schematic Diagram

The lateral view in the schematic diagram (Figure 3–1B) can be compared with the frontal view in the filmstrip (Figure 3–2A). It is clear from this comparison that the production of a phoneme is a constantly changing articulatory event. A schematic drawing is inadequate in representing an articulatory event. In addition to showing lip involvement, this diagram shows that the tongue is placed at a neutral position. This is different from the other pairs of stops, /t, d/ and /k, g/, where the tongue plays the major role in closing the oral cavity. The voicing nature of the stop /b/ is denoted by a plus sign (+) at the vocal folds.

Ultrasound

Figure 3–1C shows the tongue surface during production of /b/ as a bright white line. The tongue tip is on the right and is toward the floor of the mouth. Similar to the image of /p/, the back of the tongue is somewhat raised in the oral cavity. An air shadow can be seen above the tongue and diagonal muscle fibers can be seen below the surface of the tongue.

Electropalatograph (EPG)

Similar to the phoneme /p/, there is limited tongue/palate contact for the EPG image of /b/ in Figure 3–1D. In this image the tongue touches the most posterior lateral margins of the palate. There is no contact with the central regions of the palate. Gibbon, Lee, and Yuen (2007) found that the extent of tongue/palate contact for the production of /b/ was significantly correlated with the extent of contact for the surrounding vowels. Similar to the phoneme /p/, the primary oral mechanisms involved in shaping the oromusculature to produce a /b/ are the lips and the soft palate (see Figures 3–1A and 3–1B).

DYNAMIC IMAGES OF THE ARTICULATORY AND ACOUSTIC CHARACTERISTICS OF /b/

In order to obtain a comprehensive view of the production of this consonant, the dynamic aspects of the production of /b/ are shown in a filmstrip, spectrogram, and EPG images.

/b/ in Word-Initial and Word-Final Contexts: "bib"

Filmstrip: /bɪb/ "bib"

The phoneme /b/ is at the initial and final positions of the word /bɪb/. The first nine frames in Figure 3–2A show the lips closed. A slight trace of acoustic energy begins at frame 4, indicating that, unlike voiceless stops, voiced stops emit acoustic energy prior to the opening at the point of contact. This articulatory phenomenon contributes to negative voice onset time (-VOT). Frame 10 shows the opening of the lips and, at that point, the nature of the acoustic tracing changes from a low frequency, low amplitude /b/ to a high frequency, high amplitude /ɪ/. The maximal opening of the vowel /ɪ/ can be seen sustained in frames 12, 13, and 14. Then the lips gradually close for production of the final target /b/.

Sound Spectrogram: /bɪb/ "bib"

The voiced-labial stop consonant /b/ is presented in the initial and final positions with the vowel /ɪ/ in the medial position in the word "bib" in Figure 3–2B. The vowel /ɪ/, which is known to have high second formant frequencies, is presented in the context of the consonant /b/ in order to maximize the visual effect of the formant transitions. The voicing nature of the initial /b/ is signaled by two factors: a 180-msec negative voice onset time and a rising first formant for the

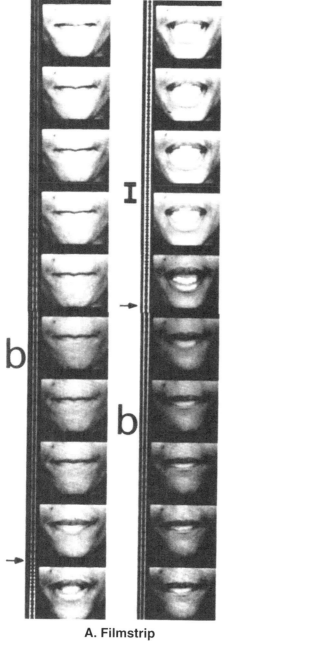

A. Filmstrip

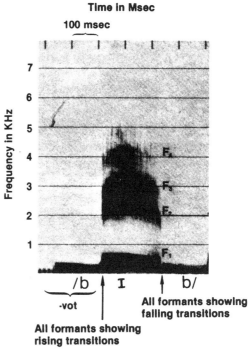

B. Spectrogram

Figure 3–2. Dynamic images of /b/ in the word-initial and word-final contexts: "bib." *continues*

vowel /ɪ/. The rising first and second formants indicate low energy (below 2000 Hz) for the plosive burst of the phoneme /b/ in the initial position. The falling F1 accommodates the voicing characteristic of the final /b/. The falling F2 accommodates the labial place of articulation. All of the formants except the F1 show a bowlike configuration. This indicates that, although an isolated vowel /ɪ/ may contain a steady state resembling

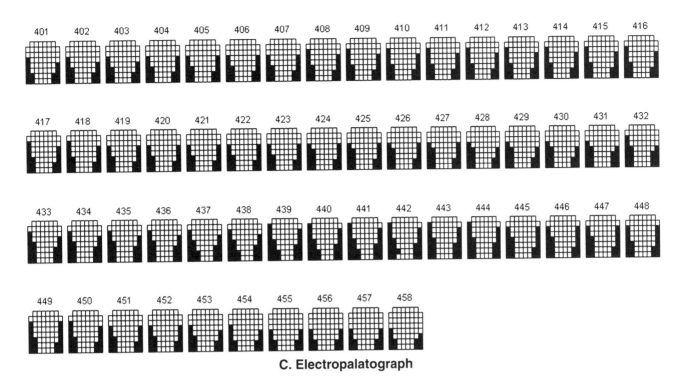

C. Electropalatograph

Figure 3–2. *continued*

a straight line, the formants in this sound spectrogram change drastically because of the nature of the features of the preceding and following consonants.

Electropalatograph: /bɪb/ "bib"

Figure 3-2C presents tongue/palate contact for the word "bib." Throughout this word the EPG frames have some tongue/palate contact along the lateral margins. There is more contact than for the word "pop" (see Chapter 2) as the vowel /ɪ/ "bib" has more contact than the vowel /ɑ/ in "pop". The coarticulatory influences of the vowel /ɪ/ extend through the production of the word-initial and word-final /b/ consonants.

/b/ in Within-Word Context: "baby"

Filmstrip: /beɪbɪ/ "baby"

This filmstrip shows the production of /b/ at the initial and medial positions. The initial position /b/ seems to be longer in duration than the medial position /b/.

Prior to lip opening (in the seventh frame), there are at least six frames showing articulatory gestures prior to the plosive burst (Figure 3-3A). At the medial position, however, there are only three frames showing complete lip closure prior to lip opening (in frame 20). This allows us to conclude a longer duration for this stop at the initial position than at the medial position. It may also be noted that the initial position /b/ is part of the stressed syllable /beɪ/, whereas the medial position /b/ is part of the unstressed syllable /bɪ/. The consonant in the stressed syllable has a longer duration than the consonant in the unstressed syllable.

Sound Spectrogram: /beɪbɪ/ "baby"

The phoneme /b/ is contrasted at the initial and medial positions in the word "baby." The vowel following /b/ at the initial position is /eɪ/ and the vowel following /b/ at the medial position is /ɪ/. The + voicing nature of the consonant /b/ is indicated by the presence of negative voice onset time (of approximately 100 msec) and a rising F1 for the vowel /eɪ/

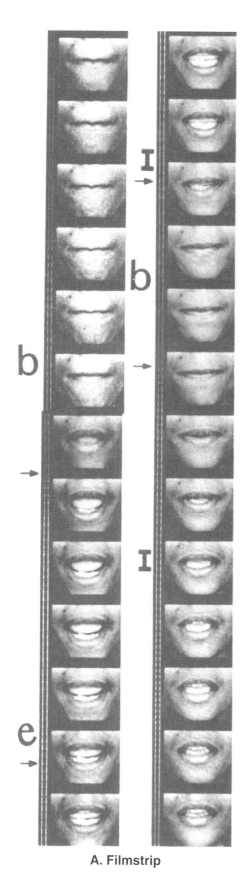

b

b

e

A. Filmstrip

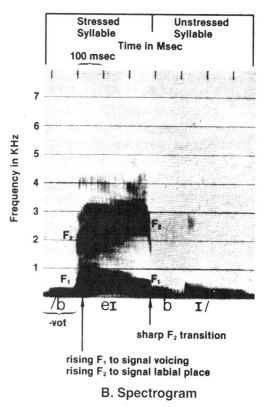

B. Spectrogram

Figure 3–3. Dynamic images of /b/ in the within-word context: "baby." *continues*

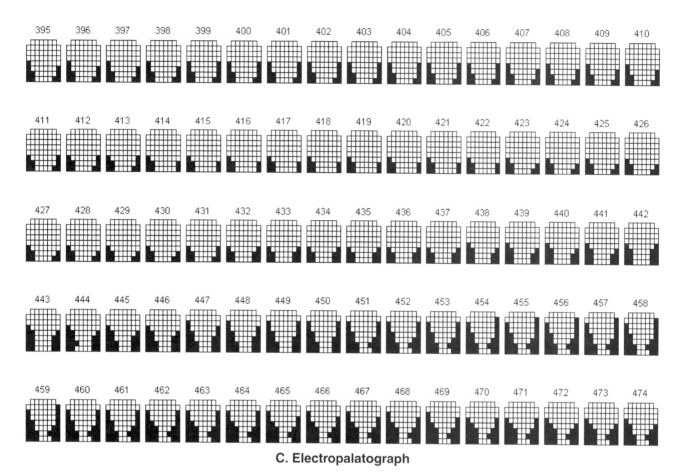

C. Electropalatograph

Figure 3–3. *continued*

(Figure 3–3B). The rising F2 signals the low-frequency energy of the plosive burst (below 2000 Hz). In the first half of the vowel segment, the formant frequencies of the vowel /e/ are evident, and in the second half of the vowel segment, the formant frequencies of the vowel /ɪ/ are evident. The sharply dropping transition of the F2 signals the onset of low-frequency labial energy (below 2000 Hz). The vowel following the medial position /b/ shows short duration, a rising F2, and low amplitude characteristics, all of which imply the weakness or unstressing of the second syllable in the word "baby."

Electropalatograph: /beɪbi/ "baby"

The word /beɪbi/[1] "baby" is presented in Figure 3–3C. The first /b/ was identified to extend from frames 395

to 416 by using information about voice onset time from the simultaneous spectrogram to facilitate identification. Using the same technique, the second /b/ was identified to extend from frames 447 to 460. In both cases, there is limited tongue contact along the lateral margins of the palate for the production of /b/. There is slightly more contact during the second production of /b/ due to the coarticulatory influence of the vowel /i/.

INTRA- AND INTERSPEAKER VARIABILITY FOR /b/

Electropalatographic images enable consideration of intra- and interspeaker variability.

---

[1]/beɪbi/ is the Australian English pronunciation of "baby."

EPG images of productions of /b/ by children with cleft palate are provided in order to compare production with the typical adult's EPG images of /b/.

Interspeaker Variability for /b/ in Speakers with Impaired Speech

Children with Cleft Palate

Gibbon and Crampin (2002) described the production of /p, b, m/ for 27 Scottish-English speaking adults and children aged 5 to 62 years who had a history of cleft palate and produced compensatory speech errors. Fifteen productions of words containing the bilabial consonants were produced by each speaker. Three speakers were described as frequently producing "labial-lingual double articulations (LLDAs)" (p. 40): speaker P (aged 9;07), speaker L (aged 9;10), and speaker J (aged 12;6). Each of the three speakers produced LLDAs during production of /b/. Figure 3–4 illustrates the cumulative maximum contact EPG frames for the production of /b/ by these three Scottish English-speaking children (P, L, J). Black shading indicates that the electrode was contacted at least 80% of the time over five productions of words containing /b/. Evidence of production at both alveolar and velar edges of the palate is apparent for each of these three speakers.

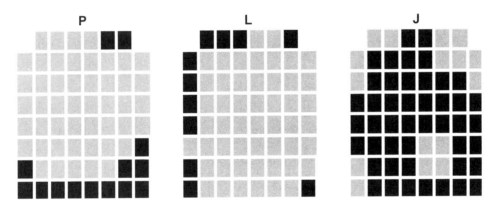

Figure 3–4. Cumulative maximum contact EPG frames for the production of /b/ by three Scottish English-speaking children (P, L, J) with cleft palate (adapted from Gibbon & Crampin, 2002, Figure 4, p. 45).

Chapter 4

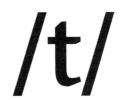

The consonant /t/ is a voiceless alveolar stop.

Place of articulation: alveolar

Voicing: voiceless

Advancement: front

Labiality: nonlabial

Sonorancy: nonsonorant (obstruent)

Continuancy: noncontinuant (stop)

Sibilancy: nonsibilant

Nasality: nonnasal (oral)

STATIC IMAGES OF THE ARTICULATORY CHARACTERISTICS OF /t/

The static images of /t/ are presented via a photograph, schematic diagram, ultrasound, and electropalatograph images (Figure 4–1).

Photograph

In this photograph (Figure 4-1A), the mouth is open and the tongue is touching the alveolar ridge to create closure of the airstream to produce /t/.

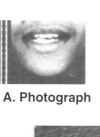

A. Photograph

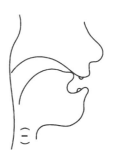

B. Schematic diagram

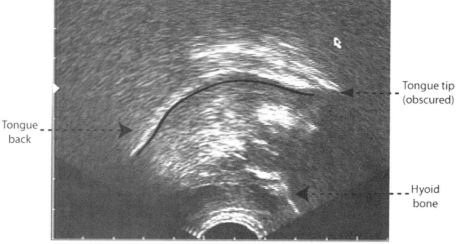

C. Ultrasound

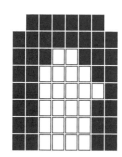

D. Electropalatograph (EPG) (single frame)

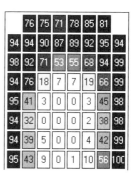

E. Electropalatograph (EPG) (cumulative frame)

Figure 4–1. Static images of the articulatory characteristics of /t/.

Schematic Diagram

In the lateral view of the production of the consonant /t/, the tongue contacts the alveolar ridge behind the upper teeth (Figure 4-1B). This view also does not demonstrate the sides of the tongue contacting the lateral margins of the palate along the teeth. The tongue's contact with the palate causes complete closure and a complete stoppage of the airstream in the oral cavity. The lack of voicing of this consonant is symbolically represented at the source (the vocal folds) by a minus sign.

Ultrasound

The bright white line on the ultrasound image in Figure 4-1C shows the tongue surface during production of /t/. The tongue tip is on the right and is raised toward the alveolar ridge. Approximately 1 cm of the tongue tip is obscured from view because of the acoustic shadow of the jaw (Stone, 2005). The back of the tongue is somewhat raised in the oral cavity. An air shadow can be seen above the tongue and diagonal muscle fibers can be seen below the surface of the tongue.

Electropalatograph (EPG)

The EPG image of /t/ (Figure 4-1D) presents as a horseshoe shape, with the tongue contacting the palate along the margins of the teeth. There is tongue/palate contact across the alveolar ridge (first two rows) with lateral bracing along the sides of the teeth (first and last columns).

The cumulative EPG image (Figure 4-1E) represents productions of /t/ by eight speakers over a total of 475 words. The darker the shading the more often that part of the palate was contacted by the tongue. The numbers indicate the percentage of contact with each EPG electrode. The number 95 in the lower left square indicates that that electrode was contacted 95% of the time by the eight speakers over the 475 words when producing /t/. The darker shading suggests that overall the speakers had horseshoe-shaped tongue contact with the palate.

Gibbon, Yuen, Lee, and Adams (2007) compared 15 typical English-speaking adults' productions of /t/, /d/, and /n/. They found that:

- /t/ and /d had similar spatial patterns
- /t/ and /d/ had more contact than /n/
- In almost every instance, /t/, /d/, and /n/ had 100% tongue/palate contact on the EPG palate at either row 1, row 2, or both
- In almost every instance, /t/, /d/, and /n/ had 0% tongue/palate contact on the EPG palate at the four electrodes at the center of the palate from row 5 to row 8
- /t/ (88%) and /d/ (83%) were more likely to have bilateral constriction compared with /n/ (55%). Bilateral constriction was defined as "100% contact at both the left-most column and the right-most column" of electrodes on the EPG palate (Gibbon et al., 2007, p. 84).

DYNAMIC IMAGES OF THE ARTICULATORY AND ACOUSTIC CHARACTERISTICS OF /t/

In order to obtain a comprehensive view of the production of this consonant, the dynamic aspects of the production of /t/ are shown in a filmstrip, spectrogram, and EPG images in two words containing /t/ in different word positions (Figures 4-2 and 4-3).

/t/ in Word-Initial and Word-Final Contexts: "tat"

Filmstrip: /tæt/ "tat"

The phoneme /t/ is at the initial and final positions of the word "tat" /tæt/. The wide lip opening starts at the first frame of the filmstrip (Figure 4-2A). In the third frame the tongue is seen touching the alveolar ridge. The following vowel /æ/ shows a front-low tongue position with wide and open lips, accompanied by considerable excursion of the mandible. The vowel is used in the stressed position and, hence, can be seen sustained from frames 7 through 13. Starting with

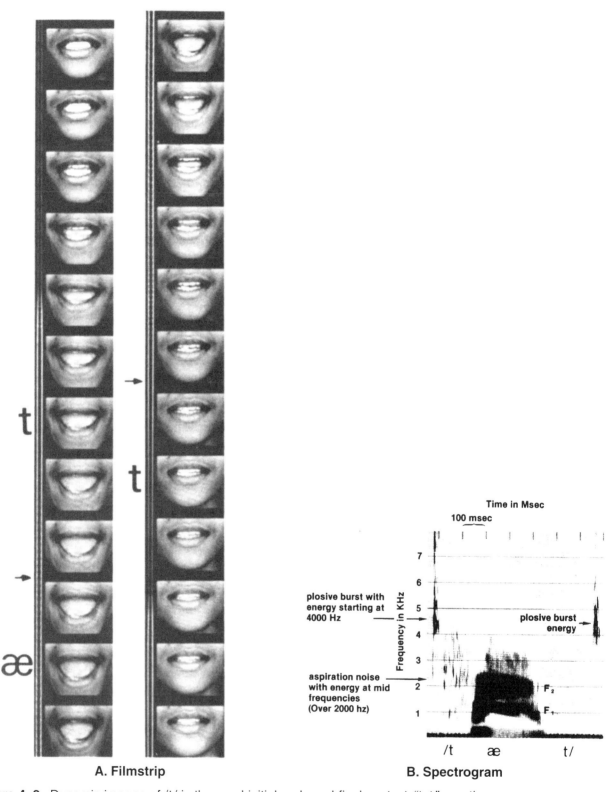

A. Filmstrip

B. Spectrogram

Figure 4–2. Dynamic images of /t/ in the word-initial and word-final context: "tat." *continues*

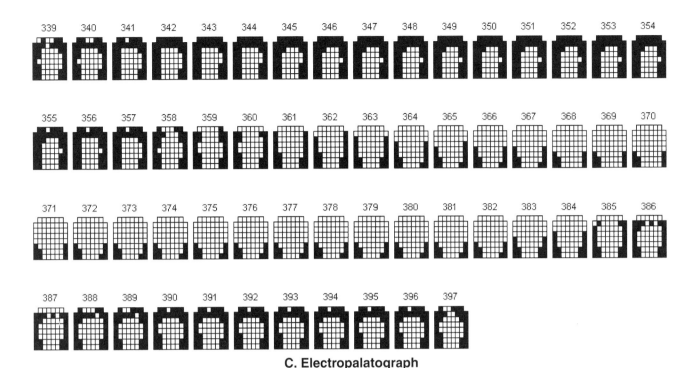

C. Electropalatograph

Figure 4–2. *continued*

frame 14, the tip of the tongue begins to rise and continues to do so until complete contact is made with the alveolar ridge in frame 16. The remaining eight frames show the process of complete closure to accomplish the necessary durational cue for the final-voiceless-stop consonant /t/.

Sound Spectrogram: /tæt/ "tat"

The phoneme /t/ is presented in both the initial and final positions in the word "tat" in the sound spectrogram (Figure 4–2B). The initial and final plosive bursts for /t/ show a clear difference from the plosive bursts for the voiceless-labial stop /p/. The plosive burst for /p/ has energy concentrated below 2000 Hz, whereas the plosive burst for the voiceless-front stop /t/ in both the initial and final positions is above 2000 Hz. Allophonic variation for English voiceless stops described for /p/ is also clearly applicable to /t/. Hence, there exists a presence of aspiration noise (over 100 msec), mostly concentrated above 2000 Hz, for the voiceless stop /t/ in the initial position. At the final position, the aspiration noise is absent and a 200-msec silence is followed by a plosive burst. The

speaker has the option of releasing or not releasing the final stop.

Electropalatograph: /tæt/ "tat"

The dynamic series of EPG palates for the production of the word "tat" is presented in Figure 4–3C. The word "tat" was extracted from the sentence "I see a tat again." Within this sentence, the word "tat" took 0.288 seconds to produce. The first frame of closure for the first /t/ is 340, and the last frame before release is 357. The typical horseshoe shape for /t/ is clearly depicted in frames 340 to 357 and again in frames 388 to 396. The vowel /æ/ (frames 358–345) has limited tongue/palate contact, concentrated toward the velar region of the palate (see Chapter 29).

/t/ in Within-Word Context: "kitty"

Filmstrip: /kɪtɪ/ "kitty"

The phoneme /t/ is at the within-word position of the word "kitty" /kɪtɪ/. Because the medial vowel and

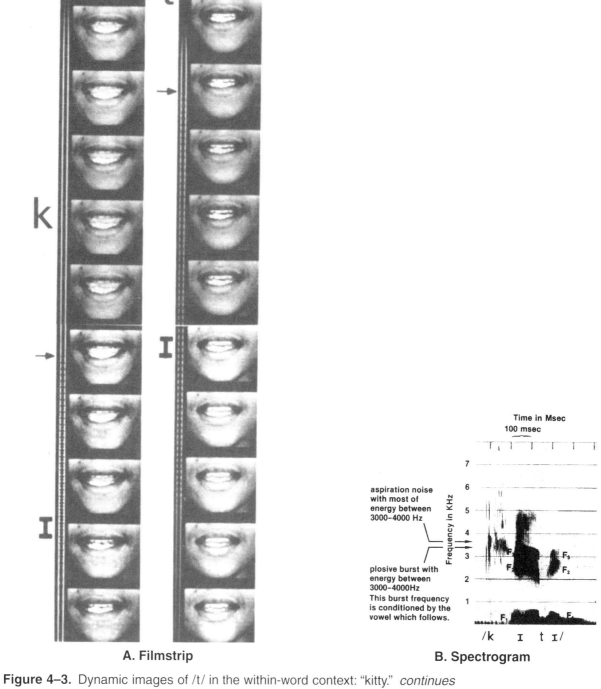

A. Filmstrip

B. Spectrogram

Time in Msec
100 msec

Frequency in KHz

aspiration noise with most of energy between 3000–4000 Hz

plosive burst with energy between 3000–4000Hz This burst frequency is conditioned by the vowel which follows.

/k ɪ t ɪ/

Figure 4–3. Dynamic images of /t/ in the within-word context: "kitty." *continues*

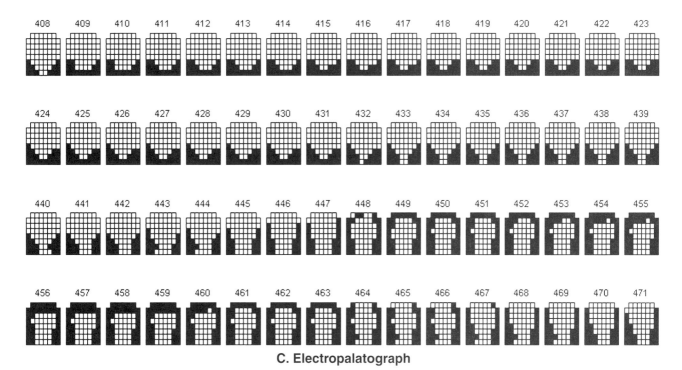

C. Electropalatograph

Figure 4–3. *continued*

the final vowel are both /ɪ/, the lips assume a wide and narrow shape for the production of /t/ (Figure 4–3A).

Sound Spectrogram: /kɪtɪ/ "kitty"

The phoneme /t/ is presented in the within-word position in the word "kitty." The stop function for /t/ at the medial position in Figure 4–3B shows a clear difference from the plosive bursts for the voiceless-velar stop /k/ at the initial position. The stop function for the voiceless-front stop /t/ at the medial position is above 2000 Hz and clearly denotes the absence of explosion which is present at the initial position /k/. Also, the back stop /k/ shows energy in the frequency domain of the second formant of the adjacent vowel /ɪ/. The coarticulatory influence of this stop on the following vowel is mainly in terms of its high-frequency energy. Therefore, the vowel formants for /ɪ/ show falling transition.

Electropalatograph: /kɪti/ "kitty"

Figure 4–3C represents the lingualpalatal contact for the production of the word /kɪti/[1] "kitty." The first frame of closure for /k/ is frame 409 and the /k/ is released at frame 432. The /k/ sound is characterised by velar tongue contact evident by dark shading on the lower part of the image of the palate (see Chapter 6). The vowel /ɪ/ (see Chapter 27) extends from frame 432 to 448. The coarticulatory influences of /t/ on the vowel /ɪ/ are evident in frames 443 to 448. Tongue palate closure for /t/ extends from frame 449 until 463. The contact pattern for /t/ is similar to a horseshoe shape with the tongue contacting the palate along the entire lateral margins with the teeth. The frames 464 to 474 represent the coarticulatory period between /t/ and the vowel /i/. The final frames (475–487) represent tongue/palate contact for the vowel /i/.

---

[1]/kɪti/ is the Australian English pronunciation of "kitty."

INTRA- AND INTERSPEAKER VARIABILITY FOR /t/

Electropalatographic images enable consideration of inter-speaker variability. First, variability between speakers of English is considered; then EPG images of children's productions of /t/ are provided. Next, variability between the English production of /t/ and the production of /t/ by speakers of other languages are compared. Finally, variability between productions of /t/ by speakers with differing types of speech impairment is presented.

Intra- and Interspeaker Variability in the Production of /t/ by Eight Typical English-Speaking Adults

Four typical adult males (M1–M4) and four typical adult females (F1–F4) produced nonsense syllables containing /t/ three times. The nonsense syllables were created with /t/ in syllable-initial and syllable-final positions in vowel contexts taken at the extremes of the vowel quadrilateral.

Maximum Contact Frames for Eight Typical English-Speaking Adults

In order to demonstrate both inter- and intraspeaker variability the maximum contact frame for the second production of each nonsense syllable for each speaker is provided in Figure 4–4. In almost every instance there is evidence of a horseshoe shape of tongue/ palate contact where the tongue touches the alveolar ridge and the lateral margins of the palate. In cases where there is limited contact on the lateral margins (such as for M2), it is hypothesized that the tongue was touching the teeth, and contact with the EPG palate was not registered. Alternate models of EPG palates that register contact with the teeth (e.g., Schmidt, 2007; Wrench, 2007) would provide data to test this hypothesis.

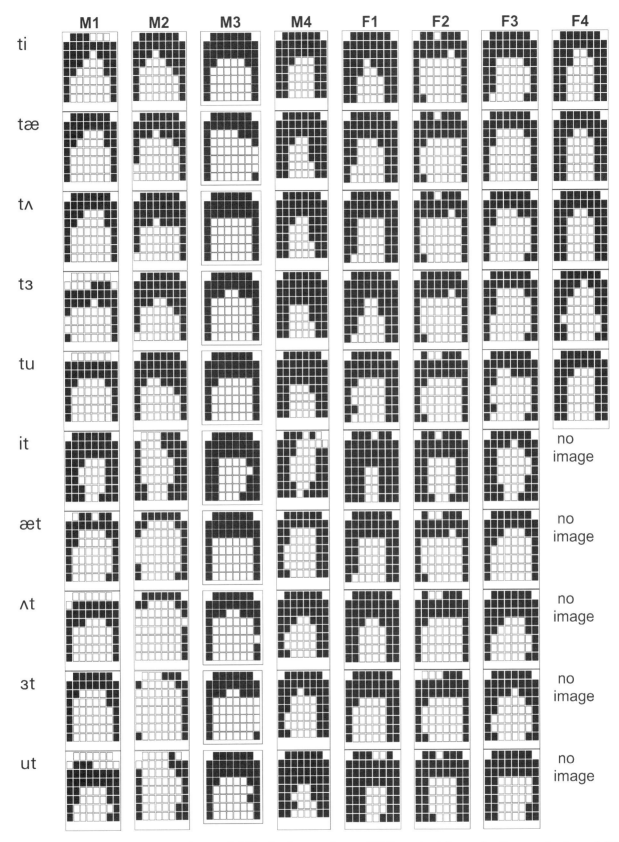

Figure 4–4. Intra- and interspeaker variability in the maximum EPG contact frame for the production of /t/ by eight typical English-speaking adults. *continues*

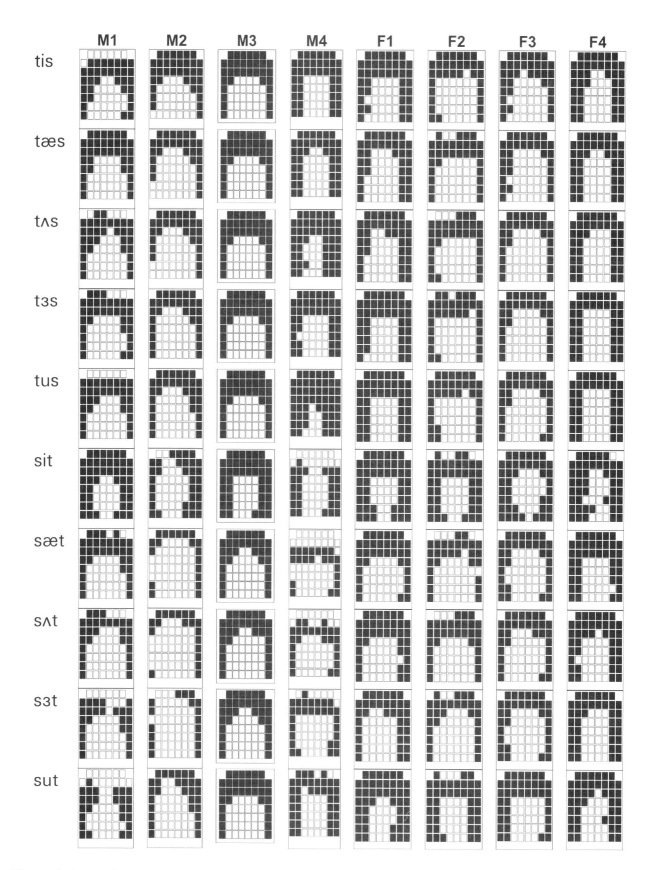

Figure 4–4. *continues*

	M1	**M2**	**M3**	**M4**	**F1**	**F2**	**F3**	**F4**

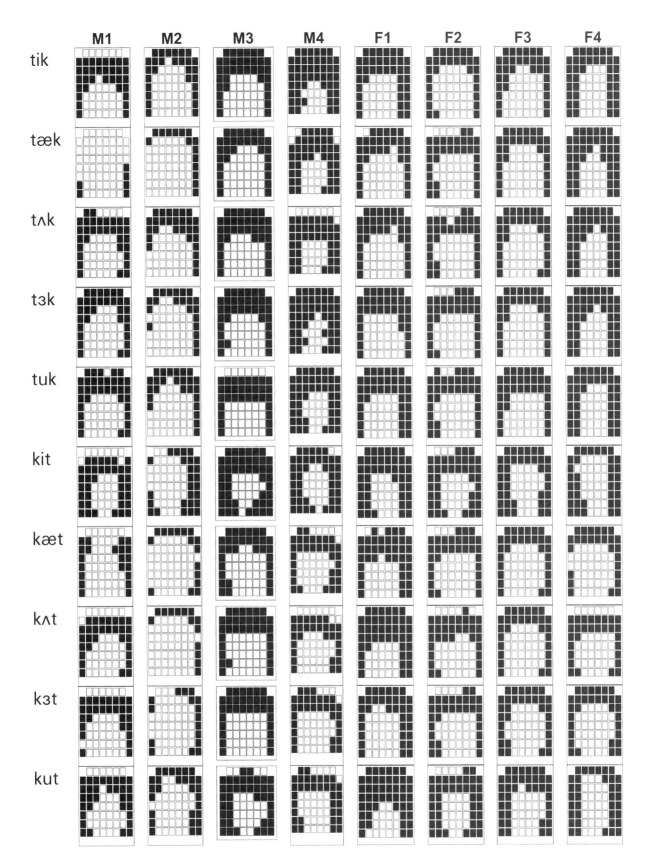

Figure 4–4. *continued*

Cumulative EPG Frames for Eight Typical English-Speaking Adults

Cumulative EPG patterns for /t/ were generated from 60 maximum contact frames (with the exception of F4) for each of the eight typical adults described above (see Figure 4-4). Each electrode on a cumulative maximum contact display has a number, corresponding to the percentage of contact over the 60 productions. The darker the shading, the more contact. In Figure 4-5 each speaker's cumulative maximum contact display is a horseshoe shape; however, there are differences in the number of rows contacted on the alveolar ridge, the width of the lateral bracing. For example, F1 had a more contact across her alveo-

lar ridge than M2 as she consistently contacted the first 3 rows of electrodes. F4 had wider lateral bracing than M2.

Interspeaker Variability in the Production of /t/ by Other English-Speaking Adults

British English-Speaking Adults

Liker, Gibbon, Wrench, and Horga (2007) created cumulative maximum contact EPG frames for /t/ for the purpose of comparing production of /t/ with the occlusion phase of /tʃ/. Seven British English speakers, four females and three males, produced /t/ in VCV

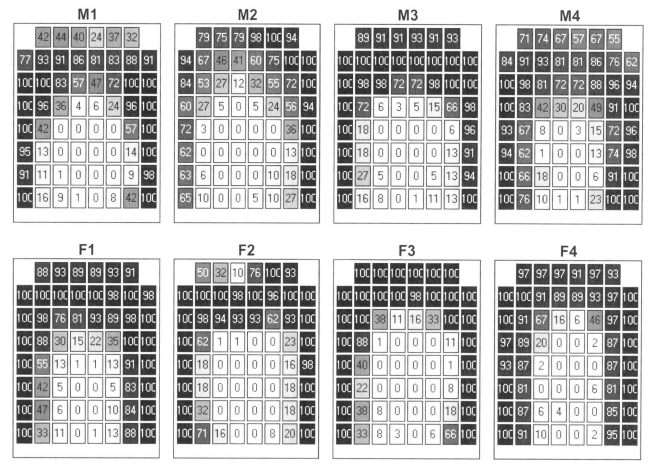

Figure 4–5. Cumulative EPG frames demonstrating intra- and interspeaker variability for the production of /t/ by eight typical English-speaking adults.

sequences in differing combinations with the vowels /a, i, u/, producing a total of 630 tokens of /t/. Figure 4-6 represents cumulative EPG frames for the production of /t/ by these seven British English-speaking adults. A black square indicates that there was at least 67% contact for that electrode.

Australian English-Speaking Adults

McAuliffe, Ward, and Murdoch (2006a) described the speech of 15 typical Australian-English speaking people in order to provide a comparison with the speech of people with Parkinson's disease. The typical speakers were divided into two groups. The seven aged controls were males and were aged between 50 and 79 years (mean = 67.71). Seven of the young controls were female and the eighth was male. The young control group was aged between 23 to 31 years (mean =

25.63). Figure 4-7 demonstrates two cumulative maximum contact EPG frames for productions of /t/ in the contexts /ti/ and /ta/. The participants were asked to produce these words in a sentence " I saw a _____ today" 10 times. In Figure 4-7, a black square indicates that that electrode was contacted at least 67% of the time. McAuliffe et al. found that there was no significant difference in the amount of tongue/palate contact between the aged and young control groups for the production of /t/.

In another study of one typical Australian English-speaking adult, McAuliffe, Ward, and Murdoch (2007) present an individual representative frame for the production of /t/. Figure 4-8 is an individual representative frame for 10 repetitions of /t/ produced by a typical adult Australian-English speaker. A black square indicates that there was at least 67% contact for that electrode.

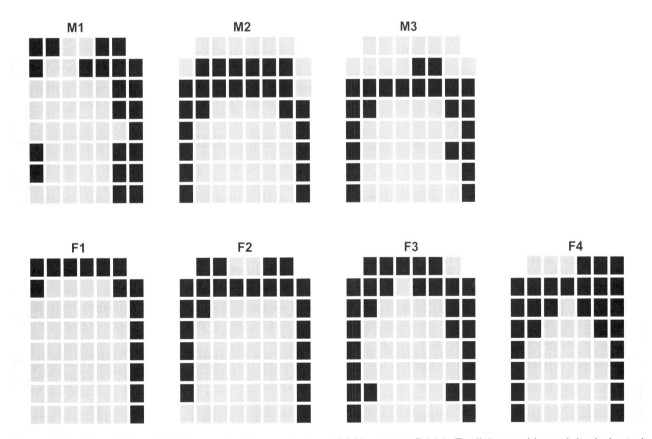

Figure 4–6. Cumulative EPG frames for the production of /t/ by seven British English-speaking adults (adapted from Liker et al., 2007, Figure 3, p. 188).

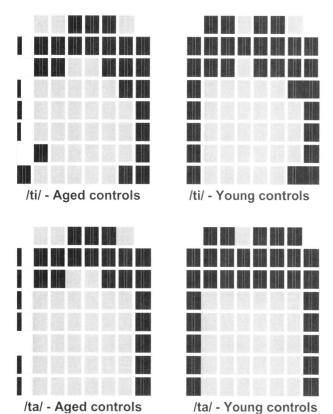

Figure 4–7. Cumulative maximum contact EPG frames for the production of /t/ by 15 Australian English-speaking adults (adapted from McAuliffe et al., 2006a, Figure 3, p. 10).

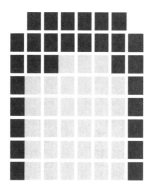

Figure 4–8. Individual representative EPG frame for the production of /t/ by one Australian English-speaking adult (adapted from McAuliffe et al., 2007, Figure 1, p. 16).

Another study of typical Australian English-speaking adults' productions of /t/ was conducted by Cheng, Murdoch, Goozée, and Scott (2007). The six male and six female adult participants, aged between 23 and 38 years, produced /t/ in CV and CVC words that were embedded within a phrase. Each phrase was produced five times, resulting in 10 productions of /t/ per speaker. Figure 4–9 provides a cumulative maximum contact frame for the production of /t/ by the adults. In Figure 4–9, a black square indicates that that electrode was contacted at least 67% of the time.

Interspeaker Variability in the Production of /t/ by English-Speaking Children

Scottish English-Speaking Children

Gibbon, McNeill, Wood and Watson (2003) provided images of the production of /t/ for a typical 12-year-old Scottish-English speaking child from the dissertation by McNeill (2001). Figure 4–10 demonstrates a cumulative maximum contact EPG frame for 11 productions of /t/. A black square indicates that that electrode was contacted at least 67% of the time. The child's production of /t/ has a similar horseshoe shape to the adults' productions shown above.

Australian English-Speaking Children

Cheng et al. (2007) described typical speech production for 36 children. There were six males and six females in each of the following age groups: 6 to 7 years, 8 to 11 years, and 12 to 17 years. The participants produced /t/ in CV and CVC words that were embedded within a phrase. Each phrase was produced five times, resulting in 10 productions of /t/ per speaker. Figure 4–11 provides a cumulative maximum contact frame for the production of /s by the children. In Figure 4–11, a black square indicates that that electrode was contacted at least 67% of the time. Although it appears that there was a midline groove (as required for production of /s/) in the production of /t/ by the 8- to 11-year-olds, the unshaded electrode was contacted 63% of the time by the participants. Cheng et al. found evidence for the maturation of the speech motor system and described this maturation as nonlinear and nonuniform.

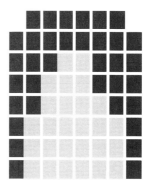

Figure 4–9. Cumulative maximum contact EPG frames for the production of /t/ by 12 typical Australian English-speaking adults (adapted from Cheng et al., 2007, Figure 1).

Figure 4–10. Cumulative maximum contact EPG frames for the production of /t/ by a typical 12-year-old Scottish English-speaking child (adapted from Gibbon et al., 2003, Figure 2, p. 56).

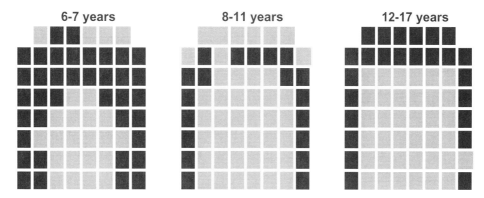

Figure 4–11. Cumulative maximum contact EPG frames for the production of /t/ by 36 typical Australian English-speaking children (adapted from Cheng et al., 2007, Figure 1).

Interspeaker Variability for /t/ in Languages Other than English

Greek-Speaking Adults

Nicolaidis (2004) described the speech of one typical Modern Standard Greek-speaking adult in order to provide comparative data for the speech of four Greek-speaking people with hearing impairment. Figure 4–12 demonstrates two cumulative maximum contact EPG frames for productions of /t/ in the contexts /ata/ and /iti/. The female participant was asked to produce these phoneme combinations ten times in a dysyllabic word of the form /pVtV/ within a carrier phrase. In Figure 4–12, a black square indicates the electrode was contacted at least 60% of the time. Again, tongue/palate contact for production of /t/ resembles a horseshoe shape; however, there is slightly more contact for this Greek speaker than for the English speakers described above.

Japanese-Speaking Adults

Figure 4–13 demonstrates the cumulative EPG pattern for /t/ in /ata/ that was generated from maximum contact frames of five typical adult Japanese speakers

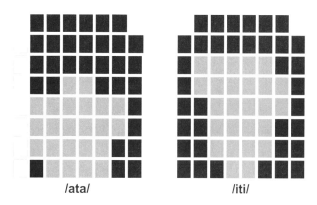

/ata/   /iti/

Figure 4–12. Cumulative maximum contact EPG frames for the production of /t/ by one Greek-speaking adult (adapted from Nicolaidis, 2004, Figure 1, p. 8).

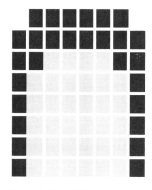

Figure 4–13. Cumulative EPG frames for the production of /t/ by five Japanese-speaking adults (adapted from Fujiwara, 2007, Figure 1b, p. 67).

(Fujiwara, 2007). A black square indicates that there was at least 67% contact for that electrode. The production of /t/ by these speakers is similar in shape to productions of /t/ by English speakers.

Norwegian-Speaking Adults

Moen and Simonsen (2007) compared the production of /t, d/ with the Norwegian sounds /ʈ, ɖ/. Figure 4–14 demonstrates the cumulative maximum contact EPG frames for /t, d/ produced by four typical adult East Norwegian speakers (AN, HS, IM, RE). The sounds were produced in four contexts: word-initial and word-final position with a closed and open vowel. The words were produced 10 times each in a carrier phrase. A black square indicates that there was at least 67% contact for that electrode across the 80 tokens. Although there are some differences between the amount of tongue/palate contact for the Norwegian versus the English productions of /t, d/, all speakers produced a horseshoe shape of tongue/palate contact.

Interspeaker Variability for /t/ Speakers with Impaired Speech

Adults with Parkinson's Disease

McAuliffe, Ward, and Murdoch (2006a) described the speech of nine Australian-English speaking people

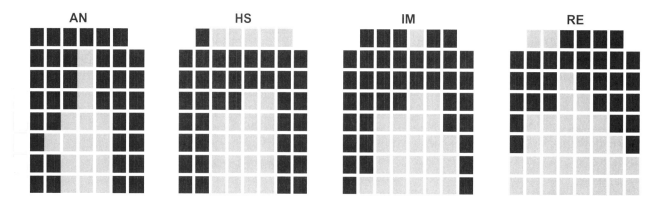

AN   HS   IM   RE

Figure 4–14. Cumulative EPG frames for the production of /t, d/ by four Norwegian-speaking adults (AN, HS, IM, RE) (adapted from Moen & Simonsen, 2007, Figure 3, p. 123).

diagnosed with Parkinson's disease. Figure 4–15 demonstrates two cumulative maximum contact EPG frames for productions of /t/ in the contexts /ti/ and /ta/. The participants were asked to produce these words in a sentence " I saw a _____ today" 10 times. In Figure 4–15, a black square indicates that that electrode was contacted at least 67% of the time. McAuliffe et al. indicated that the people with Parkinson's disease had "reductions in the amplitude of lingual movement, or articulatory undershoot" (p. 16).

Figure 4–15. Cumulative maximum contact EPG frames for the production of /t/ by nine English-speaking adults with Parkinson's disease (adapted from McAuliffe et al., 2006a, Figure 3, p. 10).

Adults with Hearing Impairment

Nicolaidis (2004) described tongue/palate contact for four adults with hearing impairment aged between 23 to 26 years and spoke typical Modern Standard Greek. Each of the four people produced /t/ in the contexts /ata/ and /iti/ within a disyllabic word form in a carrier phrase. The speakers were judged to have limited or no difficulty producing /t/ both from a perceptual and tongue/palate contact. In contrast, the speakers had difficulty producing other lingual sounds including /k, s, n, l/ which are discussed in subsequent chapters.

Children with Cleft Palate

Gibbon, Ellis, and Crampin (2004) described the production of /t, d, k, g/ for 15 Scottish-English speaking children who had repaired cleft palate. Perceptually, all children had correct production of /k, g/ but generally /t, d/ were perceived as being incorrect, predominantly as a palatal or velar sound. Figure 4–16 demonstrates cumulative tongue/palate contact for the production of /t, d/ across 10 words produced by each of the four of the speakers. In Figure 4–16, a black square indicates that that electrode was contacted at least 80% of the time. It can be seen that speakers C9 and C15 had velar tongue placement, whereas speakers C6 and C12 had alveolar + velar placement. This

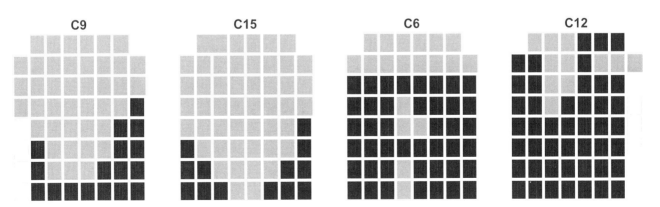

Figure 4–16. Maximum contact EPG frames for the production of /t, d/ by four Scottish English-speaking children with repaired cleft palate (adapted from Gibbon et al., 2004, Figure 1, p. 396).

placement was likened to undifferentiated gestures, or whole tongue gestures (Gibbon, 1999b) produced by children with speech impairment that involved almost the whole tongue touching the palate.

Children with Speech Impairment

Gibbon, Stewart, Hardcastle, and Crampin (1999) described the speech of an 8-year-old Scottish-English speaking boy named Robbie. Robbie had difficulty producing a range of consonants. Figure 4–17 demon-

strates the maximum contact EPG frame for production of /t/ in the phrases "a top" and "a tip." The /t/ sounds were transcribed by a speech-language pathologist as sounding like a [k]. Both images are very different, both from one another, and from the typical production of /t/ indicated in the previous figures. The major difference was due to the velar contact with the palate. Gibbon et al. (1999) describe Robbie's successful intervention using the EPG and his subsequent normalization of both his tongue/palate contacts and his increased speech intelligibility.

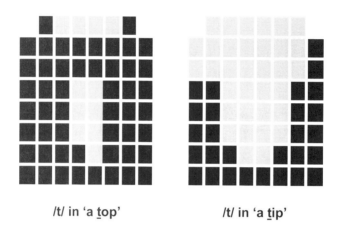

/t/ in 'a top'   /t/ in 'a tip'

Figure 4–17. Maximum contact EPG frames for the production of /t/ in "a top" and "a tip" by an 8-year-old Scottish English-speaking child with speech impairment (adapted from Gibbon et al., 1999, Figures 4a, 4b, p. 327).

Chapter 5

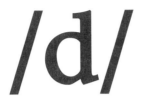

The consonant /d/ is a voiced alveolar stop.

Place of articulation: alveolar

Advancement: front

Voicing: voiced

Labiality: nonlabial

Sonorancy: nonsonorant (obstruent)

Continuancy: noncontinuant (stop)

Sibilancy: nonsibilant

Nasality: nonnasal (oral)

STATIC IMAGES OF THE ARTICULATORY CHARACTERISTICS OF /d/

The static images of /d/ are presented via a photograph, schematic diagram, ultrasound and electropalatograph images (Figure 5–1).

Photograph

In this photograph (Figure 5–1A), the mouth is open and the tongue can be seen touching the alveolar ridge to create closure of the airstream to produce /d/.

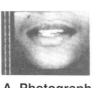

A. Photograph

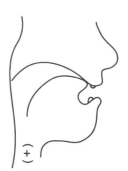

B. Schematic diagram

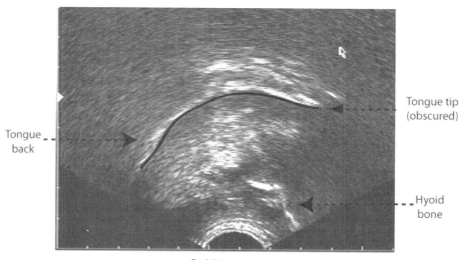

C. Ultrasound

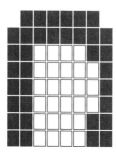

D. Electropalatograph (EPG) (single frame)

E. Electropalatograph (EPG) (cumulative frame)

Figure 5–1. Static images of the articulatory characteristics of /d/.

Schematic Diagram

The schematic diagram (Figure 5–1B) shows the tip of the tongue contacting the roof of the mouth directly behind the upper teeth. The roof of the mouth can be divided at the center, with front toward the lips and back toward the pharyngeal wall. The phoneme /d/ is clearly a front consonant, because the tongue contacts the hard palate at the front. This view does not also demonstrate the sides of the tongue contacting the lateral margins of the palate along the teeth. The tongue's contact with the palate causes complete closure and a complete stoppage of the airstream in the oral cavity. The voicing of this consonant is symbolically represented at the source (the vocal folds) by a plus sign.

Ultrasound

Figure 5–1C shows an ultrasound image of the production of /d/. Underneath the bright white line is the tongue surface. The tongue tip is on the right and is raised toward the alveolar ridge. The acoustic shadow of the jaw obscures approximately 1 cm of the tongue tip (Stone, 2005). The back of the tongue is somewhat raised in the oral cavity. Diagonal muscle fibers can be seen below the surface of the tongue and an air shadow can be seen above the tongue.

Electropalatograph (EPG)

Similar to /t/, the EPG image of /d/ (Figure 5–1D) is a horseshoe shape, with the tongue contacting the palate along the margins of the teeth. The evident asymmetry is not relevant. There is tongue/palate contact across the alveolar ridge with lateral bracing along the sides of the teeth. The cumulative EPG image (Figure 5–1E) represents productions of /d/ by eight speakers over a total of 480 words. The darker the shading the more often that part of the palate was contacted by the tongue. The numbers indicate the percentage of contact with each EPG electrode. The number 85 in the lower left square indicates that that electrode was contacted 85% of the time by the 8 speakers over the 480 words when producing /d/.

Gibbon, Yuen, Lee, and Adams (2007) compared 15 typical English-speaking adults' productions of /t/, /d/, and /n/. They found that:

- /d/ and /t/ had similar spatial contact patterns
- /d/ and /t/ had more contact than /n/
- In almost every instance, /d/, /t/, and /n/ had 100% tongue/palate contact on the EPG palate at either row 1, row 2, or both
- In almost every instance, /d/, /t/, and /n/ had 0% tongue/palate contact on the EPG palate at the four electrodes at the center of the palate from row 5 to row 8
- /d/ (83%) and /t/ (88%) were more likely to have bilateral constriction compared with /n/ (55%). Bilateral constriction was defined as "100% contact at both the left-most column and the right-most column" of electrodes on the EPG palate (Gibbon et al., 2007, p. 84).

DYNAMIC IMAGES OF THE ARTICULATORY AND ACOUSTIC CHARACTERISTICS OF /d/

In order to obtain a comprehensive view of the production of this consonant, the dynamic aspects of the production of /d/ are shown in a filmstrip, spectrogram, and EPG images (Figure 5–2).

/d/ in Word-Initial and Word-Final Contexts: "did"

Filmstrip: /dɪd/ "did"

The phoneme /d/ was presented at the initial and final positions in the word /dɪd/. Because of the voicing characteristic of this phoneme, a considerable duration of low-frequency acoustic energy is emitted throughout, prior to the plosive burst (which begins at the eighth frame). The flat lip position and outward jaw movement at the beginning of the filmstrip are the result of the influence of the vowel /ɪ/. This vowel requires flat, relatively unopen lips and an extended jaw. This influence of one phoneme on another (coarticulation) is germane to the understanding of phonetics.

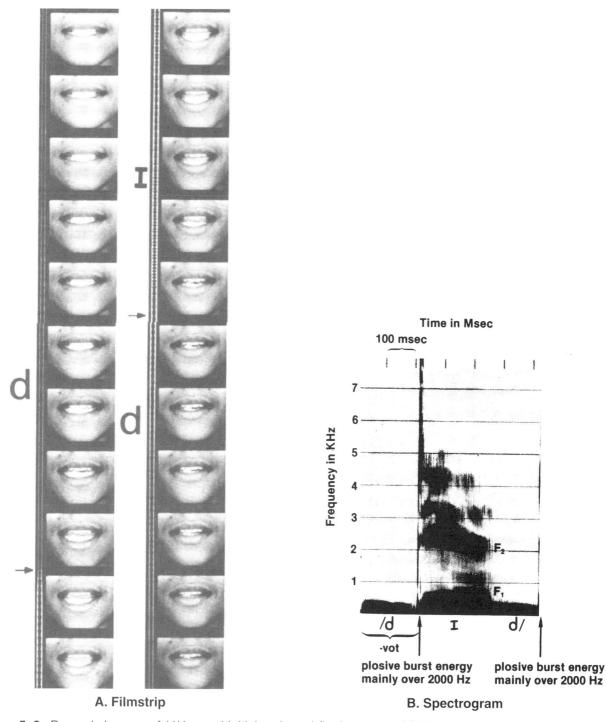

A. Filmstrip B. Spectrogram

Figure 5–2. Dynamic images of /d/ in word-initial and word-final contexts: "did." *continues*

Sound Spectrogram: /dɪd/ "did"

The phoneme /d/ is contrasted in the initial and final positions with the vowel /ɪ/ in the medial position in the word "did." A 180-msec negative voice onset time and rising F1 signal the (+) voicing feature for the phoneme /d/ in the initial position. The front nature of this consonant is indicated by the presence of most

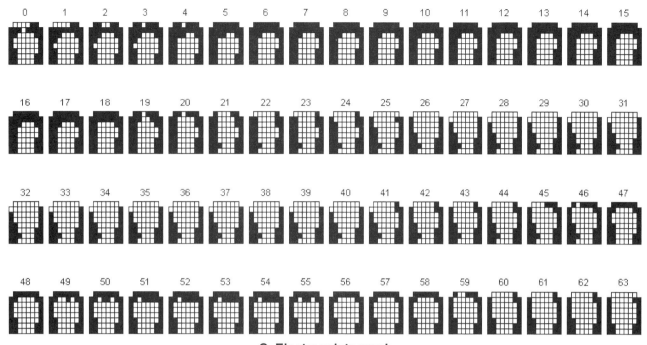

C. Electropalatograph

Figure 5–2. *continued*

of its plosive burst energy over 2000 Hz. Because of the high-frequency plosive burst energy and high-frequency second formant energy for the vowel /ɪ/, there is little formant transition. The /d/ at the final position again has its predominant energy at and above 2000 Hz. The plosive burst is preceded by a silence of approximately 175 msec.

Electropalatograph: /dɪd/ "did"

Figure 5-2C represents the lingualpalatal contact for the production of the word "did." The first frame of closure for /d/ is frame 1 and the /d/ is released beginning at frame 19. The /d/ sound is recognizable by the horseshoe-shaped activation of electrodes corresponding to the tongue's contact with the lateral margins of the palate. The vowel /ɪ/ (see Chapter 27) extends from frame 19 to 46. The coarticulatory influences of /d/ on the vowel /ɪ/ are evident throughout the vowel phase. Tongue palate closure for the word-final /d/ extends from frame 47 until 58.

/d/ in Word-Initial and Within-Word Context: "daddy"

Filmstrip: /ˈdædɪ/ "daddy"

The word /ˈdædɪ/ represents the phoneme /d/ at the initial and medial positions. In Figure 5–3A the absence of the voicing characteristic of /d/ is shown by the presence of low-frequency acoustic energy (-VOT) parallel to frames 2 through 6 and prior to the opening of the point of contact. The point of contact for /d/ is at the front of the roof of the mouth. The influence of the front low-unrounded vowel /æ/ can be seen from the very first frame by the front excursion of the mandible and the relatively unrounded lip opening.

Sound Spectrogram: /ˈdædɪ/ "daddy"

The voiced-front stop consonant /d/ is contrasted in this module at the initial and medial positions in the

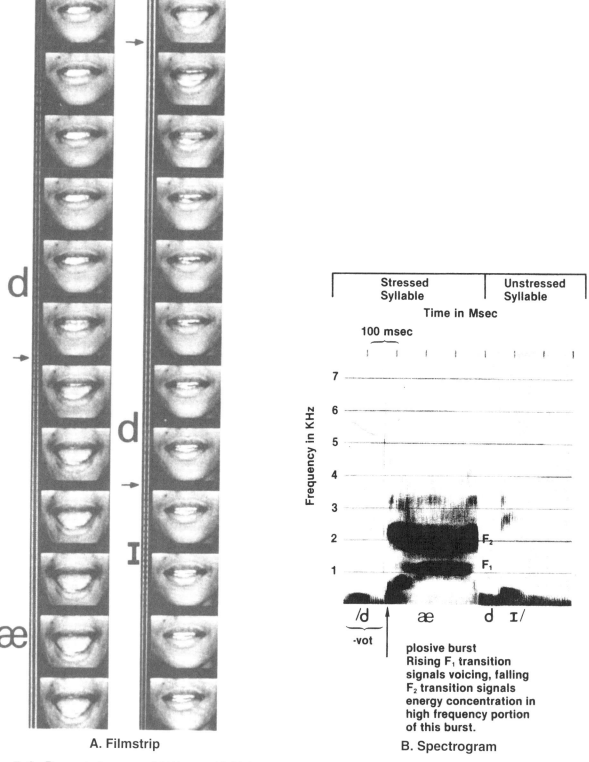

A. Filmstrip

B. Spectrogram

Within the spectrogram:

Stressed Syllable   Unstressed Syllable

Time in Msec

100 msec

Frequency in KHz

/d   æ   d   ɪ/

-vot

plosive burst
Rising F_1 transition
signals voicing, falling
F_2 transition signals
energy concentration in
high frequency portion
of this burst.

Figure 5–3. Dynamic images of /d/ in word-initial and within-word contexts: "daddy." *continues*

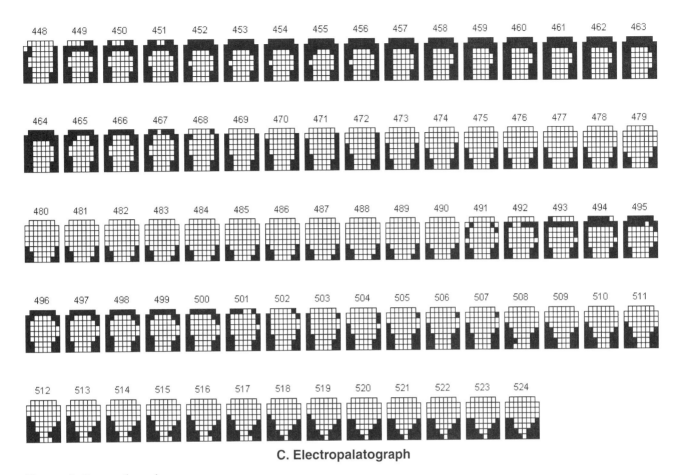

C. Electropalatograph

Figure 5–3. *continued*

word "daddy." At the initial position, it is followed by the vowel /æ/ and at the medial position by the vowel /ɪ/. The (+) voicing nature of this phoneme /d/ is indicated by a 150-msec negative voice onset time as well as a clear rising F1. The plosive burst shows traces of energy mostly over 2000 Hz, and consequently the second formant of the vowel /æ/, which has a center frequency at about 1800 Hz, shows a falling transition. A comparison of this spectrogram representing /d/ with that of Module 7 shows that the two vowels /æ/ and /ɪ/ have opposite transition tendencies. In the word "daddy," the phoneme /d/ at the medial position is followed by the high-front vowel /ɪ/, which in English is an unstressed vowel. A contrast of stressing can clearly be established by comparing the duration and energy characteristics of the first and second syllables. The first syllable in the word "daddy" is stressed, and

this is manifested by long duration (about 450 msec). The unstressing of the second syllable is manifested by relatively short duration (about 300 msec). In addition, the energy distribution across these two syllables is skewed. Most of the energy is concentrated in the first syllable, as denoted by the relative darkness of markings.

Electropalatograph: /ˈdædi/ "daddy"

The dynamic series of EPG palates for the production of the word /ˈdædi/[1] "daddy" is presented in Figure 5–3C. The word "daddy" was extracted from the sentence "I see a daddy again." Within this sentence, the word "daddy" took 0.376 seconds to produce. The first frame of closure for the first /d/ is 449, and the last frame before release is 466. The typical horseshoe

---

[1]/dædi/ is the Australian English pronunciation of "daddy."

shape for /d/ is clearly depicted in frames 449 to 466. The second /d/ extends from frames 493 to 500; however, this time there is not complete closure demonstrated around the entire lateral margins of the palate. It is hypothesized that the tongue may have been touching the teeth on the right hand side of the palate. The vowel /æ/ (frames 467–492) has limited tongue/palate contact, concentrated toward the velar region of the palate (see Chapter 29); where as /i/ (frames 500–524) has more tongue palate contact (see Chapter 26). Both vowels are influenced by coarticulation with the alveolar consonant /d/.

INTRA- AND INTERSPEAKER VARIABILITY FOR /d/

Electropalatographic images enable consideration of intra- and interspeaker variability. First, variability between speakers of English are considered. Next, variability between the English and Norwegian productions of /d/ is compared. Finally, variability between productions of /d/ by children with differing types of speech impairment is considered.

Intra- and Interspeaker Variability in the Production of /d/ by Eight Typical English-Speaking Adults

Four typical adult males (M1–M4) and four typical adult females (F1–F4) produced nonsense syllables containing /d/ three times. The nonsense syllables were created with /d/ in syllable-initial and syllable-final positions in five vowel contexts taken at the extremes of the vowel quadrilateral.

Maximum Contact Frames for Eight Typical English-Speaking Adults

In order to demonstrate both inter- and intraspeaker variability the maximum contact frame, the second production of each nonsense syllable for each speaker is provided in Figure 5–4. In almost every instance there is evidence of a horseshoe shape of tongue/palate contact where the tongue touches the alveolar ridge and the lateral margins of the palate. In cases where there is limited contact on the lateral margins (such as for M2 and M3), it is hypothesized that the tongue was touching the teeth, and contact with the EPG palate was not registered.

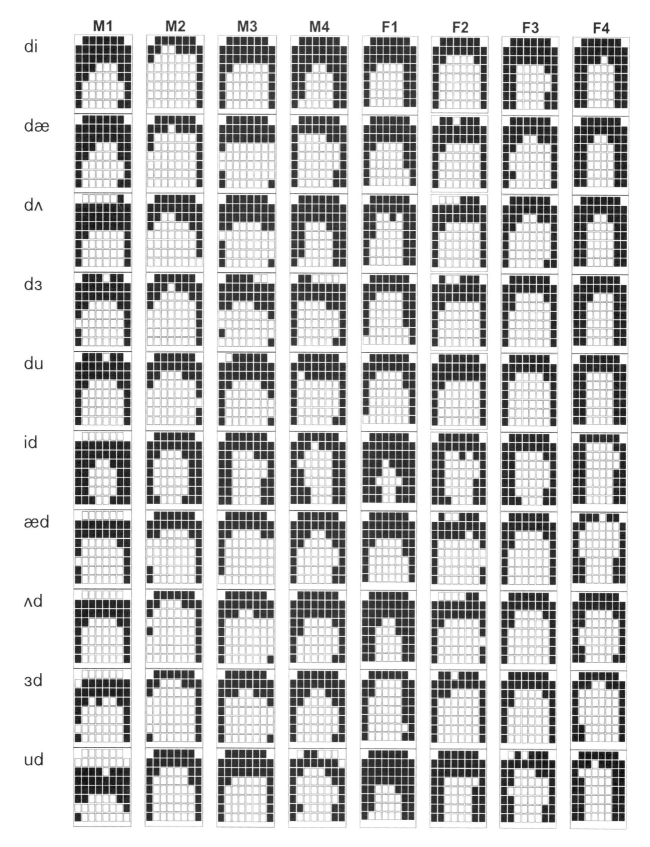

Figure 5–4. Intra- and interspeaker variability in the maximum EPG contact frame for the production of /d/ by eight typical English-speaking adults. *continues*

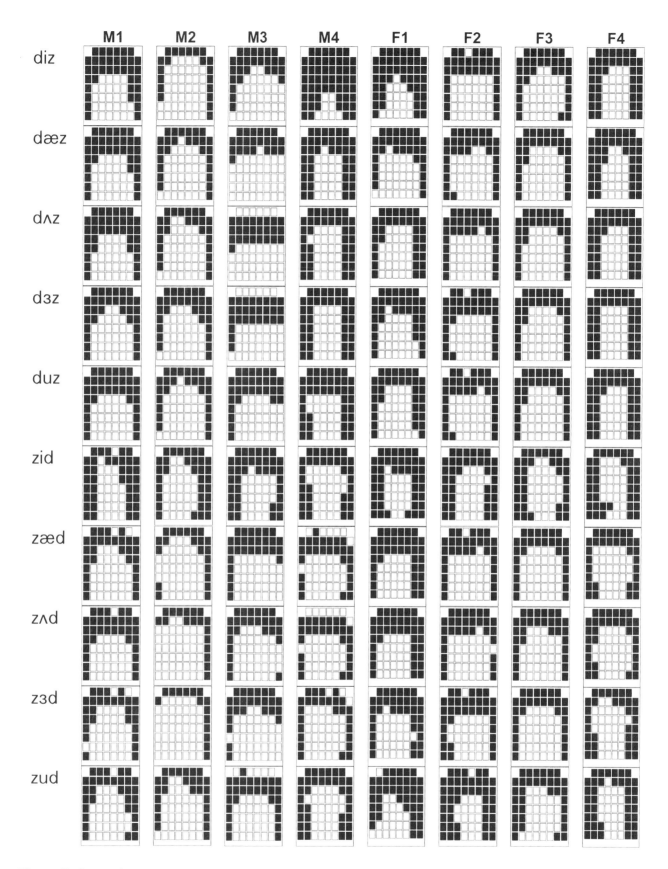

Figure 5–4. *continues*

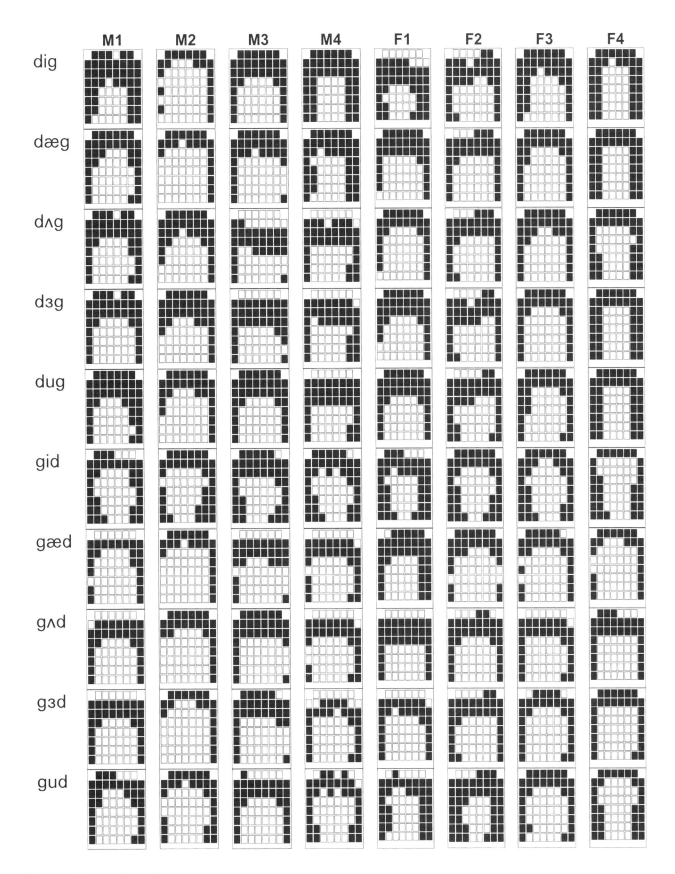

Figure 5–4. *continued*

Cumulative EPG Frames for Eight Typical English-Speaking Adults

Cumulative EPG patterns for /d/ were generated from 60 maximum contact frames (with the exception of F4) for each of the eight typical adults (Figure 5-5). The percentage of contact with each EPG electrode is displayed using shading and numbers. The darker the shading the more often that part of the palate was contacted by the tongue. A horseshoe shape is evident in each of the cumulative EPG images of /d/, with tongue/palate contact across the alveolar ridge and along the sides of the teeth.

Interspeaker Variability for /t/ in Languages Other Than English

Norwegian

Moen and Simonsen (2007) compared the production of /t, d/ with the Norwegian sounds /ʈ, ɖ/. Figure 5-6 demonstrates the cumulative maximum contact EPG frames for /t, d/ produced by four typical adult East Norwegian speakers (AN, HS, IM, RE). The sounds were produced in four contexts: word-initial and word-final position with a close and open vowel. The words were produced 10 times each in a carrier

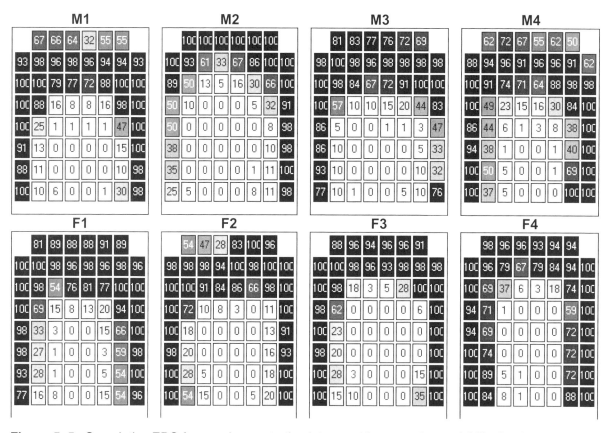

Figure 5–5. Cumulative EPG frames demonstrating intra- and interspeaker variability for the production of /d/ by eight typical English-speaking adults.

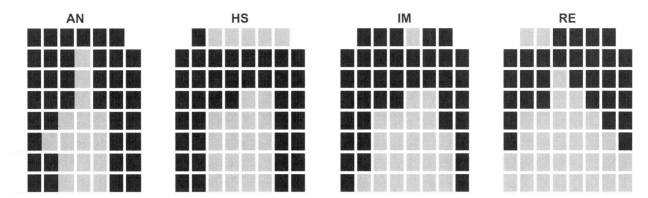

Figure 5–6. Cumulative EPG frames for the production of /t, d/ by four Norwegian-speaking adults (AN, HS, IM, RE) (adapted from Moen & Simonsen, 2007, Figure 3, p. 123).

phrase. A black square indicates that there was at least 67% contact for that electrode across the 80 tokens. Although there are some differences between the amount of tongue/palate contact for the Norwegian versus the English productions of /t, d/, all speakers produced a horseshoe shape of tongue/palate contact.

Interspeaker Variability for /d/ in Speakers with Impaired Speech

Children with Speech Impairment

Gibbon, Stewart, Hardcastle, and Crampin (1999) described the speech of an 8-year-old Scottish-English speaking boy named Robbie. Robbie had difficulty producing a range of consonants. Figure 5–7 demonstrates the maximum contact EPG frame for production of /d/ in the word "dish." The /d/ was transcribed by a speech-language pathologist as sounding like a [g]. The major difference from Robbie's production and the typical adult production is the lack of alveolar contact and the presence of velar tongue/palate contact. Gibbon et al. (1999) describe Robbie's successful intervention using the EPG and his subsequent normalization of both his tongue/palate contacts and his increased speech intelligibility.

Children with Cleft Palate

Gibbon, Ellis, and Crampin (2004) described the production of /t, d, k, g/ for 15 Scottish-English speaking

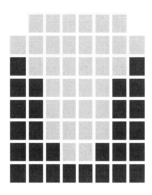

"d̲ish"

Figure 5–7. Maximum contact EPG frame for the production of /d/ in "dish" by an 8-year-old Scottish English-speaking child with speech impairment (adapted from Gibbon et al., 1999, Figure 4c, p. 327).

children who had repaired cleft palate. Perceptually, all children had correct production of /k, g/ but generally /t, d/ were perceived as being incorrect, predominantly as a palatal or velar sound. Figure 5–8 demonstrates cumulative tongue/palate contact for the production of /t, d/ across 10 words produced by each of the four of the speakers. In Figure 5–8, a black square indicates that that electrode was contacted at least 80% of the time. It can be seen that speakers C9 and C15 had velar tongue placement, whereas speakers C6 and C12 had alveolar + velar placement. This placement was likened to undifferentiated gestures, or whole tongue gestures (Gibbon, 1999) produced by children

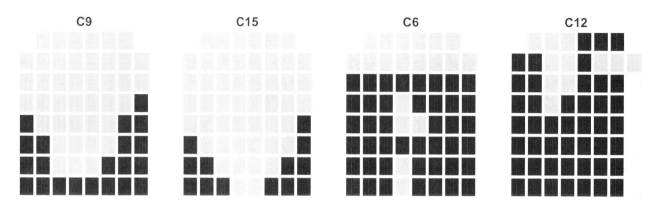

Figure 5–8. Maximum contact EPG frames for the production of /t, d/ by four Scottish English-speaking children with repaired cleft palate (adapted from Gibbon et al., 2004, Figure 1, p. 396).

with speech impairment that involved almost the whole tongue touching the palate.

Children with Perceptually Correct Productions

Gibbon (1999) described the phenomenon of "undifferentiated lingual gestures" in the speech of children with articulation/phonological disorders. One example that was provided was of a child, D8, who was diagnosed with an articulation/phonological disorder, but did have perceptually correct production of /d/. The EPG image, shown in Figure 5-9, demonstrates that D8's tongue/palate contact was not similar to that of a typical child or adult's production of /d/. Gibbon (1999b, p. 389) indicated "This EPG configuration suggests not only an abnormally high tongue body position but also an abnormally convex tongue body surface shape for an alveolar target." Understanding motoric capabilities of children, during both perceptually cor-

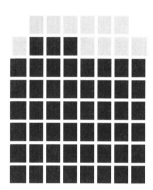

Figure 5–9. Maximum contact EPG frame for the *perceptually correct* production of /d/ in "shed" by a Scottish English-speaking child with speech impairment (adapted from Gibbon, 1999b, Figure 4, p. 389).

rect and perceptually incorrect productions of speech sounds will enable SLPs to develop more appropriate and targeted intervention goals for these children.

Chapter 6

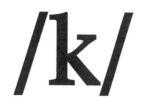

The consonant /k/ is a voiceless alveolar stop.

Place of articulation: velar

Advancement: back

Voicing: voiceless

Labiality: nonlabial

Sonorancy: nonsonorant (obstruent)

Continuancy: noncontinuant (stop)

Sibilancy: nonsibilant

Nasality: nonnasal (oral)

STATIC IMAGES OF THE ARTICULATORY CHARACTERISTICS OF /k/

The static images of /k/ are presented via a photograph, schematic diagram, ultrasound, and electropalatograph images (Figure 6-1).

Photograph

The photograph in Figure 6-1A was taken of the production of /k/ immediately followed by the vowel /ɪ/ in the word "kitty." Consequently, the lip shape reflects the forthcoming vowel. The movement of the tongue

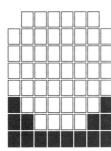

A. Photograph

B. Schematic diagram

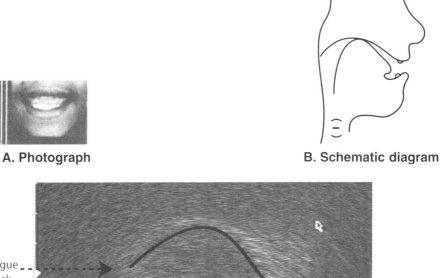

C. Ultrasound

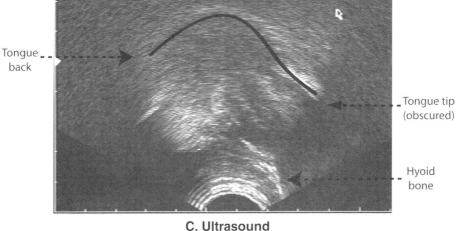

D. Electropalatograph (EPG) (single frame)

E. Electropalatograph (EPG) (cumulative frame)

Figure 6–1. Static images of the articulatory characteristics of /k/.

toward the velum is unable to be captured in a photograph of the face.

Schematic Diagram

The lateral view of the phoneme /k/ (Figure 6–1B) shows tongue contact at the back of the roof of the mouth (the velum). Because of the stop nature of this consonant, complete closure is accomplished at this point, and there is a complete stoppage of the airstream. The voiceless aspect of this consonant is symbolized by a minus sign (–) at the site of the vocal folds.

Ultrasound

Figure 6–1C shows the tongue in an ultrasound image during production of /k/. The surface of the tongue is difficult to see during production of velars (Stone, 2005), but the bulk of the tongue can be seen as an inverted U shape in the middle of the image and the tip is the brighter line pointing toward the floor of the mouth at the right of the image. The diagonal lines below the surface of the tongue are the muscle fibers.

Electropalatograph (EPG)

The EPG image of /k/ (Figure 6–1D) is shaped like a smile, with the tongue contacting the posterior and lateral margins of the hard palate. The palate design means that data are recorded up until the juncture between the hard and soft palates. It is possible that there is additional contact occurring on the soft palate. At times, the EPG image for /k/ may not have complete closure across the back of the EPG palate, particularly in the context of back vowels because closure is occurring on the soft palate.

The cumulative EPG image (Figure 6–1E) represents productions of /k/ by eight speakers over a total of 480 words. The darker the shading the more often that part of the palate was contacted by the tongue. The numbers indicate the percentage of contact with each EPG electrode. The number 99 in the lower left square indicates that that electrode was contacted 99% of the time by the eight speakers over the

480 words when producing /k/. Although the electrodes in the middle back row are shaded, Figure 6–1E shows that not all speakers have complete closure across the hard palate. It is probable that complete closure occurs on the soft palate (velum) in these instances.

DYNAMIC IMAGES OF THE ARTICULATORY AND ACOUSTIC CHARACTERISTICS OF /k/

In order to obtain a comprehensive view of the production of this consonant, the dynamic aspects of the production of /k/ are shown in a filmstrip, spectrogram, and EPG images (Figure 6–2).

/k/ in Word-Initial Context: "kitty"

Filmstrip: /kɪtɪ/ "kitty"

The criterion phoneme /k/ is in the initial position of the word /kɪtɪ/. Although it is not possible to photograph the velar contact of the tongue, the lip formation for the /k/ phoneme seems to be governed by the vowel that follows it. Because the medial vowel and the final vowel are both /ɪ/, the lips assume a wide and narrow shape.

Sound Spectrogram: /kɪtɪ/ "kitty"

The phoneme /k/ is presented in the initial position followed by the vowel /ɪ/ in the word "kitty." The phoneme /k/ is a back-voiceless stop consonant. The devoicing characteristic of this phoneme is marked by a clear absence of negative voice onset time. The aspiration nature of the voiceless stop /k/ at the initial position can be clearly seen. Aspiration noise is present for approximately 100 msec. This noise has most of its energy located between 3000 and 4000 Hz. It may be noted that, whereas the labial stops /p/ and /b/ have energy concentrations predominantly below 2000 Hz, and the front stops /t/ and /d/ have energy concentrations predominantly above 200 Hz, the back stops /k/

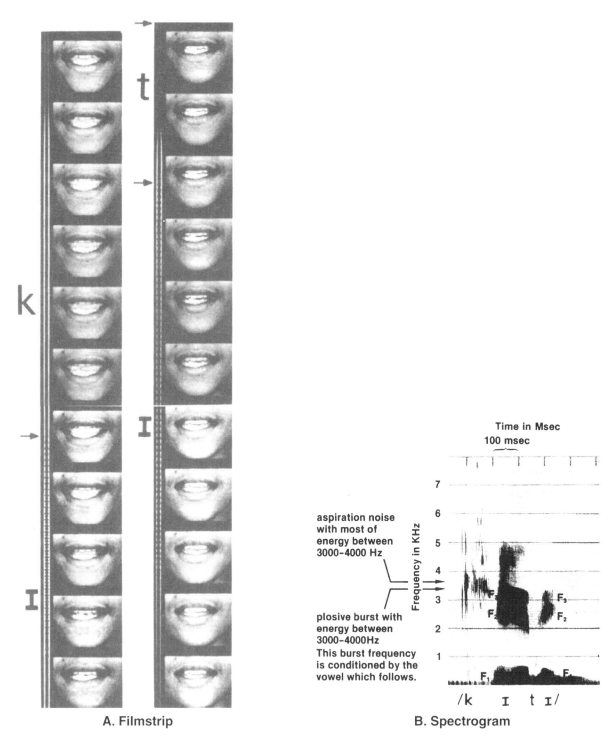

A. Filmstrip

B. Spectrogram

Figure 6–2. Dynamic images of /k/ in word-initial context: "kitty." *continues*

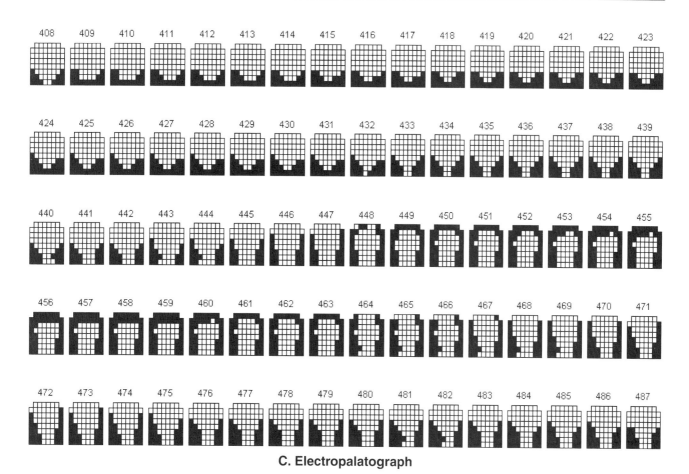

C. Electropalatograph

Figure 6–2. *continued*

and /g/ show energy in the frequency domain of the second formant of the adjacent vowel /ɪ/. The coarticulatory influence of this stop on the following vowel /ɪ/ is mainly in terms of its high-frequency energy. Therefore, the vowel formants for /ɪ/ show falling transition. This analysis is consistent with the description of lip formation in the filmstrip. Just as the lip formation of /k/ is governed by the following vowel, so is the concentration of energy.

Electropalatograph: /kɪti/ "kitty"

Figure 6-3C represents the lingualpalatal contact for the production of the word /kɪti/[1] "kitty." The first frame of closure for /k/ is frame 409 and the /k/ is released at frame 432. The /k/ sound is characterized by velar tongue contact evident by dark shading on the lower part of the image of the palate. The vowel /ɪ/ (see Chapter 27) extends from frame 432 to 448. The coarticulatory influences of /t/ on the vowel /ɪ/ are evident in frames 443 to 448. Tongue palate closure for /t/ extends from frame 449 until 463. The contact pattern for /t/ is similar to a horseshoe shape with the tongue contacting the palate along the entire lateral margins with the teeth (see Chapter 4). The frames 464 to 474 represent the coarticulatory period between /t/ and the vowel /i/. The final frames (475-487) represent tongue/palate contact for the vowel /i/.

---

[1]/kɪti/ is the Australian English pronunciation of "kitty."

INTRA- AND INTERSPEAKER VARIABILITY FOR /k/

Electropalatographic images enable consideration of intra- and interspeaker variability. First, variability between speakers of English is considered. Then EPG images of children's productions of /k/ are provided. Next, variability between the English and Greek production of /k/ are compared. Finally, variability between productions of /k/ by speakers with differing types of speech impairment is presented.

Intra- and Interspeaker Variability in the Production of /k/ by Eight Typical English-Speaking Adults

Four typical adult males (M1–M4) and four typical adult females (F1–F4) produced nonsense syllables containing /k/ three times. The nonsense syllables were created with /k/ in syllable-initial and syllable-final positions in vowel contexts taken at the extremes of the vowel quadrilateral.

Maximum Contact Frames for Eight Typical English-Speaking Adults

In order to demonstrate both inter- and intraspeaker variability in the production of /k/ the maximum contact frame for the second production of each nonsense syllable for each of the eight speakers is provided in Figure 6–3. For each production the tongue contacts the palate in the last rows of the palate, indicating velar tongue placement.

Cumulative EPG Frames for Eight Typical English-Speaking Adults

Cumulative EPG patterns for /k/ were generated from 60 maximum contact frames for each of the eight typical adults described above. Each electrode on a cumulative maximum contact display has a number, corresponding to the percentage of contact over the 60 productions (Figure 6–4). The darker the shading, the more contact. In Figure 6–4 each speaker's cumulative maximum contact display is focused around the velar regions of the palate.

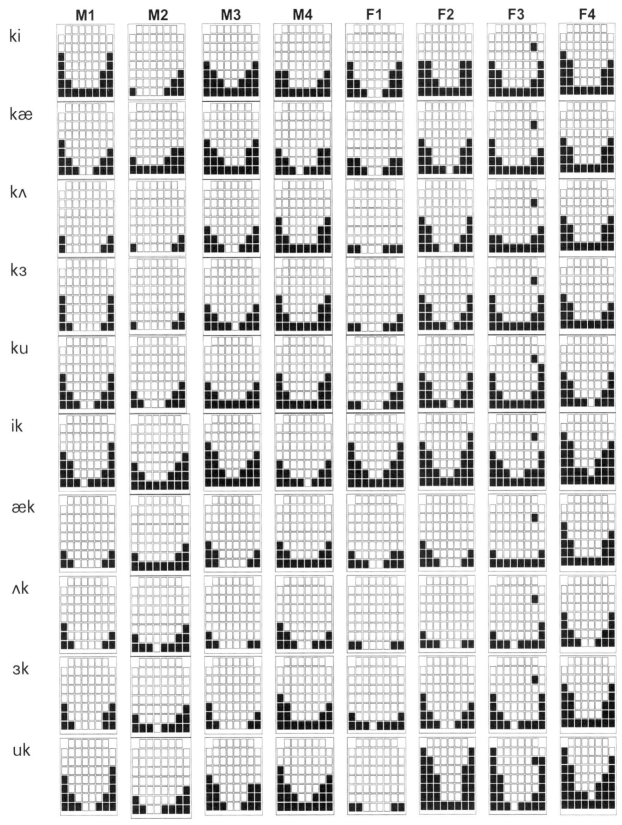

Note. F3 had one electrode in the third row that incorrectly recorded activation

Figure 6–3. Intra- and interspeaker variability in the maximum EPG contact frame for the production of /k/ by eight typical English-speaking adults. *continues*

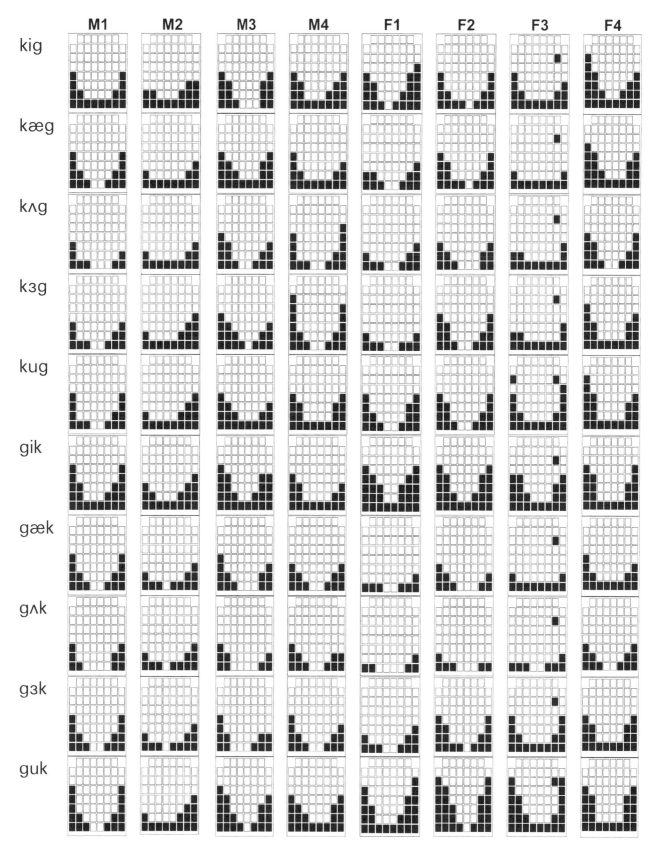

Note. F3 had one electrode in the third row that incorrectly recorded activation

Figure 6–3. *continues*

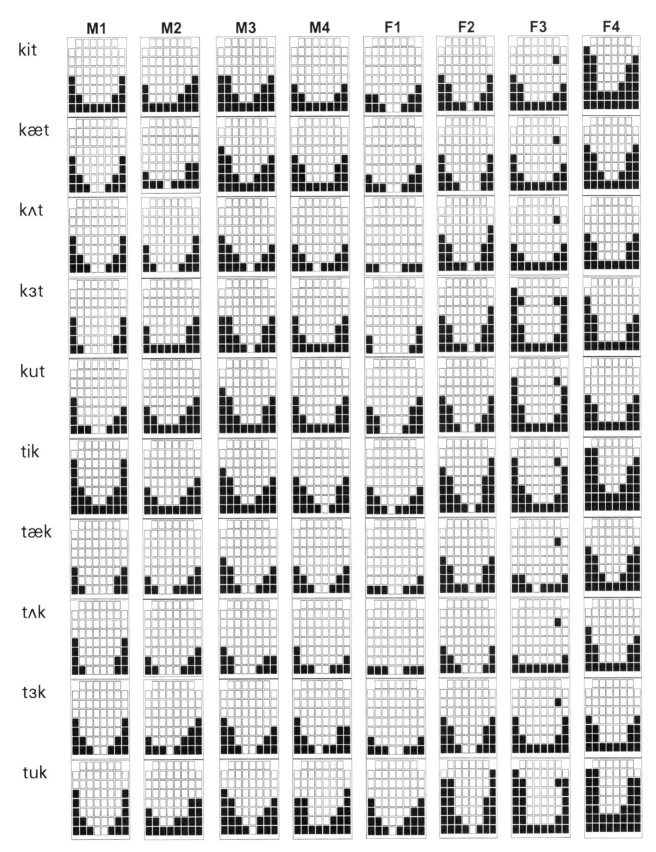

Note. F3 had one electrode in the third row that incorrectly recorded activation

Figure 6–3. *continued*

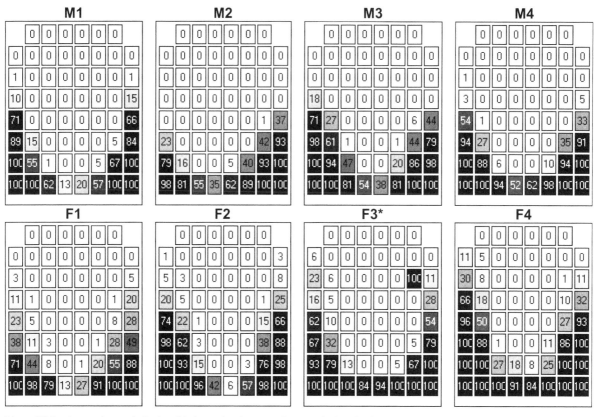

*Note. F3 had one electrode in the third row that incorrectly recorded activation.

Figure 6–4. Cumulative EPG frames demonstrating intra- and interspeaker variability for the production of /k/ by eight typical English-speaking adults.

Interspeaker Variability in the Production of /k/ by Other English-Speaking Adults

Australian English-Speaking Adults

Cheng, Murdoch, Goozée, and Scott (2007) conducted a study to describe typical speech production for 36 children and 12 adults. The six male and six female adult participants, aged between 23 and 38 years, produced /k/ in CV and CVC words that were embedded within a phrase. Each phrase was produced five times, resulting in 10 productions of /k/ per speaker. Figure 6-5 provides a cumulative maximum contact frame for the production of /k/ by the adults. In Figure 6-5, a black square indicates that that electrode was contacted at least 67% of the time. It is hypothesized that closure for the /k/ occurred on the soft palate as there is no recorded closure across the posterior section of the EPG palate.

Interspeaker Variability for /k/ in English-Speaking Children

Scottish English-Speaking Children

Gibbon, McNeill, Wood, and Watson (2003) provided images of the production of /k/ for a typical 12-year-old Scottish-English speaking child from the dissertation by McNeill (2001). Figure 6-6 demonstrates a cumulative maximum contact EPG frame for 11 productions of /k/. A black square indicates that that electrode was contacted at least 67% of the time. Her production is similar to an adultlike production of /k/.

Australian English-Speaking Children

Cheng et al. (2007) conducted a study to describe typical speech production for 36 children with six males and six females in each of the following age groups: 6 to 7 years, 8 to 11 years, and 12 to 17 years. The participants produced /k/ in CV and CVC words that were embedded within a phrase. Each phrase was produced five times, resulting in 10 productions of /k/ per speaker. Figure 6–7 provides a cumulative maximum contact frame for the production of /k/ by the children. In Figure 6-7, a black square indicates that that electrode was contacted at least 67% of the time.

Each cumulative frame has a similar array of contacted electrodes to the images of adults' productions of /k/ mentioned above.

Interspeaker Variability for /k/ in Languages Other Than English

Greek-Speaking Adults

Nicolaidis (2004) described the speech of one typical Modern Standard Greek-speaking adult in order to provide comparative data for the speech of four Greek-

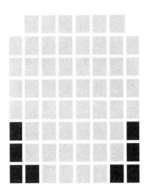

Figure 6–5. Cumulative maximum contact EPG frames for the production of /k/ by 12 typical Australian English-speaking adults (adapted from Cheng et al., 2007, Figure 1).

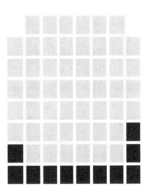

Figure 6–6. Cumulative maximum contact EPG frames for the production of /k/ by a typical 12-year-old Scottish English-speaking child (adapted from Gibbon et al., 2003, Figure 2, p. 56).

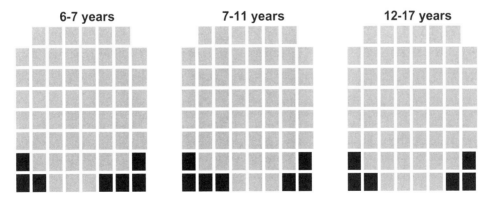

Figure 6–7. Cumulative maximum contact EPG frames for the production of /k/ by 36 typical Australian English-speaking children (adapted from Cheng et al., 2007, Figure 1, p. 380).

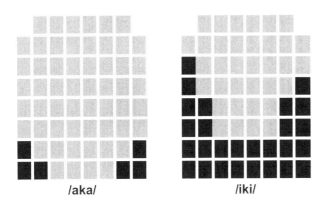

Figure 6–8. Cumulative maximum contact EPG frames for the production of /k/ by one Greek-speaking adult (adapted from Nicolaidis, 2004, Figure 1, p. 8).

speaking people with hearing impairment. Figure 6–8 demonstrates two cumulative maximum contact EPG frames for productions of /k/ in the contexts /aka/ and /iki/. The female participant was asked to produce these phoneme combinations 10 times in a dysyllabic word of the form /pVkV/ within a carrier phrase. In Figure 6–8, a black square indicates that that electrode was contacted at least 60% of the time. The coarticulatory influence of the vowel is apparent. There is much greater tongue/palate contact and more forward placement of the tongue in the context of /i/ compared with /a/.

Interspeaker Variability for /k/ in Speakers with Impaired Speech

Adults with Hearing Impairment

Nicolaidis (2004) also described the speech of three females and one male with hearing impairment aged between 23–26 years. Each spoke typical Modern Standard Greek. Each of the four people produced /k/ in the contexts /aka/ and /iki/ within the word form /pVkV/ within a carrier phrase. Each word was produced ten times. Figure 6–9 demonstrates two cumulative maximum contact EPG frames for each speaker (HI1–HI4) for productions of /k/ in the two contexts /aka/ and /iki/. In Figure 6–9, a black square indicates that that electrode was contacted at least 60% of the time. Speakers HI1 and HI2 had particular difficulty producing a /k/ in the context of a front vowel.

Speaker HI1 produced a double articulation with closure across the alveolar and velar regions of the palate. Such articulations are usually only produced by typical speakers in the context of /kt/ in words such as "tractor" and "kitkat." Speakers H3 and H4 had typical placement for the production of /k/.

Children with Cerebral Palsy

Gibbon and Wood (2003) described the speech of an 8-year-old boy (D) with congential left hemiplegia who had difficulty producing the velar consonants /k, g, ŋ/. Figure 6–10 demonstrates a cumulative maximum contact EPG frame for 16 productions of /k/ prior to intervention. A black square indicates that that electrode was contacted at least 67% of the time. This image was very similar to D's cumulative EPG frame for /t/. Gibbon and Wood (2003) indicated that intervention using EPG was successful and that D was able to produce velar sounds with similar tongue/palate contacts to those produced by a typical speaker.

Children with Down Syndrome

Gibbon et al. (2003) described the speech of a 10-year-old Scottish-English speaking girl (P) with Down syndrome. P had difficulty producing the velar consonants /k, g, ŋ/. Figure 6–11 demonstrates a cumulative maximum contact EPG frame for 16 productions of /k/ prior to intervention. A black square indicates that that electrode was contacted at least 67% of the time. This image was very similar to her cumulative EPG frame for /t/. It is clear that P's preintervention production of /k/ had limited velar contact with the palate. Gibbon et al. (2003) describe P's successful intervention using the EPG and that her velar tongue/palate contacts became more similar to those produced by a typical speaker.

Children with Cleft Palate

Gibbon, Ellis, and Crampin (2004) described the production of /t, d, k, g/ for 15 Scottish English-speaking children who had repaired cleft palate. Perceptually, all children had correct production of /k, g/. Using EPG there was 77% correct tongue placement for velar targets (/k, g/) compared with 32% for alveolar targets (/t, d/).

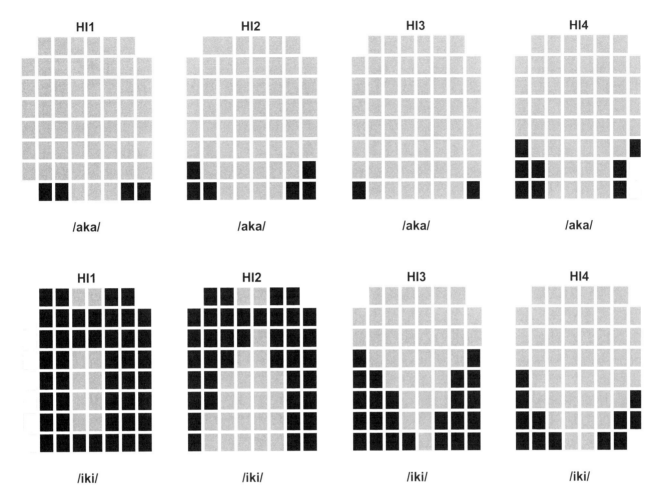

Figure 6–9. Cumulative maximum contact EPG frames for the production of /k/ by four Greek-speaking adults with hearing impairment (adapted from Nicolaidis, 2004, Figure 1, p. 8).

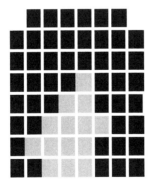

Figure 6–10. Cumulative maximum contact EPG frames for the production of /k/ by an 8-year-old child with cerebral palsy (adapted from Gibbon & Wood, 2003, Figure 1, p. 368).

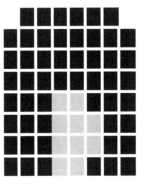

Figure 6–11. Cumulative maximum contact EPG frames for the production of /k/ by a 10-year-old Scottish English-speaking child with Down syndrome (adapted from Gibbon et al., 2003, Figure 2, p. 56).

Chapter 7

/g/

The consonant /g/ is a voiced velar stop.

Place of articulation: velar

Advancement: back

Voicing: voiced

Labiality: nonlabial

Sonorancy: nonsonorant (obstruent)

Continuancy: noncontinuant (stop)

Sibilancy: nonsibilant

Nasality: nonnasal (oral)

STATIC IMAGES OF THE ARTICULATORY CHARACTERISTICS OF /g/

The static images of /g/ are presented via a photograph, schematic diagram, ultrasound, and electropalatograph images (Figure 7-1).

Photograph

In this photograph, the mouth is open and the tongue tip can be seen behind the lower teeth. The photograph does not demonstrate the tongue touching the velum to create closure of the airstream to produce /g/.

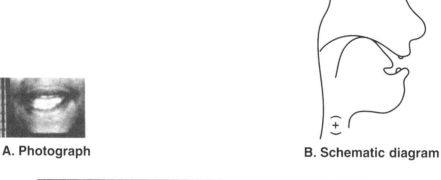

A. Photograph

B. Schematic diagram

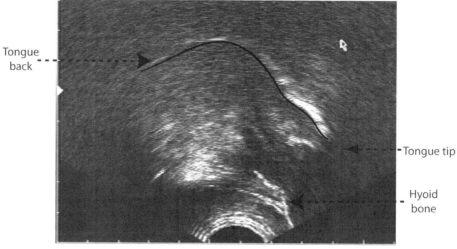

C. Ultrasound

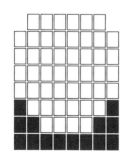

D. Electropalatograph (EPG) (single frame)

E. Electropalatograph (EPG) (cumulative frame)

Figure 7–1. Static images of the articulatory characteristics of /g/.

Schematic Diagram

The schematic diagram shows the back of the tongue touching the back of the roof of the mouth or the velum. The back of the tongue tightly contacts the velum and completely stops the flow of the airstream. The voicing feature of /g/ is denoted by the (+) at the vocal folds.

Ultrasound

In Figure 7–1C the white line extending from the middle of the right of the image and upward toward the top of the image shows the tongue surface during production of /g/. The tongue tip is toward the right of the screen. The back of the tongue is raised in the oral cavity. Stone (2005) indicates that images of velar sounds (and other sounds with steep slopes such as high vowels) are difficult to see on ultrasound. An air shadow can be seen above the tongue tip and blade and diagonal muscle fibers can be seen below the surface of the tongue.

Electropalatograph (EPG)

As for /k/, the EPG image of /g/ (Figure 7–1D) is shaped like a smile, with the tongue contacting the posterior and lateral margins of the hard palate. The palate design means that data is recorded up until the juncture between the hard and soft palates. It is possible that there is additional contact occurring on the soft palate. At times, other EPG images for /g/ may not have complete closure across the back of the EPG palate, particularly in the context of back vowels because closure is occurring on the soft palate.

The cumulative EPG image (Figure 7–1E) represents productions of /g/ by eight speakers over a total of 480 words. The darker the shading the more often that part of the palate was contacted by the tongue. The numbers indicate the percentage of contact with each EPG electrode. The number 100 in the lower left square indicates that that lateral velar electrode was contacted 100% of the time by the eight speakers over the 480 words when producing /k/.

DYNAMIC IMAGES OF THE ARTICULATORY AND ACOUSTIC CHARACTERISTICS OF /g/

In order to obtain a comprehensive view of the production of this consonant, the dynamic aspects of the production of /g/ are shown in a filmstrip, spectrogram, and EPG images.

/g/ in Word-Initial and Word-Final Contexts: "gag"

Filmstrip: /gæg/ "gag"

The phoneme /g/ is presented at the initial and final positions of the word /gæg/. Low-frequency acoustic energy prior to the burst at the initial position is less evident for the voiced stop /g/ as compared to the voiced stops /b/ and /d/. The coarticulatory influence of the vowel /æ/ on the lips can be noted throughout the filmstrip.

Sound Spectrogram: /gæg/ "gag"

The voiced-back stop phoneme /g/ is contrasted at the initial and final positions with the vowel /æ/ at the medial position in the word "gag." The (+) voicing nature of this consonant is indicated by a negative voice onset time of approximately 100 msec and a clear rising first formant. The plosive burst has energy components first at about 500 Hz and then again at around 3500 Hz. This bimodal energy distribution is characteristic of the back stop consonants /k/ and /g/. This differs from the unimodal distribution of the labials /p/ and /b/ (energy in the low frequencies, below 2000 Hz) and the front consonants /t/ and /d/ (energy over 2000 Hz). The F2 shows a falling transition, indicating the higher weight of the cues attributable to the high-frequency energy in the plosive burst for the initial position /g/, rather than the low-frequency energy. The following phoneme /g/ again is clearly produced as a voiced back stop, voicing being represented by the presence of vocal fold vibration at the base of the spectrogram as well as by the falling F1. The rising F2 signals the back place of articulation. This is analogous to the falling F2 for the initial /g/.

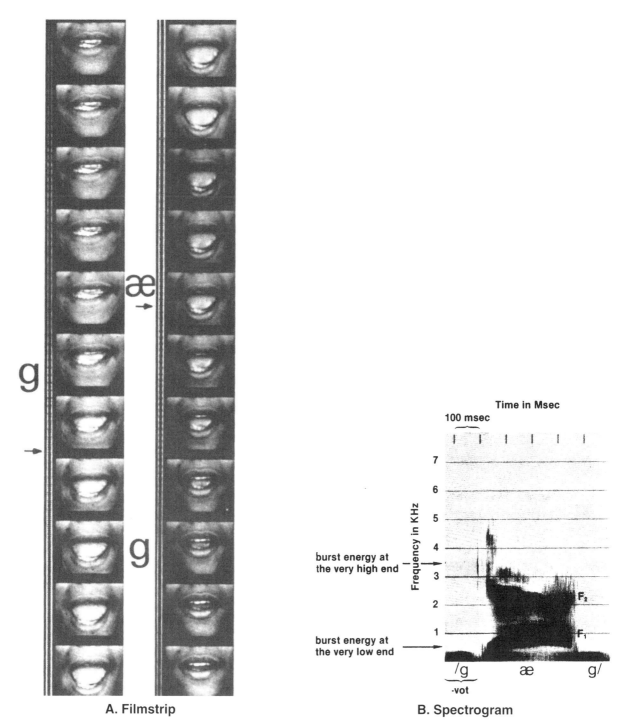

A. Filmstrip

B. Spectrogram

Figure 7–2. Dynamic images of /g/ in the word-initial and word-final contexts: "gag." *continues*

Electropalatograph: /gæg/ "gag"

Figure 7-2C presents 80 EPG frames demonstrating tongue/palate contact during the production of "gag."

Closure for the first /g/ sound commences at frame 407. Tongue contact with the velum is indicated by the black shading on the lower part of the palate. The first /g/ sound is released at frame 425. The vowel /æ/

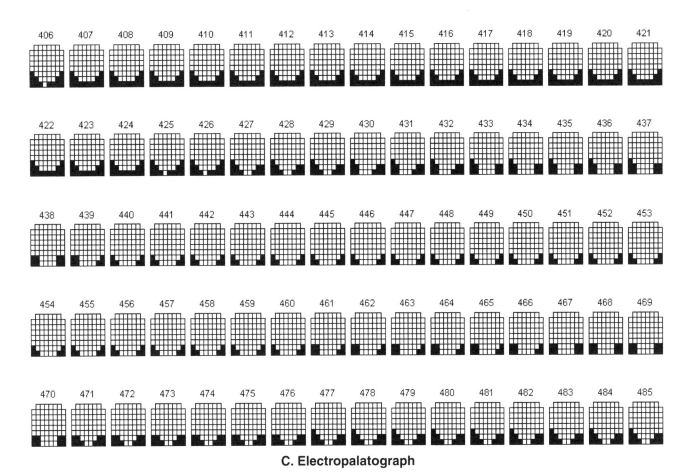

C. Electropalatograph

Figure 7–2. *continued*

is produced with an open mouth; thus there is limited tongue/palate contact from frames 425 to 470. The word-final /g/ commences at frame 471. This frame was identified using the simultaneous spectrogram to categorize the closure phase for /g/. Frame 471 also coincides with closure along the back of the palate for all but 2 electrodes. It is probable that there was complete closure for the final /g/ sound; however, the EPG palate only extends to the juncture between the hard and soft palate. It is hypothesized that complete closure occurred with tongue contact to the soft palate.

INTERSPEAKER VARIABILITY FOR /g/

Electropalatographic images enable consideration of interspeaker variability. In this chapter, variability between eight typical adult speakers is considered.

Intra- and Interspeaker Variability in the Production of /g/ by Eight Typical English-Speaking Adults

Four typical adult males (M1–M4) and four typical adult females (F1–F4) produced nonsense syllables containing /g/ three times. The nonsense syllables were created with /g/ in syllable-initial and syllable-final positions in vowel contexts taken at the extremes of the vowel quadrilateral.

Maximum Contact Frames for Eight Typical English-Speaking Adults

In order to demonstrate both inter- and intra-speaker variability the maximum contact frame for the second production of each nonsense syllable for each speaker is provided in Figure 7–3.

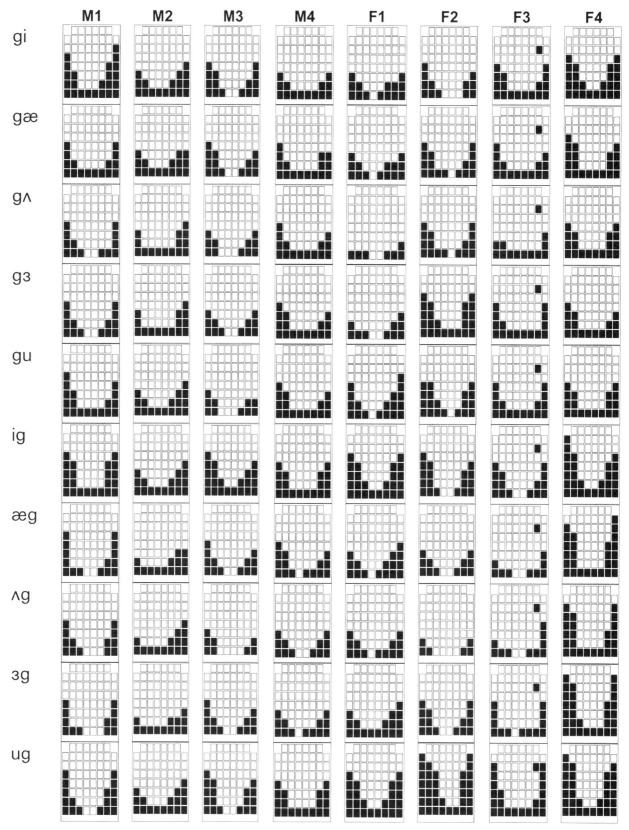

Note. F3 had one electrode in the third row that incorrectly recorded activation

Figure 7–3. Intra- and interspeaker variability in the maximum EPG contact frame for the production of /g/ by eight typical English-speaking adults. *continues*

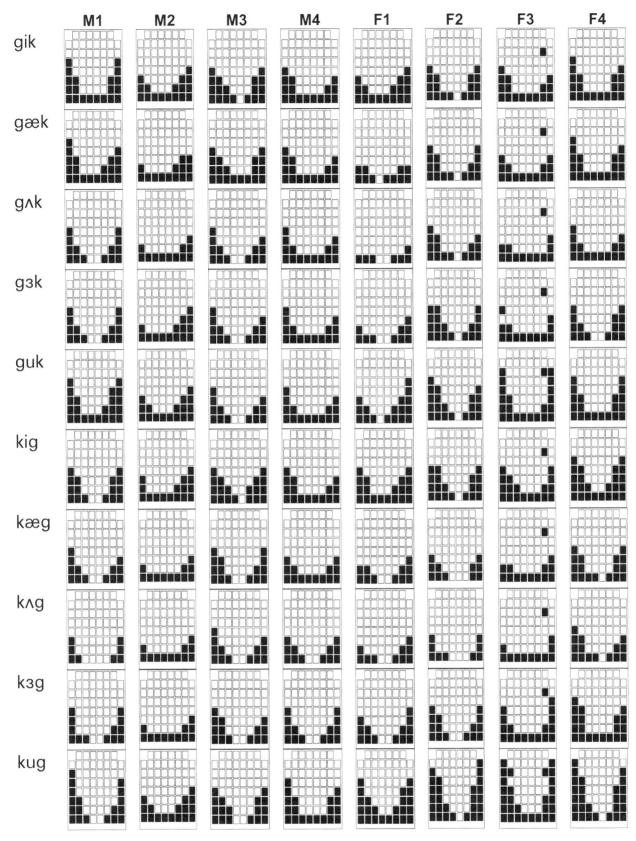

Note. F3 had one electrode in the third row that incorrectly recorded activation

Figure 7–3. *continues*

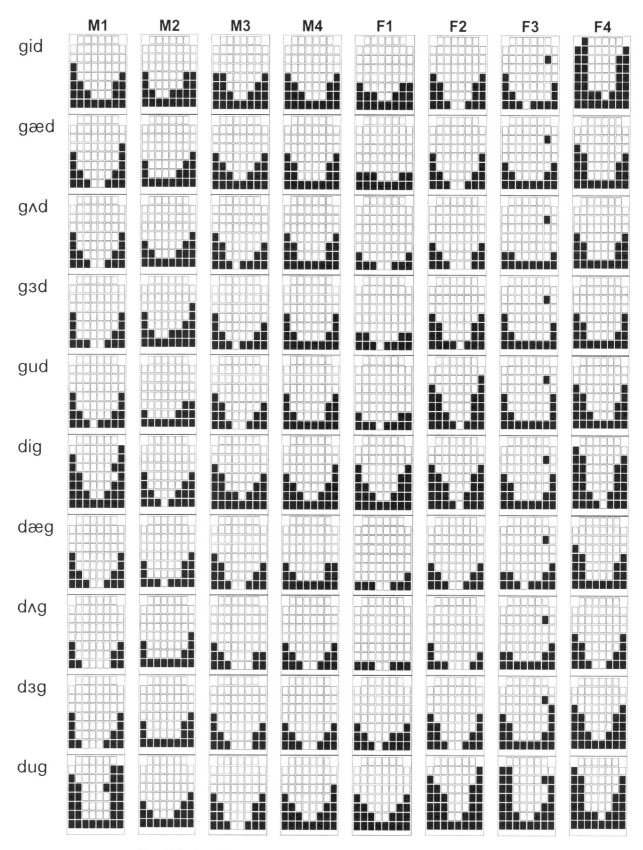

Note. F3 had one electrode in the third row that incorrectly recorded activation

Figure 7–3. *continued*

It can be observed that generally the vowel contexts /i/ and /u/ created more tongue/palate contact for the production of /g/ than the other vowel contexts. F4 frequently had more lateral contact than the other participants across many words.

Cumulative EPG Frames for Eight Typical English-Speaking Adults

Cumulative EPG patterns for /g/ were generated from maximum contact frames for each of the eight typical adults described above. Each electrode on a cumulative maximum contact display has a number, corre-

sponding to the percentage of contact over the 60 productions. The darker the shading, the more contact. In Figure 7–4 each speaker's cumulative maximum contact display has contact at the velar region of the palate. F3 has the most consistent pattern of closure across the posterior rows of electrodes during the production of /g/. It is hypothesized that when the other participants did not have observable closure across the EPG palate, there was closure occurring behind the EPG palate on the soft palate. The other factor to note in Figure 7–4 is the differing extent of contact along the lateral posterior margins of the palate for each participant.

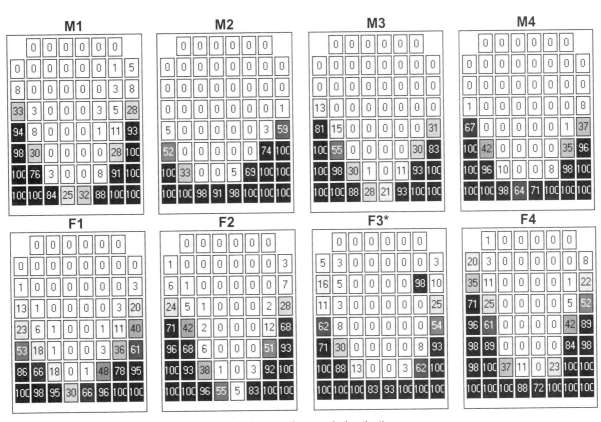

*Note. F3 had one electrode in the third row that incorrectly recorded activation.

Figure 7–4. Cumulative EPG frames demonstrating intra- and interspeaker variability for the production of /g/ by eight typical English-speaking adults.

Chapter 8

/m/

The consonant /m/ is a voiced bilabial nasal.

Place of articulation: bilabial

Advancement: front

Voicing: voiced

Labiality: labial

Sonorancy: sonorant

Continuancy: —

Sibilancy: nonsibilant

Nasality: nasal

STATIC IMAGES OF THE ARTICULATORY CHARACTERISTICS OF /m/

The static images of /m/ are presented via a photograph, schematic diagram, ultrasound, and electropalatograph images (Figure 8-1).

Photograph

In the photograph (Figure 8-1A), the lips are together to produce the bilabial sound /m/. The airstream is directed through the nose.

A. Photograph

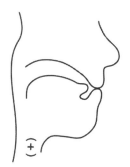

B. Schematic diagram

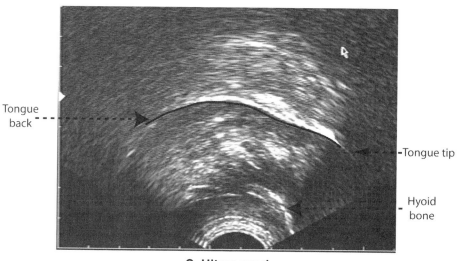

Tongue back

Tongue tip

Hyoid bone

C. Ultrasound

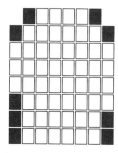

D. Electropalatograph (EPG) (single frame)

Figure 8–1. Static images of the articulatory characteristics of /m/.

Schematic Diagram

The lateral view in the schematic diagram (Figure 8–1B) can be compared with the frontal view in the film-strip. In addition to showing the lip involvement, this diagram shows that the tongue is in a neutral position. The involvement of the vocal folds in the production of /m/ is denoted by a plus sign (+). The phoneme /m/ is a nasal consonant. The lowering of the velum opens the velopharyngeal port and involves the nasal cavity in the production of this sound. The airstream is blocked in the oral cavity, but flows uninterrupted through the nasal cavity.

Ultrasound

A midsagittal ultrasound image of the tongue surface during production /m/ is shown in Figure 8–1C. Underneath the bright white line is the tongue surface. The tongue is raised compared to its resting position as described in Chapter 1; however, unlike many of the consonant sounds, the midsagittal section of the tongue in the production of /m/ is flat in configuration. The tongue tip is on the right of the image. An air shadow can be seen above the tongue and diagonal muscle fibers can be seen below the surface of the tongue. The hyoid bone is seen as the bright diagonal line at the bottom right of the image.

Electropalatograph (EPG)

Figure 8–1D demonstrates the tongue/palate contact for the production of /m/ produced in spontaneous speech. In this image there is limited contact at the alveolar and velar regions of the palate, with no contact with the central regions of the palate. Figure 8–1D should be compared with the /m/ produced in "mom" in Figure 8–2C. Within the word context, there was even less tongue/palate contact. Gibbon, Lee, and Yuen (2007) found that for eight typical adult speakers the extent of tongue/palate contact for the production of /m/ was significantly correlated with the contact

for the surrounding vowels. They also found that under experimental conditions there was significantly more tongue/palate contact for /m/ than for /b/ or /p/.

DYNAMIC IMAGES OF THE ARTICULATORY AND ACOUSTIC CHARACTERISTICS OF /m/

In order to obtain a comprehensive view of the production of this consonant, the dynamic aspects of the production of /m/ are shown in a filmstrip, spectrogram, and EPG images (Figure 8–2).

/m/ in Word-Initial and Word-Final Contexts: "mom"

Filmstrip: /mɑm/ "mom"

In Figure 8-2A, the phoneme /m/ is presented at the initial and final positions of the word /mɑm/. There are three frames at the initial position and five at the final position that show complete lip contact. The process of lip opening into the medial position vowel /ɑ/ is gradual. The long, steady state position of this vowel is denoted by the almost identical lip positions in frames 6 through 12.

Sound Spectrogram: /mɑm/ "mom"

The phoneme /m/ is contrasted in the initial and final positions in the word "mom." The band of energy below 1000 Hz weakens in the medial vowel /ɑ/, clearly showing the effect of nasalization. The labiality and voicing features for /m/ are both indicated by the presence of low-frequency energy and a rising F1 transition. The final position /m/ is indicated by a very weak F2 energy band and low-amplitude, falling first and second formant transitions.

Electropalatograph: /mʌm/ "mom"

Figure 8-2C contains EPG frames for the production of /mʌm/[1] "mom" (Figure 8-2B) in the sentence context

---

[1]/mʌm/ is the Australian English pronunciation of "mom."

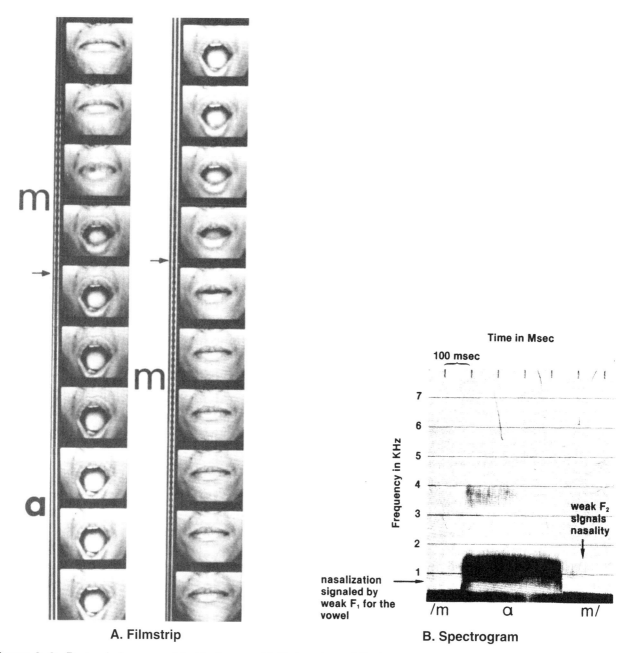

A. Filmstrip

B. Spectrogram

Figure 8–2. Dynamic images of /m/ in the word-initial and word-final contexts: "mom." *continues*

"I see a mom again." The word "mom" took 0.478 seconds to produce and is displayed in 80 EPG frames. Almost every EPG frame is exactly the same, with only one electrode contacted, demonstrating the extremely limited amount of tongue palate contact during the production of the consonant /m/ and the vowel /ʌ/. Using the simultaneous spectrogram, waveform, audio and EPG data (not shown in Figure 8–2c),

the initial /m/ was identified as extending from frames 370 to 394. The vowel /ʌ/ was identified as extending from frames 395 to 442 and the final /m/ was identified as extending from frames 443 to 465. These phoneme boundaries were not apparent from the EPG frames. It appears that the final /m/ was influenced by coarticulation with the following word "again" as there was slightly more tongue/palate contact for the final /m/.

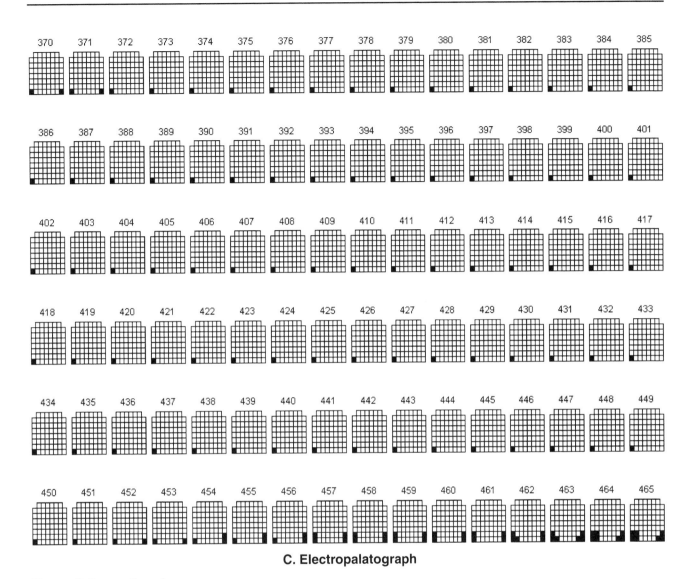

C. Electropalatograph

Figure 8–2. *continued*

INTRA- AND INTERSPEAKER VARIABILITY FOR /m/

Electropalatographic images enable consideration of intra- and interspeaker variability.

EPG images of productions of /m/ by children with cleft palate are provided to compare production with the typical adult's EPG images of /m/.

Interspeaker Variability for /m/ in Speakers with Impaired Speech

Children with Cleft Palate

Gibbon and Crampin (2002) described the production of /p, b, m/ for 27 Scottish-English-speaking adults and children aged 5 to 62 years who had a history of cleft palate and produced compensatory speech errors.

Fifteen productions of words containing the bilabial consonants were produced by each speaker. Figure 8–3 illustrates the cumulative maximum contact EPG frames for the production of /m/ by three children in the study (P [aged 9;07], L [aged 9;10], and J [aged 12;6]). Black shading indicates that the electrode was contacted at least 80% of the time over five productions of words containing /m/. These three speakers were described as frequently producing "labial-lingual double articulations (LLDAs)" (p. 40) across the bilabial targets. Figure 8–3 shows that L consistently produced LLDAs for words containing /m/; whereas J inconsistently produced LLDAs and P did not produced LLDAs for /m/. The speakers most frequently produced LLDAs during production of /b/.

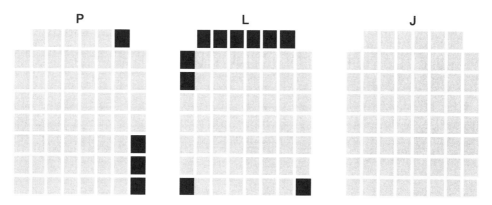

Figure 8–3. Cumulative maximum contact EPG frames for the production of /m/ by three Scottish English-speaking children (P, L, J) with cleft palate (adapted from Gibbon & Crampin, 2002, Figure 4, p. 45).

Chapter 9

/n/

The consonant /n/ is a voiced alveolar nasal.

Place of articulation: alveolar

Advancement: front

Voicing: voiced

Labiality: nonlabial

Sonorancy: sonorant

Continuancy: —

Sibilancy: nonsibilant

Nasality: nasal

STATIC IMAGES OF THE ARTICULATORY CHARACTERISTICS OF /n/

The static images of /n/ are presented via a photograph, schematic diagram, ultrasound, and electropalatograph images (Figure 9–1).

Photograph

In this photograph (Figure 9-1A), the mouth is open and the tongue can be seen touching the alveolar ridge to create closure of the airstream to produce /n/.

A. Photograph

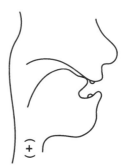

B. Schematic diagram

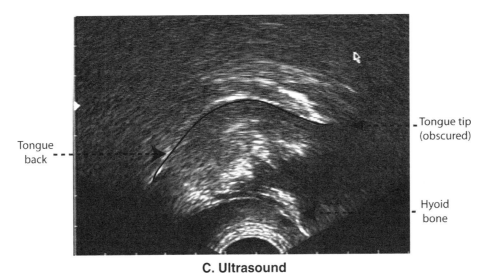

C. Ultrasound

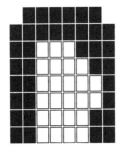

D. Electropalatograph (EPG) (single frame)

E. Electropalatograph (EPG) (cumulative frame)

Figure 9–1. Static images of the articulatory characteristics of /n/.

Schematic Diagram

The schematic diagram (Figure 9–1B) shows the tip of the tongue contacting the roof of the mouth directly behind the upper teeth. This view does not also demonstrate the sides of the tongue contacting the lateral margins of the palate along the teeth. The roof of the mouth can be divided at the center, with front toward the lips and back toward the pharyngeal wall. The phoneme /n/ is clearly a front consonant as the tongue contacts the hard palate at the front. Closure of the oral cavity at the point of contact is shown. This closure results in a stoppage of the airstream in the oral cavity. There is, however, an uninterrupted flow of air through the nasal cavity. The lowering of the velum opens the velopharyngeal port and involves the nasal cavity in the production of this sound. The vocal folds vibrate in the production of /n/, as indicated by the plus (+) voicing symbol.

Ultrasound

The bright white line on the ultrasound image in Figure 9–1C shows the tongue surface during production of /n/. Approximately 1 cm of the tongue tip (on the right of the image) is obscured from view because of the acoustic shadow of the jaw (Stone, 2005). The tongue tip is raised toward the alveolar ridge. The back of the tongue is somewhat raised in the oral cavity. An air shadow can be seen above the tongue and diagonal muscle fibers can be seen below the surface of the tongue.

Electropalatograph (EPG)

The EPG image of /n/ (Figure 9–1D) presents as a horseshoe shape, similar to the EPG image for /t/ and /d/. The tongue contacts the palate along the margins of the teeth: across the alveolar ridge and with lateral bracing along the sides of the teeth. The image is slightly asymmetrical probably due to being captured during spontaneous speech. The cumulative EPG image (Figure 9–1E) represents productions of /n/ by eight speakers over a total of 390 words. The darker the shading the more often that part of the palate was contacted by the tongue. The numbers indicate the percentage of contact with each EPG electrode. The number 71 in the lower left square indicates that that electrode was contacted 71% of the time by the eight speakers over the 395 words when producing /n/.

Gibbon, Yuen, Lee, and Adams (2007) compared 15 typical English-speaking adults' productions of /n/, /t/, and /d/. The found that:

◆ There was less contact for /n/ than for /t/ and /d/
◆ In almost every instance, /n/, /t/, and /d/ had 100% tongue/palate contact on the EPG palate at either row 1, row 2, or both
◆ In almost every instance, /n/, /t/, and /d/ had 0% tongue/palate contact on the EPG palate at the four electrodes at the center of the palate from row 5 to row 8
◆ /n/ (55%) was less likely to have bilateral constriction than /t/ (88%) and /d/ (83%). Bilateral constriction was defined as "100% contact at both the left-most column and the right-most column" of electrodes on the EPG palate (Gibbon et al., 2007, p. 84).

Additional information about the use of EPG for understanding typical adults' productions of /n/ is provided in McLeod (2006).

DYNAMIC IMAGES OF THE ARTICULATORY AND ACOUSTIC CHARACTERISTICS OF /n/

In order to obtain a comprehensive view of the production of this consonant, the dynamic aspects of the production of /n/ are shown in a filmstrip, spectrogram and EPG images in two words containing /n/ in different word positions (Figure 9–2).

/n/ in Word-Initial and Word-Final Contexts: /nʌn/ "none" or "nun"

Filmstrip: /nʌn/ "none"

The consonant phoneme /n/ is presented at the initial and final positions of the word /nʌn/. The vowel /ʌ/ is in the medial position. The first frame of the filmstrip

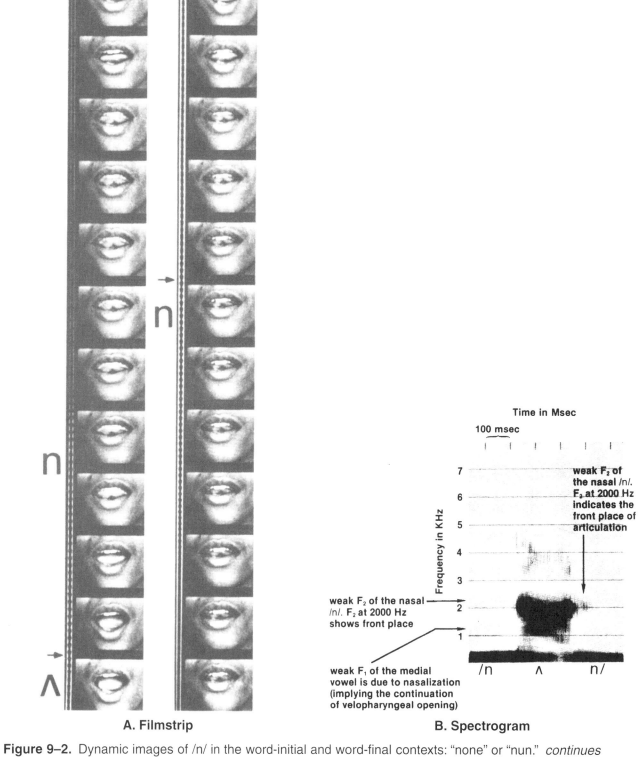

A. Filmstrip

B. Spectrogram

Figure 9–2. Dynamic images of /n/ in the word-initial and word-final contexts: "none" or "nun." *continues*

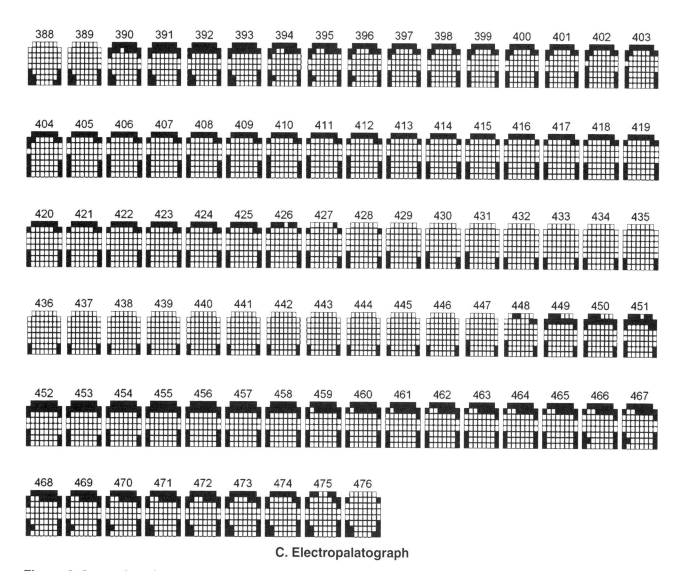

C. Electropalatograph

Figure 9–2. *continued*

shows open lips and a slight forward excursion of the tongue. In the second frame, the front body of the tongue has been slightly lifted. In the third frame, it is lifted a little more. It is evident in the fourth frame that the objective of the dynamic activity was tongue contact at the front of the roof of the mouth. This contact persists to the 10th frame. In the 10th frame, a release of the tongue from the palate can be seen.

Sound Spectrogram: /nʌn/ "none"

The phoneme /n/ is contrasted at the initial and final positions with the vowel /ʌ/ at the medial position in the word "none." The nasalization of this vowel, caused by the coarticulatory influence of the initial and final nasals, can be seen in the low amplitude of the first formant. The first formant of the vowel /ʌ/ is much lighter than the second formant. There is a faint, rising, first formant transition, signaling voicing and nasality. It is the weakness of this transition that signals nasality. The second formant of the nasal /n/ is at 2000 Hz but, again, its energy is weak. The falling F2 transition indicates the place of articulation, and the very weak presence of second formant energy at both the initial and final positions indicates the feature nasality and front place of articulation.

Electropalatograph: /nʌn/ "none"

The dynamic series of EPG palates for the production of the word "none" or "nun" is presented in Figure 9–2C. The word "nun" was extracted from the sentence "I see a nun again." Within this sentence, the word "nun" took 0.437 seconds to produce. The first frame of closure for the first /n/ is 390, and the last frame before release is 425. The first frame of closure for the second /n/ is 449, and the last frame before release is 474. The typical horseshoe shape for /n/ is not depicted in Figure 9–2C as the sides of the palate do not appear to be contacted. It is hypothesized that closure was created by the tongue touching the lateral margins of the teeth. The Reading WIN/EPG palate does not extend onto the teeth; however, the new design of these palates will enable identification of contact with the teeth (Wrench, 2007). McLeod (2006) similarly identified the incomplete closure of /n/ in many typical adult speakers' productions of /n/. The vowel /ʌ/ (frames 429–447) has limited tongue/palate contact, concentrated toward the velar region of the palate (see Chapter 34).

INTRA- AND INTERSPEAKER VARIABILITY FOR /n/

Electropalatographic images enable consideration of intra- and interspeaker variability. First, variability between eight speakers of English is considered. These images are contrasted with those of a Greek speaker. Finally, variability between productions of /n/ by speakers with hearing impairment and cleft palate is shown.

Intra- and Interspeaker Variability in the Production of /n/ by Eight Typical English-Speaking Adults

Four typical adult males (M1–M4) and four typical adult females (F1–F4) produced nonsense syllables containing /n/ three times. The nonsense syllables were created with /n/ in syllable-initial and syllable-final positions in vowel contexts taken at the extremes of the vowel quadrilateral.

Maximum Contact Frames for Eight Typical English-Speaking Adults

In order to demonstrate both inter- and intraspeaker variability the maximum contact frame for the second production of each nonsense syllable for each speaker is provided in Figure 9–3. As for the production of /t/ and /d/, many EPG images are in the form of a horseshoe shape of tongue/palate contact where the tongue touches the alveolar ridge and the lateral margins of the palate. However, there are a number of cases where there is limited contact on the lateral margins (such as for M2 and M3); it is hypothesized that the tongue was touching the teeth, and contact with the EPG palate was not registered (McLeod, 2006).

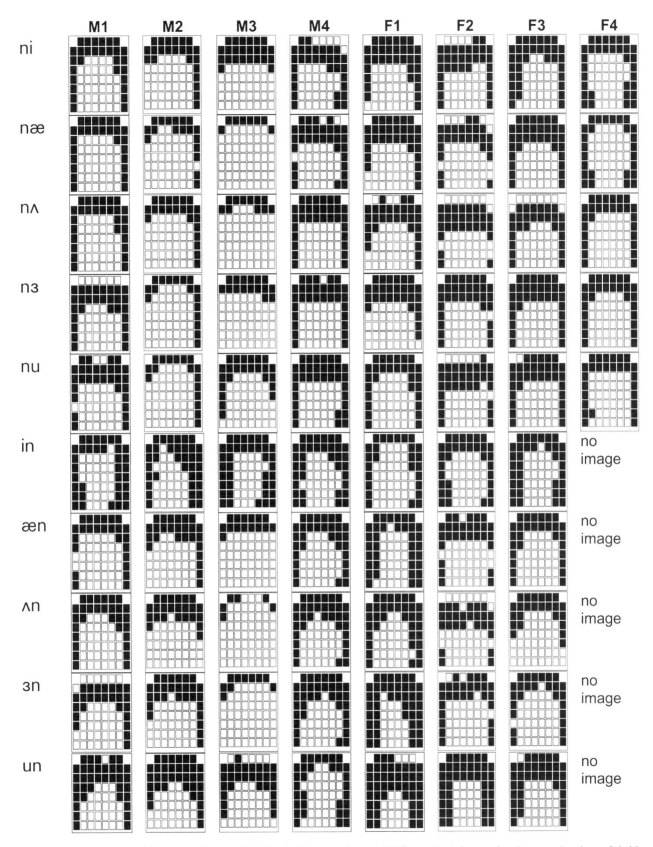

Figure 9–3. Intra- and interspeaker variability in the maximum EPG contact frame for the production of /n/ by eight typical English-speaking adults. *continues*

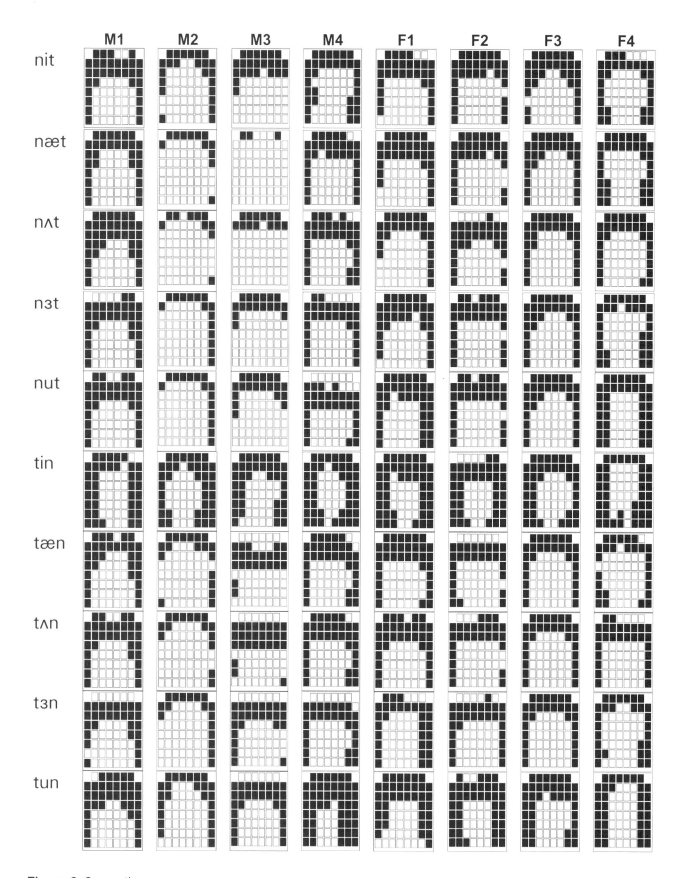

Figure 9–3. *continues*

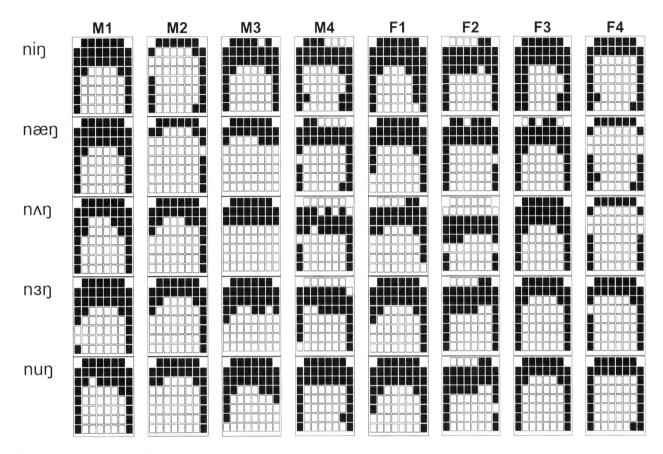

Figure 9–3. *continued*

Cumulative EPG Frames for Eight Typical English-Speaking Adults

Cumulative EPG patterns for /n/ were generated from 50 maximum contact frames (with the exception of F4) for each of the eight typical adults described above. Each electrode on a cumulative maximum contact display has a number, corresponding to the percentage of contact over the 50 productions. The darker the shading, the more contact. In Figure 9–4 each speaker's cumulative maximum contact display is a horseshoe shape; however, there are differences in the number of rows contacted on the alveolar ridge, the width of the lateral bracing. For example, M1, M4, F1, and F2 had a more contact across the alveolar ridge than the other speakers.

Interspeaker Variability for /n/ in Languages Other Than English

Greek-Speaking Adults

Nicolaidis (2004) described the speech of one typical Modern Standard Greek-speaking adult in order to provide comparative data for the speech of four Greek-speaking people with hearing impairment. Figure 9–5 demonstrates two cumulative maximum contact EPG frames for productions of /n/ in the contexts /ana/ and /ini/. The female participant was asked to produce these phoneme combinations ten times in a dysyllabic word of the form /pVnV/ within a carrier phrase. In Figure 9–5, a black square indicates that that electrode was contacted at least 60% of the time. The coarticulation

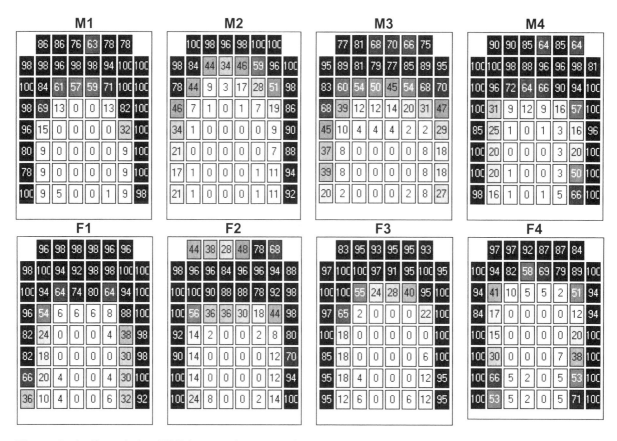

Figure 9–4. Cumulative EPG frames demonstrating intra- and interspeaker variability for the production of /n/ by eight typical English-speaking adults.

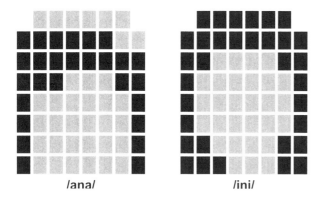

Figure 9–5. Cumulative maximum contact EPG frames for the production of /n/ by one Greek-speaking adult (adapted from Nicolaidis, 2004, Figure 1, p. 8).

with the vowel is evident in the way that the /n/ produced in the context of /a/ is produced farther back in the mouth than the /n/ produced in the context of /i/.

Interspeaker Variability for /n/ Speakers with Impaired Speech

Adults with Hearing Impairment

Nicolaidis (2004) described tongue/palate contact for four adults with hearing impairment. The three females and one male were aged between 23 to 26 years. Each spoke typical Modern Standard Greek. Each of the four people produced /n/ in the contexts /ana/ and /ini/ within the word form /pVnV/ within a carrier phrase. Each word was produced ten times. Figure 9-6 demonstrates two cumulative maximum contact EPG frames for each speaker (HI1–HI4) for productions of /n/ in the two contexts /ana/ and /ini/. In Figure 9-6, a black square indicates that that electrode was contacted at least 60% of the time. Most of the productions in Figure 9-6 are similar to the tongue/palate contact for /n/ produced by typical speakers, with the exception

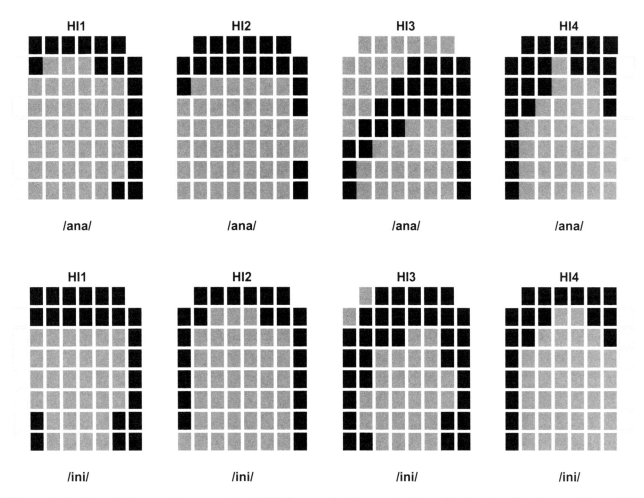

Figure 9–6. Cumulative maximum contact EPG frames for the production of /n/ by four Greek-speaking adults with hearing impairment (adapted from Nicolaidis, 2004, Figure 1, p. 8).

of HI3's production of /ana/. This production was produced asymmetrically and the closure occurred farther back in the mouth.

Children with Cleft Palate

Howard (2004) compared perceptual and instrumental analyses of speech produced by three adolescents with a history of cleft palate. Within this comprehensive research, four frames of maximum contact were provided for the production of /n/ by two of the speakers: Rachel (aged 13;1) and Beth (aged 16;1). Figure 9-7 provides the maximum contact frame for the production of /n/ by Rachael in the context of "knife." Figure 9-7 also provides three maximum contact frames for three productions of the word "banana" by Beth. Considerable variability in productions are evident. Only Beth's first production of the /n/ in "banana" is similar to typical productions of /n/. The other frames in Figure 9-7 have too much contact at the velar region of the palate.

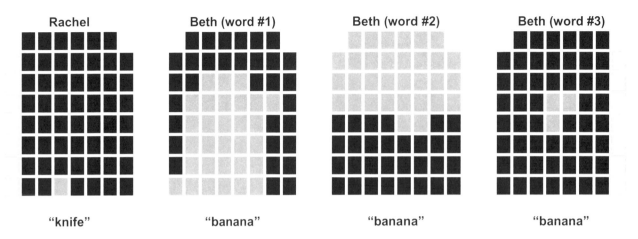

Figure 9–7. Maximum contact EPG frames for the production of /n/ by two English-speaking adolescents with a history of cleft palate (adapted from Howard, 2004, Figure 3, p. 322 and Figure 9, p. 329).

Chapter 10

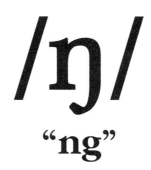

"ng"

The consonant /ŋ/ is a voiced velar nasal.

Place of articulation: velar

Advancement: back

Voicing: voiced

Labiality: nonlabial

Sonorancy: sonorant

Continuancy: —

Sibilancy: nonsibilant

Nasality: nasal

STATIC IMAGES OF THE ARTICULATORY CHARACTERISTICS OF /ŋ/

The static images of /ŋ/ are presented via a photograph, schematic diagram, ultrasound, and electropalatograph images (Figure 10-1).

Photograph

In this photograph (Figure 10-1A), the mouth is open and the tongue can be seen behind the lower teeth. The photograph does not show the tongue touching the velum to create closure of the airstream to produce /ŋ/.

A. Photograph

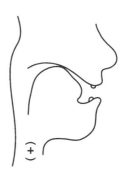

B. Schematic diagram

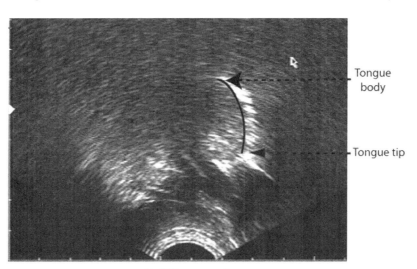

C. Ultrasound

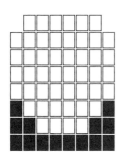

D. Electropalatograph (EPG) (single frame)

E. Electropalatograph (EPG) (cumulative frame)

Figure 10–1. Static images of the articulatory characteristics of /ŋ/.

Schematic Diagram

The schematic diagram shows the back of the tongue touching the back of the roof of the mouth or the velum. The back of the tongue contacts the velum and completely stops the flow of the airstream through the oral cavity. There is, however, an uninterrupted flow of air through the nasal cavity. The lowering of the velum opens the velopharyngeal port and involves the nasal cavity in the production of this sound. The voicing feature of /ŋ/ is denoted by the (+) at the vocal folds.

Ultrasound

Figure 10–1C shows a midsagittal ultrasound image of the tongue surface during production of /ŋ/. The tongue tip and blade is the bright white line that is almost vertical at the right of the screen. The body of the tongue is barely visible on this image. Stone (2005) indicates that steeply sloping tongue surfaces, such as in the production of velar sounds, are difficult to see on ultrasound images.

Electropalatograph (EPG)

Like the EPG images for /k/ and /g/, the EPG image for /ŋ/ (Figure 10–1D) is shaped like a smile, with the tongue contacting the posterior and lateral margins of the hard palate. Additional tongue contact may occur on the soft palate; however, the palate design means that data is only recorded up until the juncture between the hard and soft palates. At times, EPG images for /ŋ/ may not have complete closure across the back of the EPG palate, particularly in the context of back vowels because closure is occurring on the soft palate.

The cumulative EPG image (Figure 10–1E) represents productions of /ŋ/ by eight speakers over a total of 480 words. The darker the shading the more often that part of the palate was contacted by the tongue. The numbers indicate the percentage of contact with each EPG electrode. The number 100 in the lower left square indicates that that lateral velar electrode was contacted 100% of the time by the eight speakers over the 230 words when producing /ŋ/.

[1]/ˈsɜtʃɪŋ/ is the Australian English pronunciation of "searching."

DYNAMIC IMAGES OF THE ARTICULATORY AND ACOUSTIC CHARACTERISTICS OF /ŋ/

In order to obtain a comprehensive view of the production of this consonant, the dynamic aspects of the production of /ŋ/ are shown in a filmstrip, spectrogram, and EPG images (Figure 10–2).

/ŋ/ in Word-Final Context: "searching?

Filmstrip: /ˈsɜtʃɪŋ/ "searching"

The phoneme /ŋ/ is presented in the final position in the word /ˈsɜtʃɪŋ/. This filmstrip (Figure 10–2A) demonstrates the strong influence of neighboring sounds on each other. In addition, it can be seen here that the production of speech is a dynamic event. The very first frame shows rounding of the lips, which is atypical for the production of /s/. This rounding persists throughout the production of /s/. The influence of lip rounding caused by /ɜ/ and /tʃ/ can be viewed in both the backward and forward coarticulators. The example of backward coarticulation is the rounding of /s/, and the example of forward coarticulation is the rounding of /ɪ/ and /ŋ/.

Sound Spectrogram: /ˈsɜtʃɪŋ/ "searching"

The phoneme /ŋ/ is produced in the word-final position of the word "searching." The nasalization of the vowel /ɪ/, is caused by the coarticulatory influence of the final nasal, and can be seen in the low amplitude of the first formant (a phenonmenon called antiresonance). The first formant of the vowel /ɪ/ is much lighter than the second formant. There is a faint, rising, first formant transition, signaling voicing and nasality.

Electropalatograph: /ˈsɜtʃɪŋ/ "searching"

Figure 10–2C contains 135 EPG frames for the word /ˈsɜtʃɪŋ/[1] "searching." The word extends over 0.669 seconds and was produced within a sentence context. The /s/ extends from 455 to 487, the vowel /ɜ/ extends from 498 to 512, and the affricate /tʃ/ extends from 520 to

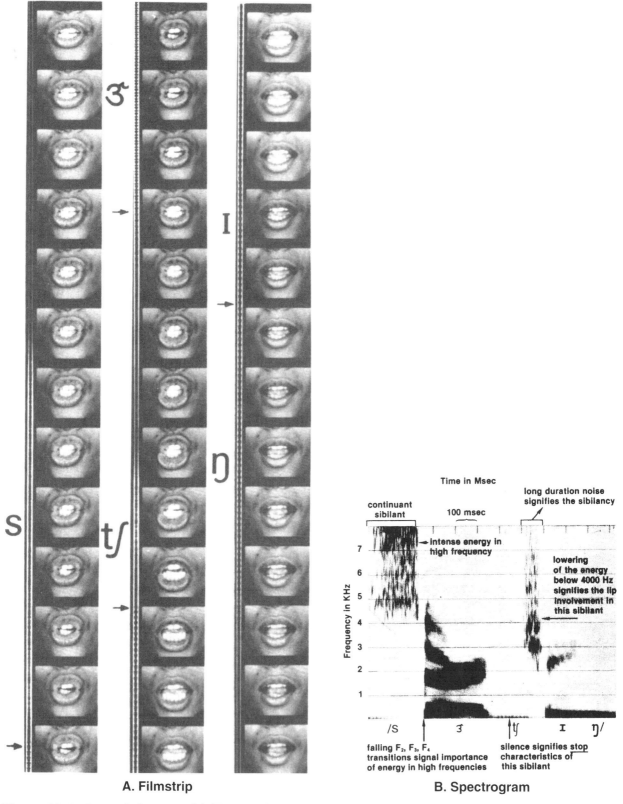

A. Filmstrip

B. Spectrogram

Figure 10–2. Dynamic images of /ŋ/ in word-final context: "searching." *continues*

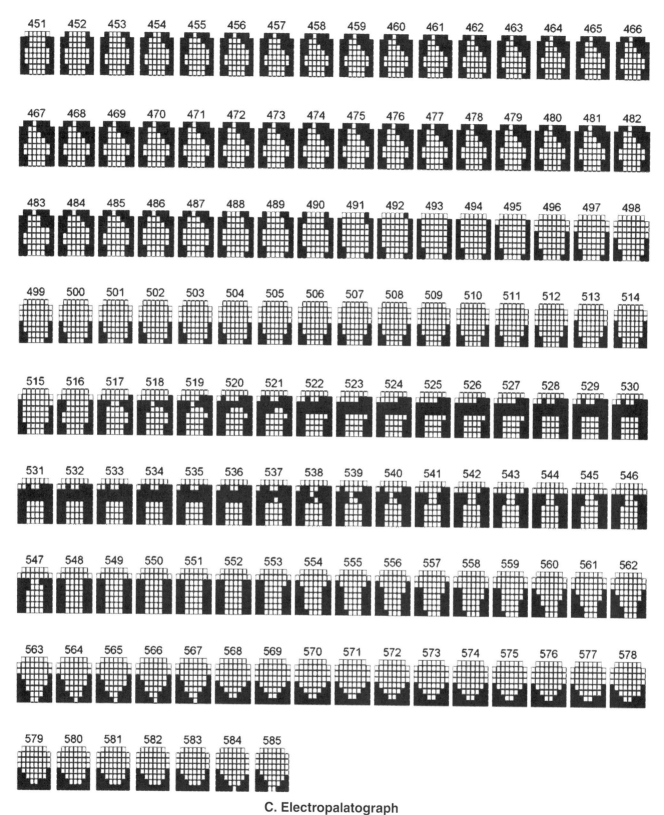

C. Electropalatograph

Figure 10–2. *continued*

547. The vowel /ɪ/ extends from 554 to 567 (identified using simultaneous spectrogram and waveform data) and the velar nasal /ŋ/ extends from 568 to 583. The frames that are unaccounted for are periods of transition between the sounds. The EPG frames that depict /ŋ/ demonstrate velar tongue placement with electrodes along the base and lower sides of the palate being contacted. The first frame of closure is frame 568 and the first frame of release appears to be frame 584. As discussed in Chapter 9, the EPG palate only extends to the juncture between the hard and soft palates; thus, it is possible that stoppage of the oral airstream extended slightly beyond frame 583.

INTRA- AND INTERSPEAKER VARIABILITY FOR /ŋ/

Electropalatographic images enable consideration of intra- and interspeaker variability. This section will concentrate on variability in the production of /ŋ/ by eight typical adults.

Intra- and Interspeaker Variability in the Production of /ŋ/ by Eight Typical English-Speaking Adults

Four typical adult males (M1–M4) and four typical adult females (F1–F4) produced nonsense syllables containing /ŋ/ three times. The nonsense syllables were created with /ŋ/ in the syllable-final position only, as /ŋ/ does not occur in the syllable initial position in English.

Maximum Contact Frames for Eight Typical English-Speaking Adults

In order to demonstrate both inter- and intraspeaker variability the maximum contact frame for the second production of each nonsense syllable for each speaker is provided in Figure 10–3. For the majority of speakers, there was lingual contact at the velar region of the palate. Three speakers (F1, F2, M4) produced /ŋ/ as /n/ on a few occasions. This could have been due to the complexity of producing the nonsense words, or dialectical variation (Horvath, 1985).

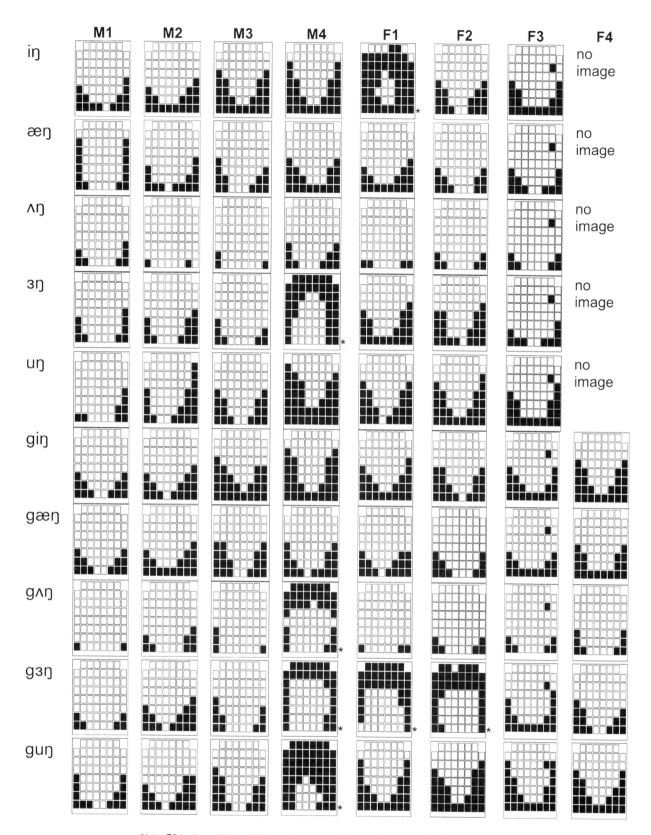

Note. F3 had one electrode in the third row that incorrectly recorded activation
* indicates that the participant produced /n/ instead of /ŋ/

Figure 10–3. Intra- and interspeaker variability in the maximum EPG contact frame for the production of /ŋ/ by eight typical English-speaking adults. *continues*

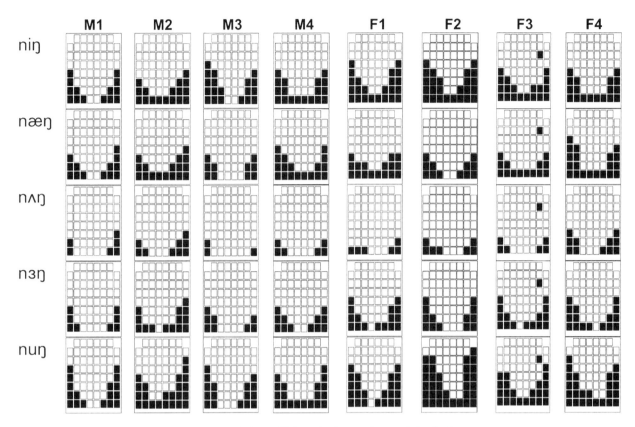

Note. F3 had one electrode in the third row that incorrectly recorded activation
* indicates that the participant produced /n/ instead of /ŋ/

Figure 10–3. *continues*

Cumulative EPG Frames for Eight Typical English-Speaking Adults

Cumulative EPG patterns for /ŋ/ were generated from maximum contact frames for each of the eight typical adults described above. Each electrode on a cumulative maximum contact display has a number, corresponding to the percentage of contact over the number of productions. The darker the shading, the more contact.

In Figure 10–4 each speaker's cumulative maximum contact display has lingual contact along the velar region of the palate. However, due to either the complexity of producing the nonsense words, or dialectical variation (Horvath, 1985), three speakers (F1, F2, M4) produced /ŋ/ as /n/ on a few occasions. This is evident by occasional tongue/palate contact on the alveolar regions of the cumulative palate.

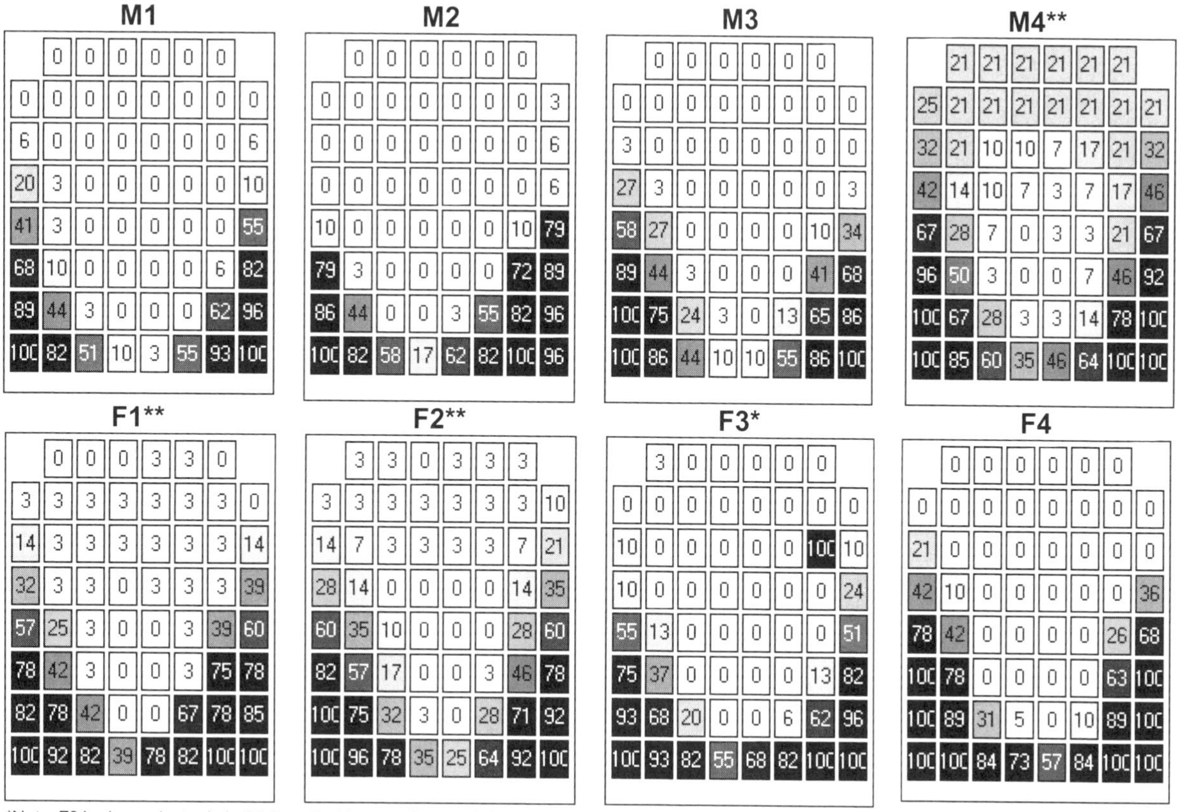

M1 **M2** **M3** **M4****

F1** **F2**** **F3*** **F4**

*Note: F3 had one electrode in third row that incorrectly recorded activation.
**F1 and F2 produced /ŋ/ as [n] once and M4 produced /ŋ/ as [n] seven times.

Figure 10–4. Cumulative EPG frames demonstrating intra- and interspeaker variability for the production of /ŋ/ by eight typical English-speaking adults.

Chapter 11

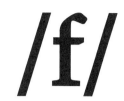

The consonant /f/ is a voiceless labiodental fricative.

Place of articulation: labiodental

Voicing: voiceless

Advancement: front

Labiality: labial

Sonorancy: nonsonorant (obstruent)

Continuancy: continuant

Sibilancy: sibilant

Nasality: nonnasal (oral)

STATIC IMAGES OF THE ARTICULATORY CHARACTERISTICS OF /f/

The static images of /f/ are presented via a photograph, schematic diagram, ultrasound, and electropalatograph images (Figure 11–1).

Photograph

In this photograph (Figure 11–1A), the upper incisors are placed on the lower lip and the airstream is channelled to create the long-duration, high-frequency sound /f/.

A. Photograph

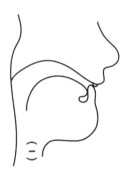

B. Schematic diagram

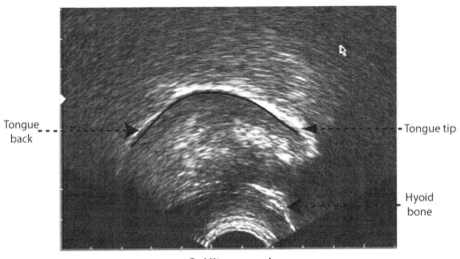

Tongue back

Tongue tip

Hyoid bone

C. Ultrasound

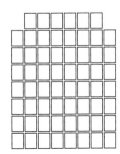

D. Electropalatograph (EPG) (single frame)

Figure 11–1. Static images of the articulatory characteristics of /f/.

Schematic Diagram

The schematic diagram (Figure 11–1B) shows the lateral view of the labiodental phoneme /f/. It also illustrates the independence of the feature labiality from the feature front/back as the tongue maintains a neutral position. The lack of voicing in the production of /f/ is symbolically represented by (–) in the vicinity of the vocal folds.

Ultrasound

A midsagittal ultrasound image of the tongue surface during production /f/ is shown in Figure 11–1C. Underneath the bright white line is the tongue surface. The tongue takes the shape of an inverted U. The tongue tip is on the right of the image, toward the floor of the mouth. An air shadow can be seen above the tongue and diagonal muscle fibers can be seen below the surface of the tongue. The hyoid bone is seen as the bright diagonal line at the bottom right of the image.

Electropalatograph (EPG)

The EPG image of /f/ in Figure 11–1D has no tongue/palate contact at all. In this figure every square corresponding to an electrode on the palate is white; whereas, if there was contact with the tongue, the squares corresponding to the electrodes would be colored black. The extent of tongue/palate contact for /f/ is influenced by the surrounding vowel. In the production of the word "fife" as illustrated in Figure 11–2C, there is some (minimal) contact with the posterior lateral margins of the palate.

DYNAMIC IMAGES OF THE ARTICULATORY AND ACOUSTIC CHARACTERISTICS OF /f/

In order to obtain a comprehensive view of the production of this consonant, the dynamic aspects of the production of /f/ are shown in a filmstrip, spectrogram, and EPG images in two words containing /f/ in different word positions (Figure 11–2).

/f/ in Word-Initial and Word-Final Contexts: "fife"

Filmstrip: /faɪf/ "fife"

The phoneme /f/ is presented at the word-initial and word-final positions in the word /faɪf/ (Figure 11–2A). The vowel-acoustic energy begins halfway through the 12th frame. In the first 11 frames the high-frequency, low-amplitude, long-duration energy associated with the initial /f/ cannot be seen in the sound track by the naked eye. The flexible lower lip against the rigid upper incisors channels the airstream and creates the long-duration, high-frequency sound /f/.

Sound Spectrogram: /faɪf/ "fife"

Figure 11–2B provides a sound spectrogram of the word "fife." The phoneme /f/ is contrasted at the initial and final positions with the vowel /aɪ/ in the medial position. The lack of any glottal vibration at the outset of this sound spectrogram precludes the presence of voicing for the phoneme /f/. Although the rising F1 may be falsely attributed to the feature (+) voicing, in this case it is caused by the labial nature of the phoneme /f/. Consequently, some low-frequency energy exists, which affects the F1. The falling F2 shows the presence of some high-frequency friction noise, although no trace of this noise can be seen on the sound spectrogram. The lack of these tracings is representative of the fact that the phoneme /f/ is extremely low in amplitude and, therefore, sometimes cannot be transmitted adequately by a microphone to a sound spectrogram. The following vowel, although a diphthong, clearly maintains the strict formant boundaries of both of the component vowels /a/ and /ɪ/. The formant frequencies of the vowel /a/ in this utterance are approximately 1000 Hz and 1500 Hz, respectively, for F1 and F2. The vowel segment /a/ occupies about three-fourths of the duration of the diphthong. The F1 makes a substantial downward glide and the F2 makes a substantial upward glide to approximate the vowel /ɪ/ at 300 Hz and 2700 Hz. The final-voiceless-labial continuant /f/ also does not show any trace of acoustic energy.

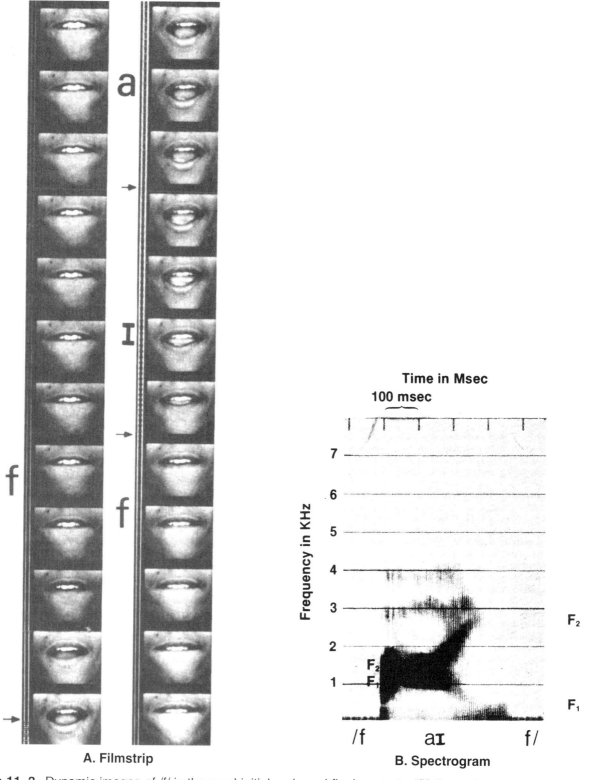

A. Filmstrip

B. Spectrogram

Figure 11–2. Dynamic images of /f/ in the word-initial and word-final contexts: "fife." *continues*

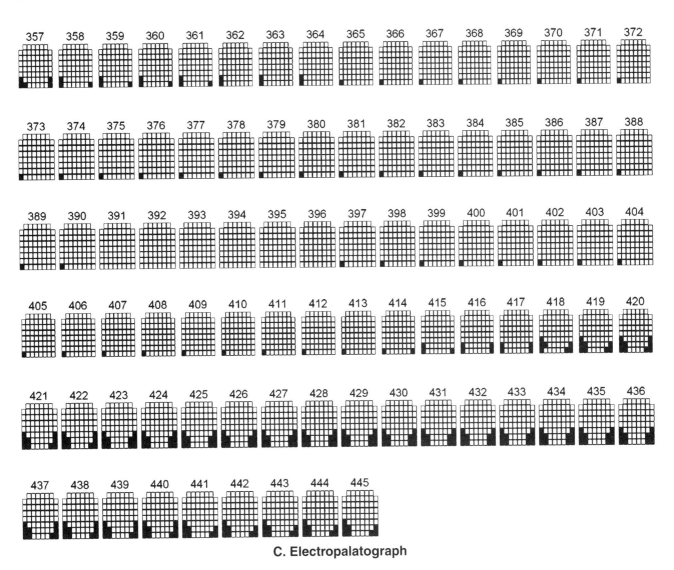

C. Electropalatograph

Figure 11–2. *continued*

Electropalatograph: /faɪf/ "fife"

The dynamic series of EPG palates for the production of the word "fife" is presented in Figure 11-2C. The word "fife" was extracted from the sentence "I see a fife again." Within this sentence context, the word "fife" took 0.440 seconds to produce. Each EPG palate in the dynamic series shows minimal tongue contact palate throughout the whole word. Using the information presented from the simultaneous sound spectrogram and waveform data (not shown in Figure 11-2C) the boundaries of the sounds were able to be identified. The first /f/ extends from 358 to 389, the diphthong /aɪ/ extends from 391 to 417, and the final /f/ extends from 420 to 445. The frames that are unaccounted for are periods of coarticulatory transition. The coarticulatory influence of the velar tongue contact in the following word ("again") is evident in that the final /f/ has greater tongue/palate contact than did the initial /f/.

Chapter 12

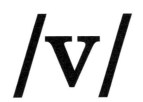

The consonant /v/ is a voiced labiodental fricative.

Place of articulation: labiodental

Advancement: front

Voicing: voiced

Labiality: labial

Sonorancy: nonsonorant (obstruent)

Continuancy: continuant

Sibilancy: sibilant

Nasality: nonnasal (oral)

STATIC IMAGES OF THE ARTICULATORY CHARACTERISTICS OF /v/

The static representations of /v/ are presented via a photograph, schematic diagram, ultrasound, and electropalatograph images (Figure 12–1).

Photograph

In this photograph (Figure 12–1A), the upper incisors are placed on the lower lip and the airstream is channelled to create the sound /v/.

A. Photograph

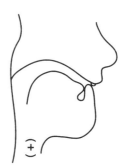

B. Schematic diagram

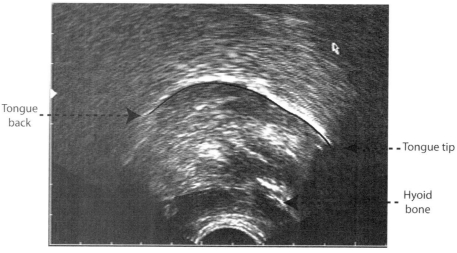

C. Ultrasound

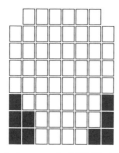

D. Electropalatograph (EPG) (single frame)

Figure 12–1. Static images of the articulatory characteristics of /v/.

Schematic Diagram

The schematic diagram (Figure 12-1B) shows the lateral view of the labiodental phoneme /v/. The tongue maintains a neutral position, illustrating the independence of the feature labiality from the feature front/back. The voicing feature in the production of /v/ is symbolically represented by (+) at the region of the vocal folds.

Ultrasound

The bright white line on the ultrasound image in Figure 12-1C shows the tongue surface during production of /v/. The tongue tip is on the right and is lowered toward the floor of the mouth. The back of the tongue is slightly raised in the oral cavity. An air shadow can be seen above the tongue and diagonal muscle fibers can be seen below the surface of the tongue.

Electropalatograph (EPG)

The EPG image of /v/ (Figure 12-1D) has limited tongue/palate contact. The contact that does occur is located at the posterior lateral corners of the palate. The extent of tongue/palate contact for /v/ is influenced by the surrounding vowels. When comparing this image to that of /f/ (Figure 11-1D) it seems that there is more contact for the voiced /v/ compared to the voiceless counterpart /f/. This needs to be verified by future research.

DYNAMIC IMAGES OF THE ARTICULATORY AND ACOUSTIC CHARACTERISTICS OF /v/

In order to obtain a comprehensive view of the production of this consonant, the dynamic aspects of the production of /v/ are shown in a filmstrip, spectrogram, and EPG images (Figure 12-2).

/v/ in Word-Initial Context: "veal"

Filmstrip: /vil/ "veal"

The criterion phoneme /v/ is at the initial position of the word /vil/ "veal." The first six frames show the lips before the labiodental closure. Frames 7 through 15 show the state of labiodental contact necessary for the production of English consonants /f/ and /v/. Frame 16 shows the beginning sign of lip opening for the vowel /i/. Frames 17 through 23 show the tongue at the front-high position for the production of the vowel /i/. Frame 24 shows the upward movement of the tongue tip for the production of the final consonant /l/. The last two frames show the tongue touching the alveolar ridge area.

Sound Spectrogram: /vil/ "veal"

Figure 12-2B presents a dynamic sound spectrogram of the word "veal." The phoneme /v/ is presented at the initial position followed by the vowel /i/ and the consonant /l/. The voicing characteristic of this continuant consonant is represented by the rising F1 of the vowel /i/, as well as by the voicing markings at the base of the sound spectrogram. Labiality can be seen represented at a very low-frequency area (1000 Hz), as well as in the rising second, third, and fourth formant transitions. The continuancy feature is mainly represented by energy at a very high-frequency region (between 7000 and 8000 Hz) for a duration of approximately 90 msec. The overall duration of this consonant is about 180 msec.

Electropalatograph: /vil/ "veal"

Figure 12-2C presents tongue/palate contact for the word "veal" in the phase "I see a veal again." The 89 EPG frames took 0.452 seconds to produce. The initial /v/ extends from frames 434 to 458, the vowel /i/ extends from 459 to 493 and the final /l/ extends from 507 to 521. The word-initial /v/ has limited tongue/palate contact; primarily centred around the posterior lateral margins of the palate. The simultaneous sound spectrogram, waveform, and audio data (not shown in

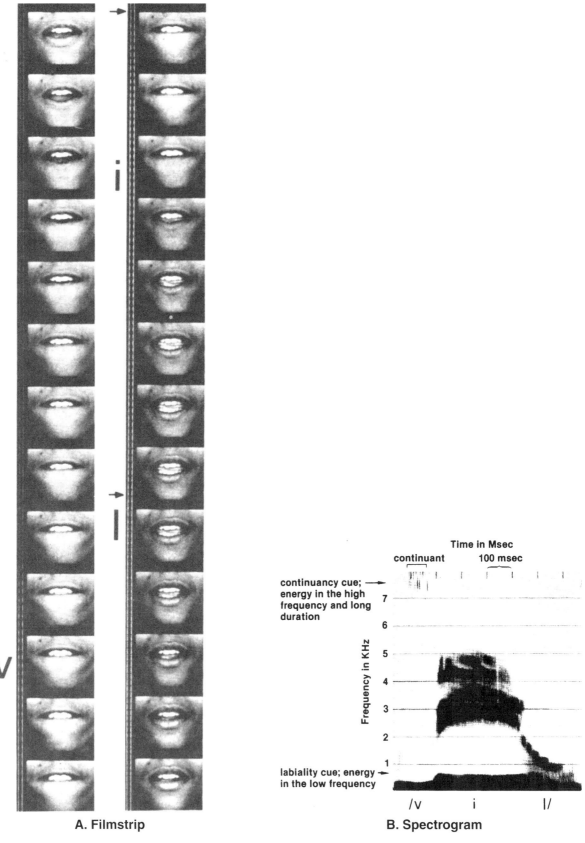

A. Filmstrip   B. Spectrogram

Figure 12–2. Dynamic images of /v/ in word-initial context: "veal." *continues*

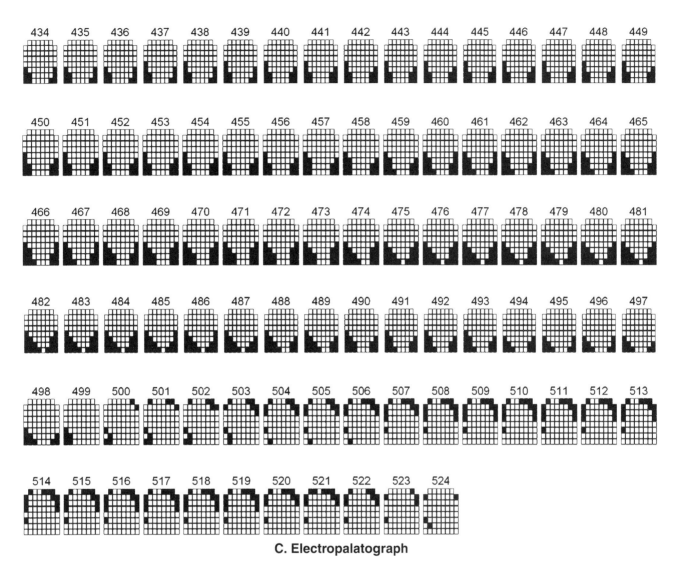

C. Electropalatograph

Figure 12–2. *continued*

Figure 12-2C) were used to identify the boundaries between /v/ and /i/ as there was no detectable difference at this point on the EPG palate trace. The EPG frames 493 to 506 represent a period of coarticulatory transition between the vowel and the /l/.

/v/ in Word-Final Context: "have"

Filmstrip: /hæv/ "have"

The filmstrip shows the continuants /h/ and /v/ at the initial and final positions, respectively, in the word /hæv/ (Figure 12-3A). The vowel /æ/ is in the medial position. In the production of this word, the articulatory gestures associated with the vowel /æ/ predominate throughout the filmstrip. Jaw excursion and unrounded lips are characteristic of this vowel. The final consonant is the voiced continuant /v/. The labiodental positioning of this consonant can be seen in the last few frames. Lip approximation can be observed beginning at the eighth frame from the bottom. Lower lip contact is made by the sixth frame from the bottom, and complete contact (with appropriate opening for the airflow) is made by the fourth frame from the bottom.

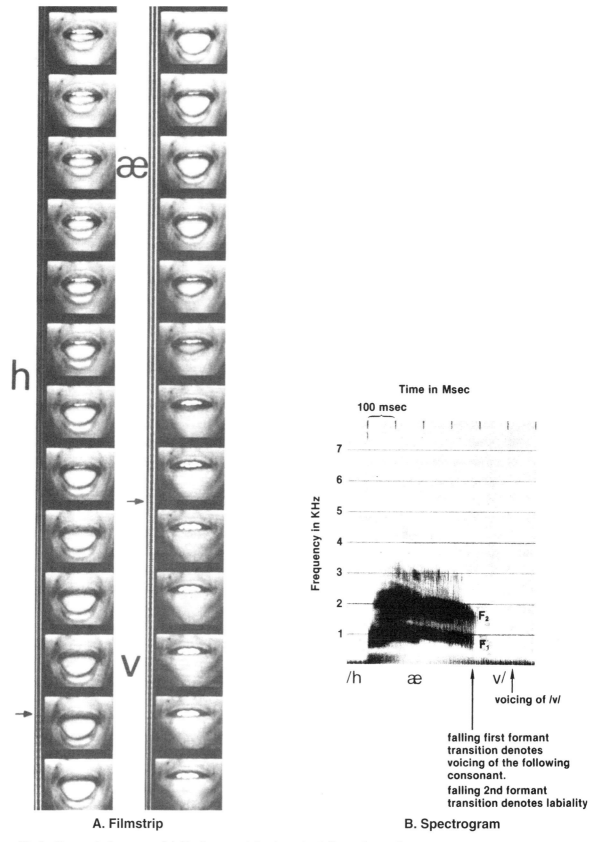

A. Filmstrip

B. Spectrogram

Figure 12–3. Dynamic images of /v/ in the word-final context: "have." *continues*

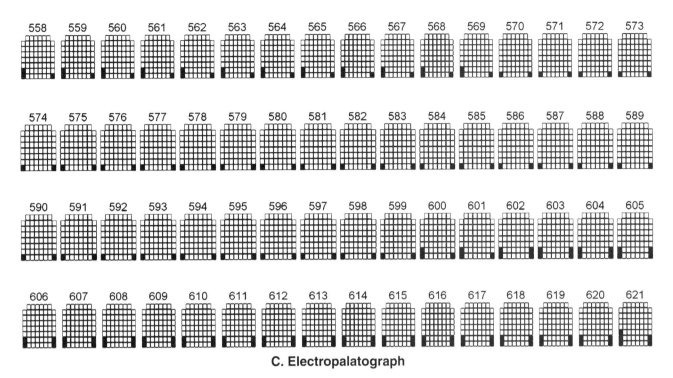

C. Electropalatograph

Figure 12–3. *continued*

Sound Spectrogram: /hæv/ "have"

The phoneme /v/ is presented at the final position in the word "have." In Figure 12-3B, labiality is indicated by the falling second formant of the preceding vowel /æ/. The feature voicing is indicated by the falling first formant of the vowel /æ/, as well as by the presence of vocal fold vibration for approximately 200 msec following the vowel formants. There is no trace of any high-frequency acoustic energy present at this final position. A comparison of this spectrogram with the one presented for the word "veal" (Figure 12-2B) shows that the feature continuancy, as represented by the presence of high-frequency noise for a long duration, is clearly seen at the initial position.

Electropalatograph: /hæv/ "have"

Figure 12-3C presents tongue/palate contact for the word "have." Throughout this word the EPG frames have limited tongue/palate contact along the posterior lateral margins. The /h/ extends from 558 to 569, the /æ/ from 570 to 599 and the /v/ from 600 to 620, detectable only by the activation of one and two electrodes, respectively. The boundaries of the consonants and vowels in this word were detected by simultaneous consideration of the EPG, waveform, and spectrogram images along with real-time audio data.

Chapter 13

/θ/

"th" (voiceless)

The consonant /θ/ is a voiceless linguodental fricative.

Place of articulation: linguodental

Advancement: front

Voicing: voiceless

Labiality: nonlabial

Sonorancy: nonsonorant (obstruent)

Continuancy: continuant

Sibilancy: nonsibilant

Nasality: nonnasal (oral)

STATIC IMAGES OF THE ARTICULATORY CHARACTERISTICS OF /θ/

The static representations of /θ/ are presented via a photograph, schematic diagram, ultrasound, and electropalatograph images (Figure 13–1).

Photograph

In this photograph (Figure 13-1A), the tongue tip is placed between the lower and upper teeth to channel the airstream to create the low energy sound /θ/.

A. Photograph

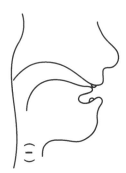

B. Schematic diagram

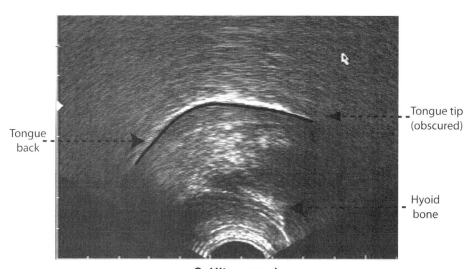

C. Ultrasound

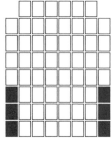

D. Electropalatograph (EPG) (single frame)

Figure 13–1. Static images of the articulatory characteristics of /θ/.

Schematic Diagram

The lateral view of the production of /θ/ (Figure 13-1B) shows the tip of the tongue placed between the upper and lower incisors. The phoneme /θ/ is a voiceless consonant. Devoicing is symbolized by a (−) in the vicinity of the vocal folds, indicating that in normal speech voicing is attributable to the vocal folds.

Ultrasound

The bright white line on the ultrasound image in Figure 13-1C shows the tongue surface during production of /θ/. The tongue is flat during production of this sound. The tongue tip is on the right and the end is slightly obscured from view because of the acoustic shadow of the jaw (Stone, 2005). Diagonal muscle fibers can be seen below the surface of the tongue.

Electropalatograph (EPG)

The EPG image of /θ/ in Figure 13-1D demonstrates limited tongue/contact during the production of this sound. Tongue contact is located at the posterior lateral margins of the palate. The extent of tongue/palate contact for /θ/ is influenced by the surrounding vowels.

DYNAMIC IMAGES OF THE ARTICULATORY AND ACOUSTIC CHARACTERISTICS OF /θ/

In order to obtain a comprehensive view of the production of this consonant, the dynamic aspects of the production of /θ/ are shown in a filmstrip, spectrogram, and EPG images (Figure 13-2).

/θ/ in Word-Initial Context: "thin"

Filmstrip

The criterion phoneme /θ/ is at the initial position of the word /θɪn/ (Figure 13-2A). In the first frame, the tongue tip can be seen securely placed between the lower and upper teeth. In frame 4 the grip of the teeth begins to relax. Frame 5 shows a complete release of the tongue tip, and frame 6 shows the tongue approximation for the vowel /ɪ/. Not unlike the phoneme /f/, the phoneme /θ/ shows very little energy. The energy is so low that it is undetectable in the sound track presented along the filmstrip. Halfway through the sixth frame the vowel energy begins, the tongue having been released from the interdental (between the upper and lower incisors) position.

Sound Spectrogram: /θɪn/ "thin"

The consonant phoneme /θ/ is presented at the word-initial position in the context of the vowel /ɪ/ in the word "thin" (Figure 13-2B). The phoneme /θ/, not unlike /f/, shows only traces of energy at a very high-frequency region (around 7000 Hz). The rising F2 transition of the vowel /ɪ/ at 2000 Hz may imply the presence of some acoustic energy at and around that frequency region. Because this phoneme does not manifest itself clearly in the acoustic domain (except when transitions are considered), it is not surprising that problems exist in the processing of this phoneme by children and adults with speech, hearing, and language deficiencies. The influence of the final nasal consonant can be seen midway through the preceding vowel /ɪ/. The weakening of the F1 for that vowel is caused by its nasalization as it is followed by /n/ in the word "thin."

Electropalatograph: /θɪn/ "thin"

Figure 13-2C presents tongue/palate contact for the word "thin." The 63 EPG frames took 0.315 seconds to produce. The initial /θ/ extends from frames 418 to 452, the vowel /ɪ/ extends from 453 to 460 and the final /n/ extends from 469 to 480. The simultaneous sound spectrogram and waveform (not shown in Figure 13-2C) were used to identify the boundaries between /θ/ and /ɪ/ as there was no detectable difference at this point on the EPG palate trace. The EPG frames 461 to 468 represent a period of coarticulatory transition between the vowel and the /n/. The word-final /n/ predominantly has contact with the tongue along the alveolar ridge and the lateral margins of the palate.

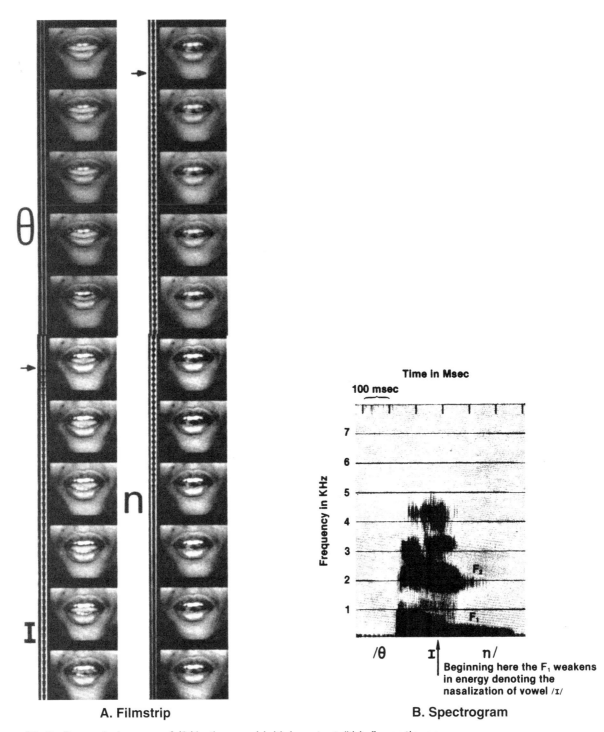

A. Filmstrip

B. Spectrogram

Figure 13–2. Dynamic images of /θ/ in the word-initial context: "thin." *continues*

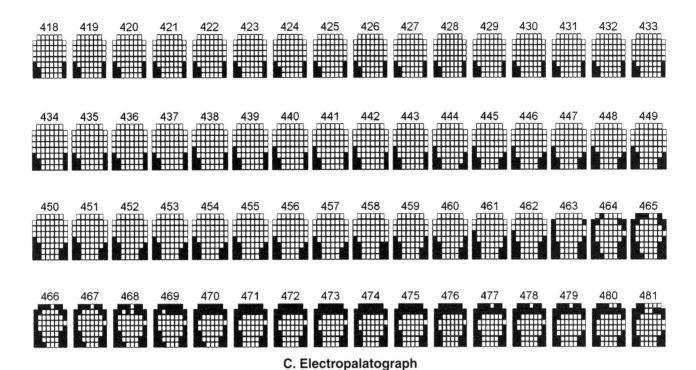

C. Electropalatograph

Figure 13–2. *continued*

/θ/ in Word-Final Context: "tooth"

Filmstrip: /tuθ/ "tooth"

The phoneme /θ/ is presented at the final position in the word "tooth" /tuθ/ (Figure 13-3A). Because of the coarticulatory influence of the vowel /u/ on the initial position /t/, signs of lip rounding can be noted from the first frame. The pretarget activity of the initial /t/ is considerably long. The plosive burst for /t/ can be seen in the sound track of frame 15. There is no acoustic energy present in the sound track prior to the 15th frame. If this were a voiced consonant, there would be low-frequency energy present prior to the burst. The coarticulatory influence of /u/ can also be seen on /θ/ in the last six frames. During the approximation of the tongue at the interdental position in the sixth frame from the end, lip rounding is attributable to the forward coarticulation of the vowel /u/. A comparison of the shape of the lips in the words "thin" and "tooth" shows that when /θ/ is followed by vowel /ɪ/, the lips are spread and less open (consistent with vowel /ɪ/); however, when /θ/ is preceded by vowel /u/, the lips are round and more open (consistent with vowel /u/).

Sound Spectrogram: /tuθ/ "tooth"

The phoneme /t/ at the initial position in Figure 13-3B is contrasted with the phoneme /θ/ at the final position in the word "tooth." Although both /t/ and /θ/ are front voiceless consonants, /t/ is a stop consonant and /θ/ is a continuant. The acoustic representation of /t/ can be seen in the presence of a plosive burst as well as aspiration noise above 3000 Hz. In contrast to the intense energy of the plosive burst and the relatively short duration of aspiration noise for /t/, the phoneme /θ/ shows practically no acoustic energy in any concentrated frequency domain. Some slight tracings of noiselike energy for /θ/ can be seen between 5000 and 8000 Hz. The duration component of that energy is approximately 150 msec, justifying the continuance characteristic of this phoneme.

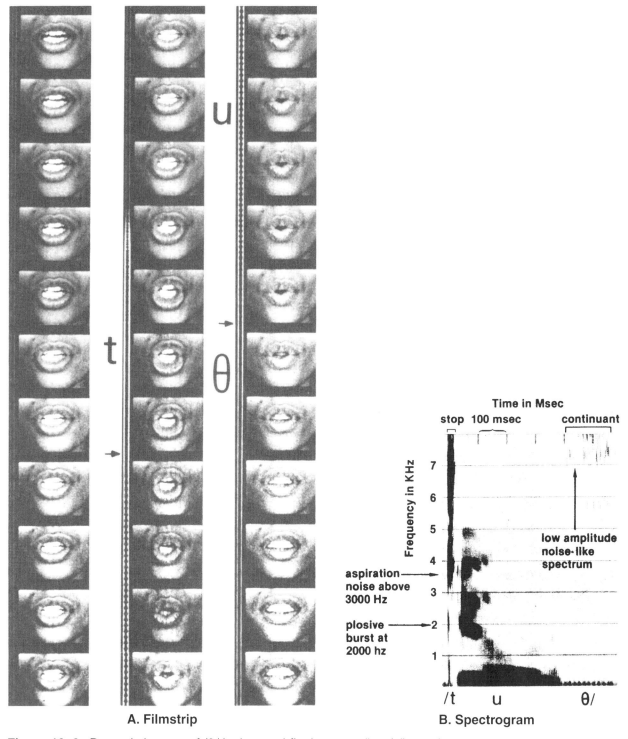

A. Filmstrip

B. Spectrogram

Figure 13–3. Dynamic images of /θ/ in the word-final context: "tooth." *continues*

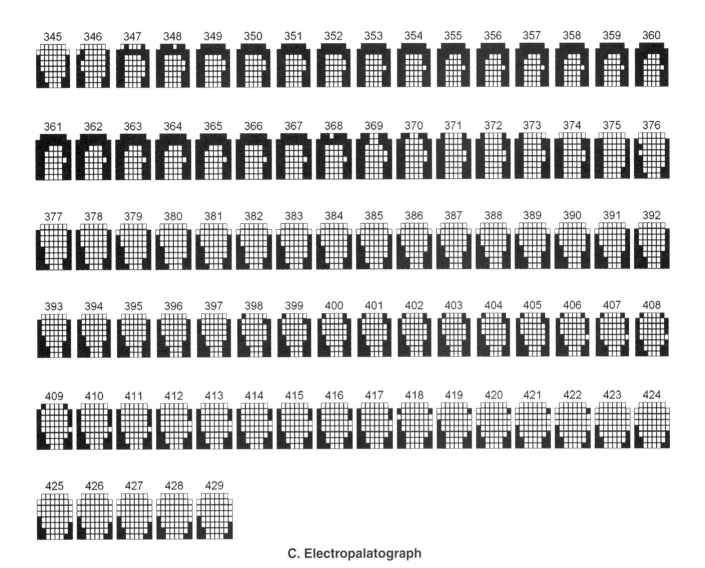

C. Electropalatograph

Figure 13–3. *continued*

Electropalatograph: /tuθ/ "tooth"

The dynamic series of EPG palates for the production of the word "tooth" is presented in Figure 13–3C and was extracted from the sentence "I see a tooth again." Within this sentence, the word "tooth" took 0.420 seconds to produce. The first frame of closure for the first /t/ is 347, and the last frame before release is 368 and /t/ is represented by the typical horseshoe shape. The vowel /u/ was identified as occurring during frames 386 to 397 by using simultaneous waveform, spectrogram, and EPG (not shown in Figure 13–3C). Using the waveform and spectrographic images, the /θ/ was identified as occurring between frames 398 and 429. The coarticulatory influence of the preceding vowel /u/ and the subsequent vowel /ə/ is evident in the different extent of tongue/palate contact during the production of /θ/. The steady state for the production of /θ/ appears to be between frames 400 and 409 where the tongue extends along the lateral margins of the palate.

Chapter 14

/ð/

"th" (voiced)

The consonant /ð/ is a voiced linguodental fricative.

Place of articulation: linguodental

Advancement: front

Voicing: voiced

Labiality: nonlabial

Sonorancy: nonsonorant (obstruent)

Continuancy: continuant

Sibilancy: nonsibilant

Nasality: nonnasal (oral)

STATIC IMAGES OF THE ARTICULATORY CHARACTERISTICS OF /ð/

The static representations of /ð/ are presented via a photograph, schematic diagram, ultrasound, and electropalatograph images (Figure 14–1).

Photograph

In this photograph (Figure 14–1A), the tip of the tongue is placed between the upper and lower incisors to produce the phoneme /ð/.

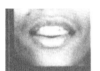

A. Photograph

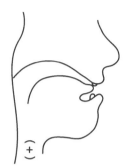

B. Schematic diagram

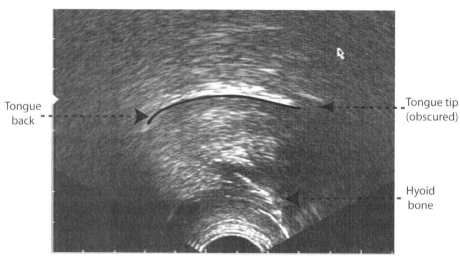

Tongue back

Tongue tip (obscured)

Hyoid bone

C. Ultrasound

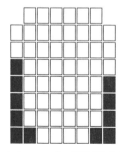

D. Electropalatograph (EPG) (single frame)

Figure 14–1. Static images of the articulatory characteristics of /ð/.

Schematic Diagram

The lateral view of the production of the phoneme /ð/ (Figure 14–1B) shows the tip of the tongue placed between the upper and lower incisors. The phoneme /ð/ is a voiced consonant. Voicing is indicated by a (+) symbol at the area of the vocal folds.

Ultrasound

A midsagittal ultrasound image of the tongue surface during production /ð/ is shown in Figure 14–1C. Underneath the bright white line is the tongue surface. The tongue is raised compared to its resting position as described in Chapter 1; however, unlike many of the consonant sounds, the midsagittal section of the tongue in the production of /ð/ is flat in configuration. The tongue tip is on the right of the image, and approximately 1cm of the tip is obscured due to the acoustic shadow of the jaw (Stone, 2005). An air shadow can be seen above the tongue and diagonal muscle fibers can be seen below the surface of the tongue. The hyoid bone is seen as the bright diagonal line at the lower right of the image.

Electropalatograph (EPG)

The EPG image of /ð/ in Figure 14–1D demonstrates limited tongue/contact during the production of this sound. Tongue contact is located along the lateral margins of the palate. The extent of tongue/palate contact for /ð/ is influenced by the surrounding vowels. When comparing this image to that of /θ/ (see Figure 13–1D) it seems that there is slightly more contact for the voiced compared to the voiceless "th." This needs to be verified by future research.

DYNAMIC IMAGES OF THE ARTICULATORY AND ACOUSTIC CHARACTERISTICS OF /ð/

In order to obtain a comprehensive view of the production of this consonant, the dynamic aspects of the production of /ð/ are shown in a filmstrip, spectrogram and EPG images.

/ð/ in Word-Initial Context; "that"

Filmstrip: /ðæt/ "that"

The phoneme /ð/ is shown in the context of the vowel /æ/ in the word /ðæt/. The first nine frames (Figures 14–2A) show the process of tongue/teeth approximation for the interdental position. The tongue first lodges in the appropriate position, and then the particular gestures are accomplished for the correct production of this sound. An opening is present for the emission of the airflow. The opening is diffuse, however, and the velocity of the air is relatively low. The sound track associated with this filmstrip shows high-frequency energy, indicating the continuancy characteristic of this consonant.

Sound Spectrogram: /ðæt/ "that"

The phoneme /ð/ is presented at the word-initial position (in Figure 14–2B) in the context of the vowel /æ/ and the consonant in the word "that." The phoneme /ð/ seems to behave like a stop consonant, except that there is a continuation of vocal fold vibration from the voiced consonant /ð/ to the vowel formants, without any stoppage of the acoustic tracing or any interruption of this tracing by a plosive burst. The duration of

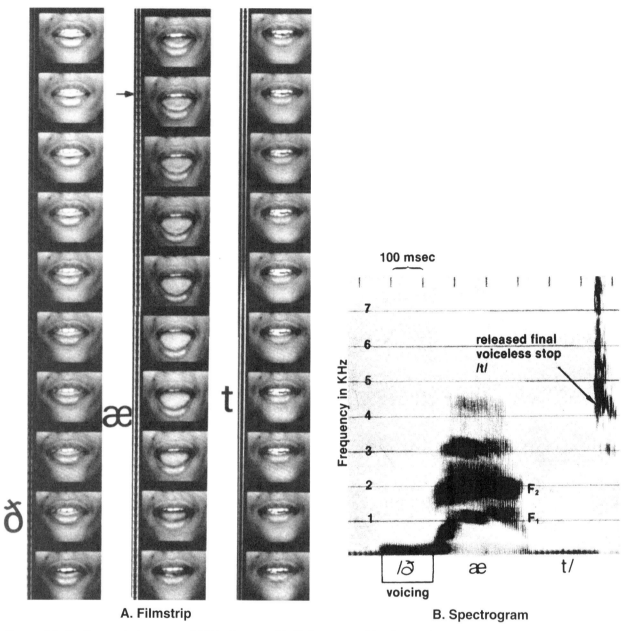

A. Filmstrip

B. Spectrogram

Figure 14–2. Dynamic images of /ð/ in the word-initial context: "that." *continues*

the voicing phenomenon is approximately 150 msec prior to the vowel transitions. The feature continuancy is also indicated by the relatively long duration of the transitional portion of the vowel (about 100 msec). In the case of the stop consonant /d/, for example, the duration of the transitional portion of the second formant of the following vowel is ordinarily shorter by about 50 msec.

Electropalatograph: /ðæt/ "that"

Figure 14-2C presents lingualpalatal contact for the word "that" as produced in a sentence. In order to identify the location of the consonants and vowel, the simultaneous audio, spectrogram, and waveform data (not shown in Figure 14-2C) were compared with the EPG frames. Frames 354 to 389 correspond to the pro-

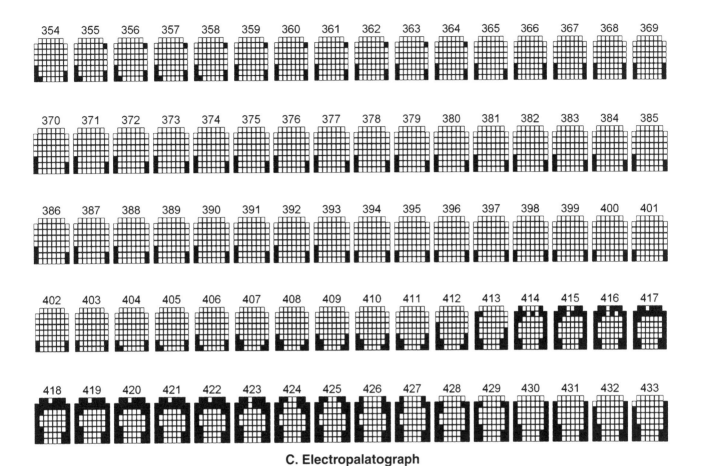

C. Electropalatograph

Figure 14–2. *continued*

duction of /ð/. There is limited tongue/palate contact for the production of /ð/. The vowel /æ/ extends from frames 390 to 413 and the closure phase for the final /t/ extends from frames 417 to 422.

/ð/ in Word-Final Context: "bathe"

Filmstrip: /beɪð/ "bathe"

The phoneme /ð/ is presented in the final position in the word /beɪð/. An examination of this filmstrip (Figure 14-3A) shows that it is difficult to pinpoint the phoneme boundaries exactly. The coarticulatory influences are overwhelming. The initial four frames show the lip closure for the /b/ phoneme. The fifth frame shows the first indication of opening for the first part of the diphthong, the vowel /e/. This gradually continues until the desired amount of opening has been reached in the seventh frame. This status is maintained through frames 8 and 9. The lips are less open for the production of the second part of the diphthong, the vowel /ɪ/. Finally, the last 10 frames show the gradually changing process that results in the production of a final-position /ð/.

Sound Spectrogram: /beɪð/ "bathe"

The phoneme /ð/ at the final position is contrasted with the phoneme /b/ at the initial position in the word "bathe." In Figure 14-3B, the voicing feature of /ð/ is indicated by the presence of voicing markers at the base of the sound spectrogram and by the falling first formant transition of the diphthong /eɪ/. The falling F2 indicates some energy for /ð/ between 1000 and 2000 Hz. The phoneme /ð/ at the final position is demonstrated acoustically, mainly in the second formant transition.

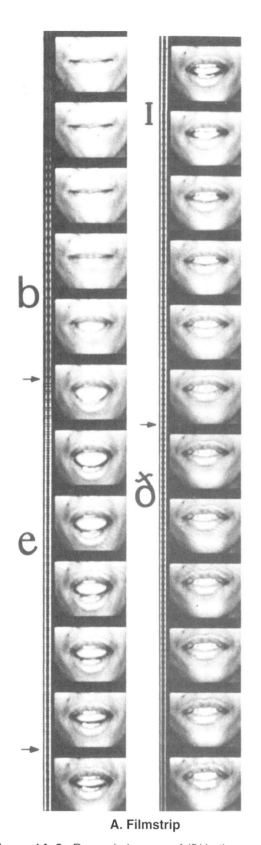

A. Filmstrip

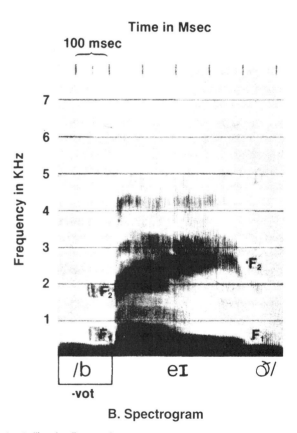

B. Spectrogram

Figure 14–3. Dynamic images of /ð/ in the word-final context: "bathe." *continues*

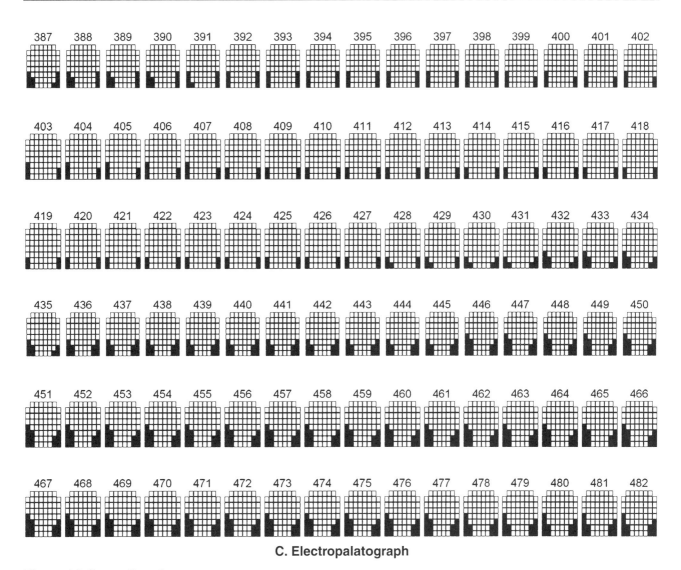

C. Electropalatograph

Figure 14–3. *continued*

Electropalatograph: /beɪð/ "bathe"

Figure 14-3C contains EPG frames for the production of "bathe" in the sentence context "I see a bathe again." The word "bathe" took 0.479 seconds to produce and is displayed in 95 EPG frames. Every EPG frame has limited tongue/palate contact, with minimal variation in the extent of contact at the posterior lateral margins of the palate. Using the simultaneous spectro- gram, waveform, audio, and EPG data (not shown in Figure 14-3C), the initial /b/ was identified as extending from frames 387 to 412. The diphthong /eɪ/ was identified as extending from frames 413 to 462. The transition point between the /e/ and /ɪ/ sounds in the diphthong occurs at approximately frame 432. The final /ð/ was identified as extending from frames 463 to 482. There was more contact for production of the /ð/ sound than for any other sound within the word "bathe."

Chapter 15

/s/

The consonant /s/ is a voiceless alveolar fricative.

Place of articulation: alveolar

Advancement: front

Voicing: voiceless

Labiality: nonlabial

Sonorancy: nonsonorant (obstruent)

Continuancy: continuant

Sibilancy: sibilant

Nasality: nonnasal (oral)

STATIC IMAGES OF THE ARTICULATORY CHARACTERISTICS OF /s/

The static images of /s/ are presented via a photograph, schematic diagram, ultrasound, and electropalatograph images (Figure 15–1).

Photograph

In this photograph (Figure 15–1A), the mouth is open and the tongue can be seen touching the alveolar ridge to create a groove through which the airstream can travel to produce /s/.

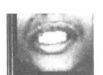

A. Photograph

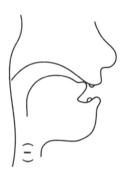

B. Schematic diagram

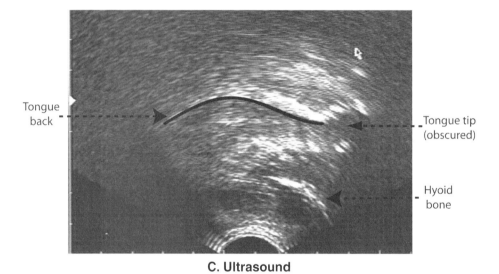

C. Ultrasound

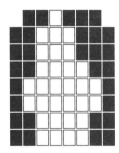

D. Electropalatograph (EPG) (single frame)

E. Electropalatograph (EPG) (cumulative frame)

Figure 15–1. Static images of the articulatory characteristics of /s/.

Schematic Diagram

The lateral view of the production of /s/ shown in this schematic diagram (Figure 15–1B) can be compared with the frontal view in the filmstrip. The tongue approximates the front portion of the roof of the mouth. This approximation is different from what has been seen for the phoneme /t/. The production of /s/ requires a steady opening (groove) for the continuant stream of the airflow. This may partially account for the designation of continuancy to /s/. The phonemes /f, v, θ, ð/ are also continuants, thereby requiring an opening at the point of contact in the oral cavity. The phonemes /s, z, ʃ, ʒ/ are sibilants because of the high turbulence (greater velocity), which requires a slightly greater opening for the much greater force of the airstream. This causes the sibilants to have much higher intensity in very high-frequency regions. This is not true for the nonsibilant continuants /f, v, θ, ð/. The phoneme /s/ is a voiceless consonant, as indicated by the minus sign in the vicinity of the vocal folds.

Ultrasound

An ultrasound of the tongue surface during production of /s/ is shown in Figure 15–1C. The tongue tip is on the right and is raised toward the alveolar ridge. Approximately 1 cm of the tongue tip is obscured from view because of the acoustic shadow of the jaw (Stone, 2005). The bright white line indicates the surface of the tongue and extends from right to left of the image. The complexity of tongue positioning for the production of /s/ is obvious: at the right of the image, the tip is raised. Next, the front of the tongue is slightly lowered, the center of the tongue is slightly raised, then the back is flattened and begins the transition toward the pharynx. An air shadow can be seen above the tongue and diagonal muscle fibers can be seen below the surface of the tongue.

Electropalatograph (EPG)

The EPG image of /s/ in Figure 15–1D presents similarly to /t, d, n/ as a horseshoe shape. The tongue contacts the palate across the alveolar ridge with lateral bracing along the lateral margins of the teeth. However, the difference between /s/ and these other alveolar sounds is that there is evidence of a groove, or inactivated electrode, on the alveolar ridge. The groove acts as a corridor for the air to move through, creating frication. Figure 15–1D is typical of the EPG image for speakers who produce /s/ with the tongue toward the roof of their mouth. A broader groove is often apparent for those who produce /s/ with their tongue placed behind their lower teeth.

Differentiation in the production of /s/ is evident in the cumulative EPG frame in Figure 15–1E. This figure represents the cumulation of 470 productions of /s/ by 8 typical adults. The middle two columns of the first two rows of the cumulative frame are much lighter than for the rest of the horseshoe shape. This corresponds with differing tongue placement and width of the groove for different speakers.

DYNAMIC IMAGES OF THE ARTICULATORY AND ACOUSTIC CHARACTERISTICS OF /s/

In order to obtain a comprehensive view of the production of this consonant, the dynamic aspects of the production of /s/ are shown in a filmstrip, spectrogram, and EPG images (Figures 15–2).

/s/ in Word-Initial and Word-Final Contexts: "sauce"

Filmstrip: /sɔs/ "sauce"

The criterion phonemes are the initial and final /s/ in the word /sɔs/ shown in Figure 15–2A. The first four frames show the alveolar contact of the tongue. Frame 5 shows the release of the tongue tip from the alveolar contact and the beginning of lip rounding for the vowel /ɔ/. A sustained state of the vowel /ɔ/ persists between frames 7 and 14. Beyond frame 15, the lips begin to approximate the final /s/, and by frame 19, the tip of the tongue has again made a contact in the vicinity of the alveolar ridge. Frames 19 through 24 show the steady state of the consonant /s/.

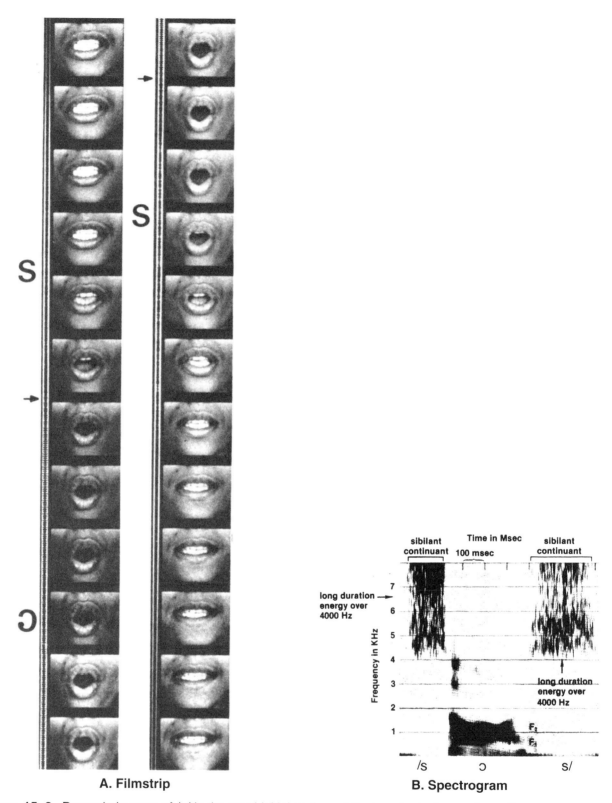

A. Filmstrip **B. Spectrogram**

Figure 15–2. Dynamic images of /s/ in the word-initial and word-final contexts: "sauce." *continues*

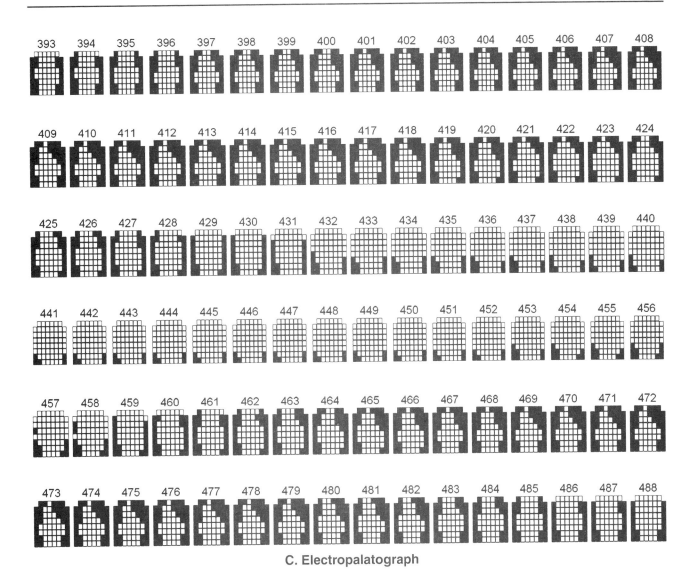

C. Electropalatograph

Figure 15–2. *continued*

Sound Spectrogram: /sɔs/ "sauce"

Figure 15–2B represents the sound spectrogram of the phoneme /s/. This phoneme is contrasted at the word-initial and word-final positions with the vowel /ɔ/ at the medial position in the word "sauce." The phoneme /s/ is a voiceless consonant and devoicing is indicated by the lack of any vocal fold vibration prior to the vowel formants. The phoneme /s/ is also sibilant, as indicated by the long-duration, hissing noise repre-sented in the high-frequency domain. The duration for the initial sibilant is approximately 200 msec and, for the final sibilant, about 300 msec. The phoneme /s/ is a front consonant, represented by the absence of energy below 4000 Hz, as well as by the total concentration of energy between 4000 and 8000 Hz. Both the F1 and F2 show falling transitions because of their efforts to approximate the energy in the high-frequency domain.

Electropalatograph: /sɔs/ "sauce"

The dynamic series of EPG palates for the production of the word "sauce" is presented in Figure 15–2C. The word "sauce" was extracted from the sentence "I see a sauce again." Within this sentence, the word "sauce" took 0.475 seconds to produce. The typical EPG shape for /s/ is clearly depicted in frames 401 to 423 and again in frames 465 to 479. This typical shape is similar to the horseshoe shape for /t/ and /d/, but with a groove, or opening for the air to pass through causing frication. In these series of images, the groove is located at the third electrode on the first row of the palate. The vowel /ɔ/ (frames 432–458) has limited tongue/palate contact, concentrated toward the velar region of the palate (see Chapter 35). The coarticulatory phases between the /s/ and the vowel occurs during frames 424 to 431 and 459 to 464.

INTRA- AND INTERSPEAKER VARIABILITY IN THE PRODUCTION OF /s/

Electropalatography enables consideration of intra- and interspeaker variability. Firstly, intra- and interspeaker variability between speakers of English is presented. Next, production of /s/ by speakers of other languages is compared with English productions. Finally, productions of /s/ by speakers with speech impairment is discussed.

Intra- and Interspeaker Variability in the Production of /s/ by Eight Typical English-Speaking Adults

Four typical adult males (M1–M4) and four typical adult females (F1–F4) who spoke Australian English produced nonsense syllables containing /s/ three times. The nonsense syllables were created with /s/ in syllable-initial and syllable-final positions in vowel contexts taken at the extremes of the vowel quadrilateral.

Maximum Contact Frames for Eight Typical English-Speaking Adults

In order to demonstrate intra- and interspeaker variability the maximum contact frame for the second production of each nonsense syllable for each speaker is provided in Figure 15–3. Figure 15–3 presents a wide range of productions by these eight typical English-speaking adults. Each production was judged by two speech-language pathologists as an adultlike /s/. In almost every instance there is evidence of a horseshoe shape of tongue/palate contact where the tongue touches the alveolar ridge and the lateral margins of the palate. In almost every instance, there is evidence of a central groove for the air to pass through to create a sibilant sound. Some speakers have wider grooves, such as M3. At times, it appears that there is no groove, such as F1's production of /sʌʃ/. Astute viewers can consider the impact of different vowel contexts and word position on the extent of tongue/palate contact for /s/ production for each speaker.

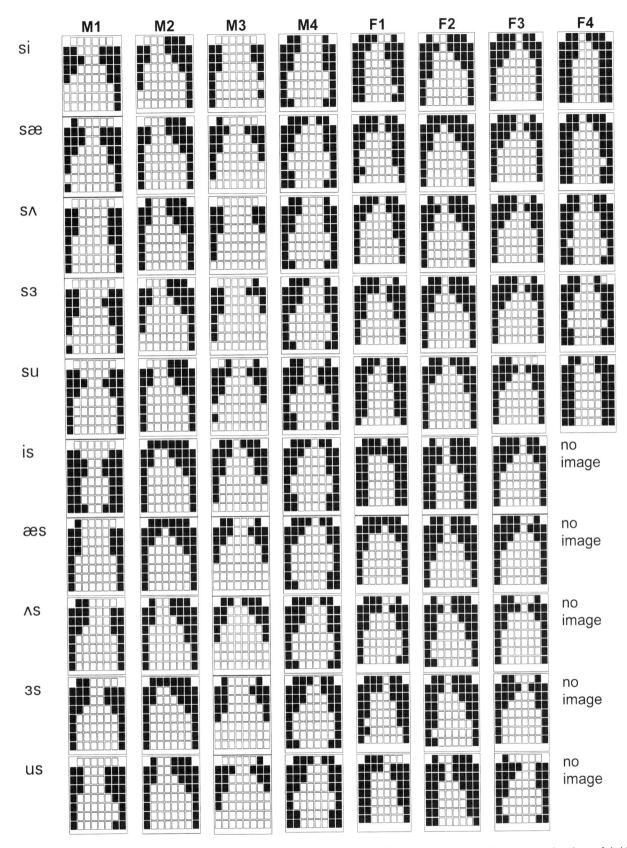

Figure 15–3. Intra- and interspeaker variability in the maximum EPG contact frame for the production of /s/ by eight typical English-speaking adults. *continues*

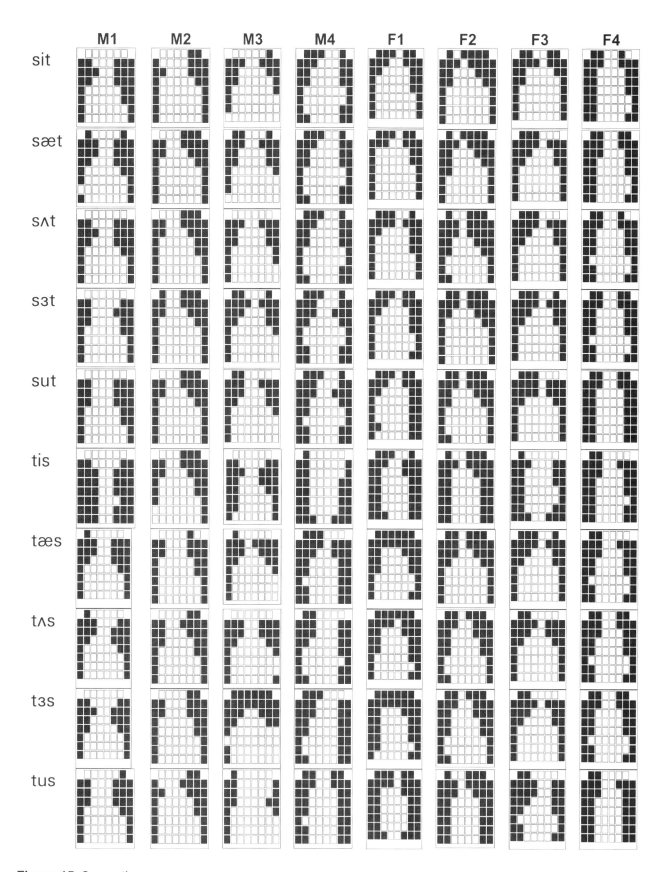

Figure 15–3. *continues*

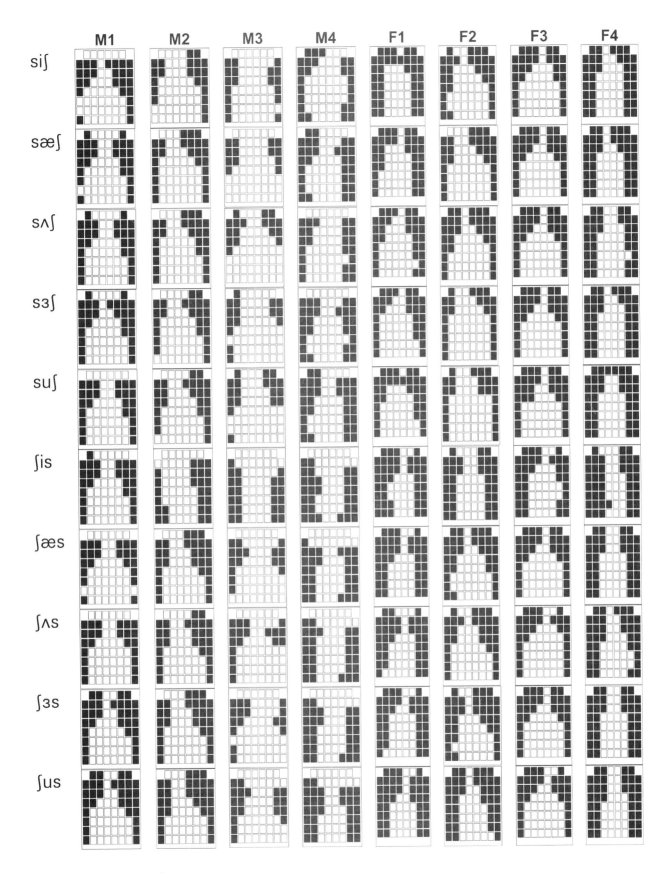

Figure 15–3. *continued*

167

Cumulative EPG Frames for Eight Typical English-Speaking Adults

Cumulative EPG patterns for /s/ were generated from 60 maximum contact frames (with the exception of F4) for each of the eight typical adults described above (Figure 15-4). Each electrode on a cumulative maximum contact display has a number, corresponding to the percentage of contact over the 60 productions. The darker the shading, the more contact. In Figure 15-4 each speaker's cumulative maximum contact display is a horseshoe shape with a groove; however, there are differences in the width and length of the groove, the number of rows contacted on the alveolar ridge, the width of the lateral bracing.

/Interspeaker Variability in the Production of /s/ by Other English-Speaking Adults

English-Speaking Adults

McLeod, Roberts, and Sita (2006) considered tongue/palate contact for the production of /s/ and /z/ for 10 English speakers from a variety of dialects including American, Canadian, English, Scottish, and Australian. Figure 15-5 demonstrates that each speaker had alveolar contact, lateral bracing and most had a midline groove for both /s/ and /z/; however, each speaker produced a unique shape for the production of /s/. McLeod et al. (2006) also indicated that the length and width of the groove across all of the words produced

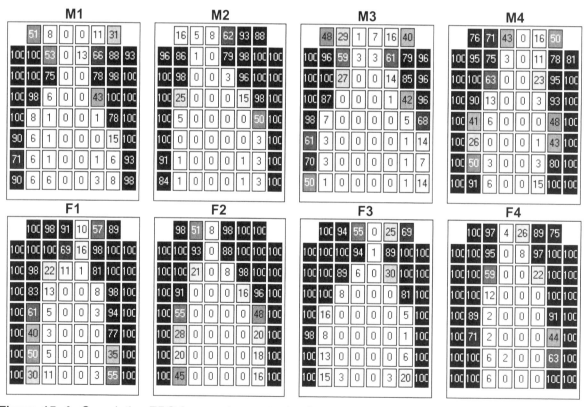

Figure 15–4. Cumulative EPG frames demonstrating intra- and interspeaker variability for the production of /s/ by eight typical English-speaking adults.

Speaker	P1	P2	P3	P4	P5	P6	P7	P8	P9	P10
Gender	**F**	**F**	**M**	**M**	**F**	**M**	**M**	**F**	**F**	**M**
Accent	Scottish	Canadian	Northern-Midland USA	Canadian	Australian	Scottish	Northern-Inland USA	Canadian	Canadian	Scottish
Most common /s/										
Second most common /s/										

Figure 15–5. Two most common maximum contact EPG frames for the production of /s/ by 10 typical English-speaking adults (adapted from McLeod et al., 2006, Figure 2, p. 57).

by the participants ranged from 0 to 3 electrodes. A statistical comparison was undertaken between tongue/palate contact for the production of /s/ and /z/. There was a complex interaction between coarticulation with the vowel, word position, and word context (nonsense syllable and real word). However for three measures (alveolar palatal contact, medial groove width, medial groove length) there was significantly greater contact for /z/ compared to /s/ in word-initial position, but not in word-final position.

Australian English-Speaking Adults

McAuliffe, Ward, and Murdoch (2006) described the speech of 15 typical Australian English-speaking people to provide a comparison with the speech of people with Parkinson's disease. The typical speakers were divided into two groups. The seven aged controls were males and were aged between 50 and 79 years (mean = 67.71). Seven of the young controls were female and the eighth was male. The young control group was aged between 23 to 31 years (mean = 25.63). Figure 15-6 demonstrates two cumulative maximum contact EPG frames for productions of /t/ in the contexts /si/ and /sa/. The participants were asked to produce these words in a sentence " I saw a _____ today" 10 times. In Figure 15-6, a black square indicates that that electrode was contacted at least 67% of the time. Unlike for the production of /l/ and /t/, McAuliffe et al. found a significant difference in the amount of tongue/palate contact between the aged and young control groups for the production of /s/.

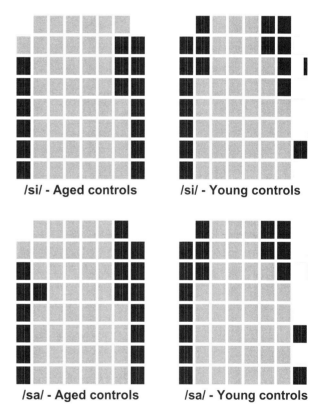

/si/ - Aged controls /si/ - Young controls

/sa/ - Aged controls /sa/ - Young controls

Figure 15–6. Cumulative maximum contact EPG frames for the production of /s/ by 15 Australian English-speaking adults (adapted from McAuliffe et al., 2006a, Figure 2, p. 9).

There was significantly more tongue/palate contact during the production of /s/ for the young compared with the aged control group.

Cheng, Murdoch, Goozée, and Scott (2007) conducted a study to describe typical speech production for 36 children and 12 adults. The six male and six female adult participants, aged between 23 and 38 years, produced /s/ in CV and CVC words that were embedded within a phrase. Each phrase was produced five times, resulting in 10 productions of /s/ per speaker. Figure 15-7 provides a cumulative maximum contact frame for the production of /s by the adults. In Figure 15-7, a black square indicates that that electrode was contacted at least 67% of the time. Cumulatively, these 12 adults had a wide midline groove of 3 electrodes.

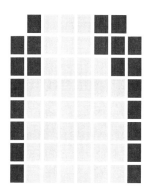

Figure 15–7. Cumulative maximum contact EPG frames for the production of /s/ by 12 typical Australian English-speaking adults (adapted from Cheng et al., 2007, Figure 1, p. 380).

English-Speaking Children

Australian English-Speaking Children

Cheng et al. (2007) also described typical speech production for 36 children. There were six males and six females in each of the following age groups: 6 to 7 years, 8 to 11 years, and 12 to 17 years. As for the adults described above, the children produced /s/ in CV and CVC words that were embedded within a phrase. Each phrase was produced five times, resulting in 10 productions of /s/ per speaker. Figure 15-8 provides a cumulative maximum contact frame for the production of /s/ by the children. In Figure 15-8, a black square indicates that that electrode was contacted at least 67% of the time. Cheng et al. found evidence for the maturation of the speech motor system and described this maturation as nonlinear and nonuniform.

Summary of English-Speaking Children

Roberts, McLeod, and Sita (2002) collected images of tongue/palate contact for typical children and adults as well as for those with speech impairment. Figure 15-9 has been adapted from the summary of Roberts et al. (2002) and demonstrates three images of typical children's productions of /s/. In each image there is evidence of a midline groove to act as a corridor for the airstream to produce /s/.

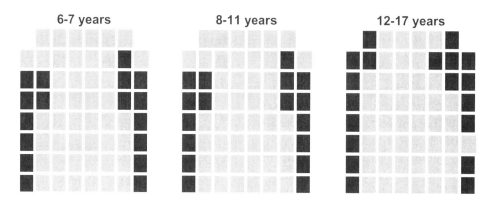

Figure 15–8. Cumulative maximum contact EPG frames for the production of /s/ by 36 typical Australian English-speaking children (adapted from Cheng et al., 2007, Figure 1, p. 380).

Interspeaker Variability in the Production of /s/ in Languages Other Than English

German-Speaking Adults

Fuchs, Brunner, and Busler (2007) described the production of voicing contrasts in German fricatives. Figure 15-10 demonstrates the cumulative maximum contact EPG frame for /s/ produced by one typical adult German male (Fuchs et al., 2007). A black square indicates that there was at least 60% contact for that electrode across the words containing /s/ in initial,

medial and final position. The groove is toward the right of the palate, similar to the production of /s/ by the Canadian female speaker (P2) in McLeod et al. (2006) shown in Figure 15-5.

Greek-Speaking Adults

Nicolaidis (2004) described the speech of one typical Modern Standard Greek-speaking adult in order to provide comparative data for the speech of four Greek-speaking people with hearing impairment. Figure 15-11 demonstrates two cumulative maximum contact EPG

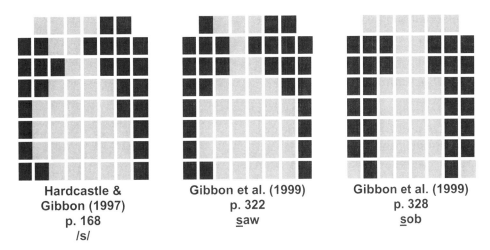

Hardcastle &
Gibbon (1997)
p. 168
/s/

Gibbon et al. (1999)
p. 322
s̲aw

Gibbon et al. (1999)
p. 328
s̲ob

Figure 15–9. Cumulative EPG frame for the production of /s/ by three English-speaking children (adapted from the summary in Roberts et al., 2002, Figure 3, p. 160).

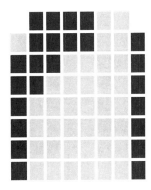

Figure 15–10. Cumulative EPG frame for the production of /s/ by one German-speaking adult (adapted from Fuchs et al., 2007, Figure 3, p. 97).

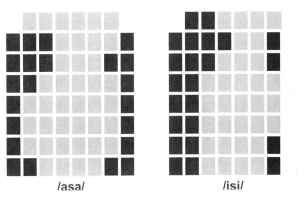

/asa/   /isi/

Figure 15–11. Cumulative maximum contact EPG frames for the production of /s/ by one Greek-speaking adult (adapted from Nicolaidis, 2004, Figure 1, p. 8).

frames for productions of /s/ in the contexts /asa/ and /isi/. The female participant was asked to produce these phoneme combinations ten times in a dysyllabic word of the form /pVsV/ within a carrier phrase. In Figure 15–11, a black square indicates the electrode was contacted at least 60% of the time. The groove is wider in the context of the /a/ vowel than the /i/ vowel.

Polish-Speaking Adults

Guzik and Harrington (2007) studied three typical Polish speakers' production of /s/ in the context of a consonant cluster [s#s] (see Figure 15–12). A black square indicates that there was at least 50% contact for that electrode at the "temporal midpoint." Again, a midline groove is a feature of the Polish production of /s/.

Putonghua-Speaking Adults

Stokes and Zhen (1998) studied one typical Putonghua speaker's production of fricatives and affricates. Putonghua is modern standard Chinese, previously known as Mandarin. The study of Stokes and Zhen included /s, ʂ, ç, ʐ, ts, tsʰ, tʂʰ, tç, tçʰ/. Figure 15–13 demonstrates the maximum contact pattern for /s/. They described the speaker's production of /s/ as "characterized by a narrow groove (one electrode wide), very little other contact in the middle of the palate, and a lateral seal. The pattern is similar to English . . . " (pp. 74–75).

Interspeaker Variability for /s/ in Speakers with Impaired Speech

English-Speaking Adults with Parkinson's Disease

McAuliffe, Ward, and Murdoch (2006) described the speech of nine people diagnosed with Parkinson's disease. Figure 15–14 demonstrates two cumulative maximum contact EPG frames for productions of /s/ in the contexts /si/ and /sa/. The participants were asked to produce these words in a sentence " I saw a _____ today" 10 times. In Figure 15–14, a black

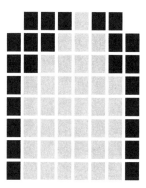

Figure 15–13. Cumulative EPG frame for the production of /s/ by one Putonghua-speaking adult (adapted from Stokes & Zhen, 1998, Figure 5, p. 74).

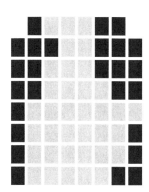

Figure 15–12. Cumulative EPG frame for the production of /s/ by three Polish-speaking adults (adapted from Guzik & Harrington, 2007, Figure 3, p. 112).

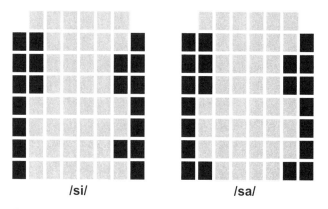

/si/   /sa/

Figure 15–14. Cumulative maximum contact EPG frames for the production of /s/ by nine English-speaking adults with Parkinson's disease (adapted from McAuliffe et al., 2006a, Figure 2, p. 9).

square indicates that that electrode was contacted at least 67% of the time. McAuliffe et al. indicated that the people with Parkinson's disease had "reductions in the amplitude of lingual movement, or articulatory undershoot" (p. 16).

Adults with Hearing Impairment

Nicolaidis (2004) described tongue/palate contact for four adults with hearing impairment. The three females and one male were aged between 23 to 26 years. Each spoke typical Modern Standard Greek. Each of the four people produced /s/ in the contexts /asa/ and /isi/ within the word form /pVsV/ within a carrier phrase. Each word was produced ten times. Figure 15–15

demonstrates two cumulative maximum contact EPG frames for each speaker (HI1–HI4) for productions of /s/ in the two contexts /asa/ and /isi/. In Figure 15–15, a black square indicates that that electrode was contacted at least 60% of the time. In each cumulative frame a central groove was evident albeit of differing widths.

Children with Cleft Palate

Lee, Gibbon, Crampin, Yuen, and McLennan (2007) described J, and eight-year-old Scottish English-speaking boy, who was born with a unilateral cleft lip and palate. Lee et al. (2007) provided dynamic images for J's production of /s/ in two different phrases, "a seat" and

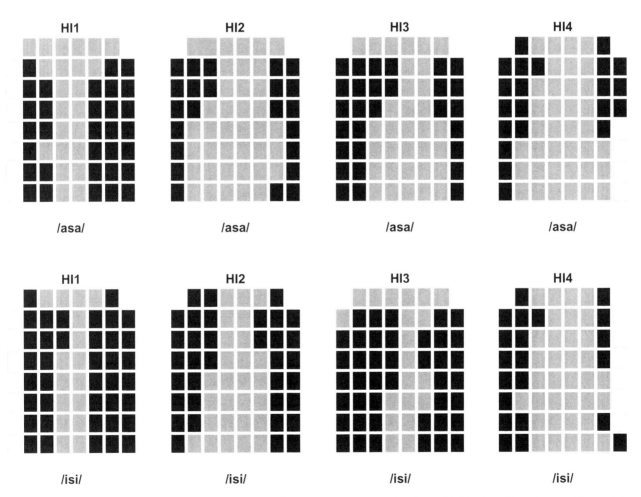

Figure 15–15. Cumulative maximum contact EPG frames for the production of /s/ by four Greek-speaking adults with hearing impairment (adapted from Nicolaidis, 2004, Figure 1, p. 8).

"a sob." The maximum contact for the production of /s/ in these two words is illustrated in Figure 15-16. His production in "a seat" was described as "retraction" and in "a sob" was described as an "open pattern" (p. 61).

Howard (2004) compared perceptual and instrumental analyses of speech produced by three adolescents with a history of cleft palate. Within this comprehensive research, one frame of maximum contact was provided for the lateralized production of /s/ by Beth (age 16;1) in the context of "sock." Additionally a composite contact frame was provided for the production of /s/ by Danny (age 13;10). Figure 15-17 includes both images. Beth's lateralized production of /s/ is characterized by alveolar + velar tongue/palate contact with no central groove. In comparison, although Danny has a central groove, it occurs at the velar, rather than the alveolar position of the palate.

Children and Adults with Lateral Lisps

Lateral productions of /s/ and /z/, are often resistant to traditional speech-language pathology intervention (Gibbon & Hardcastle, 1987). EPG patterns for sounds heard as lateralised /s/ and /z/ are surprisingly diverse (Dent, 2001). Roberts, McLeod, and Sita (2002) collated published EPG images of productions of /s/ and /z/ that described as lateralized. These were redrawn for the purposes of the *Speech Sounds: A Pictorial Guide to Typical and Atypical Speech* (Figure 15-18) so that they were comparable with the other EPG images in the text. The main feature of the productions in Figure 15-18 is that the groove is absent. Air is therefore forced over the sides of the tongue rather than through the groove. For most of these EPG images, there is greater palatal contact than for normal productions with the exception of four productions that had less contact.

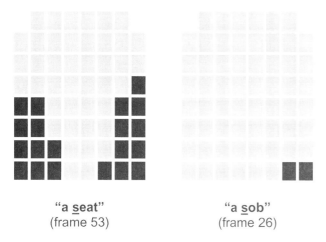

"a <u>s</u>eat"
(frame 53)

"a <u>s</u>ob"
(frame 26)

Figure 15–16. Maximum contact EPG frames for the production of /s/ by one Scottish English-speaking boy with a history of cleft lip and palate (adapted from Lee et al., 2007, Figure 1, p. 61).

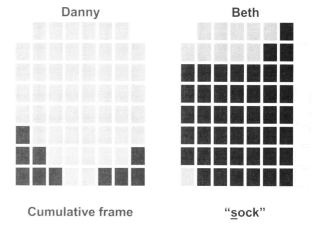

Danny

Beth

Cumulative frame

"<u>s</u>ock"

Figure 15–17. Maximum contact EPG frames for the production of /s/ by two English-speaking adolescents with a history of cleft palate (adapted from Howard, 2004, Figure 4, p. 324 and Figure 8, p. 329).

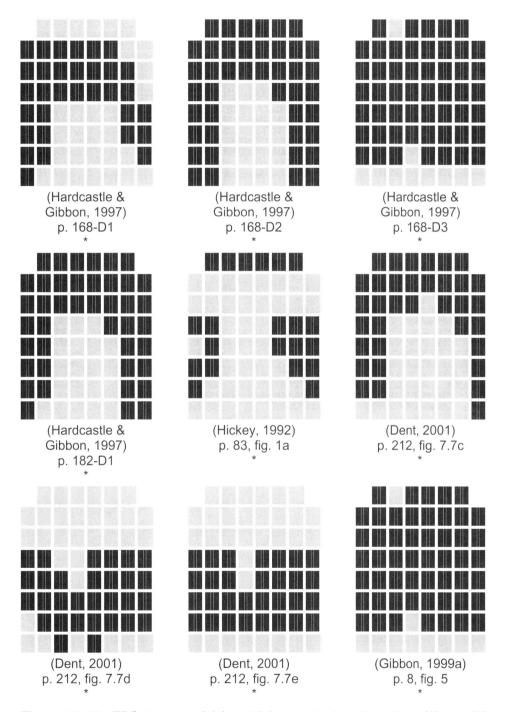

Figure 15–18. EPG images of /s/ and /z/, perceived as lateralized [ɬ] and [ɮ] (adapted from Roberts et al., 2002, Figure 5, p. 161). (*context unknown) *continues*

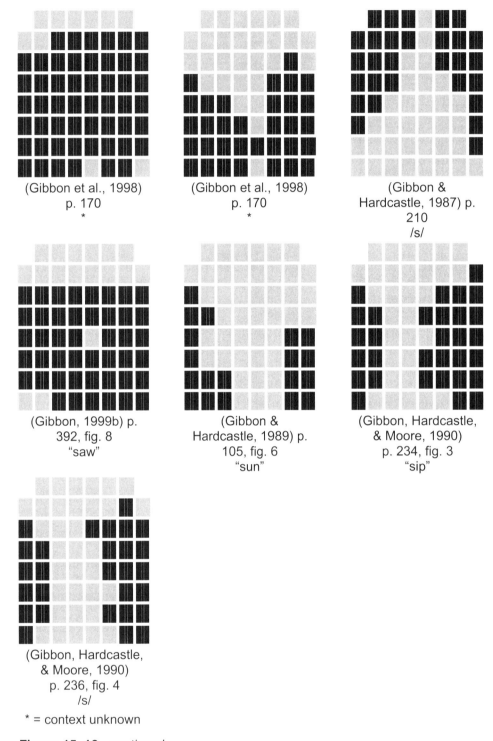

(Gibbon et al., 1998)
p. 170
*

(Gibbon et al., 1998)
p. 170
*

(Gibbon &
Hardcastle, 1987) p.
210
/s/

(Gibbon, 1999b) p.
392, fig. 8
"saw"

(Gibbon &
Hardcastle, 1989) p.
105, fig. 6
"sun"

(Gibbon, Hardcastle,
& Moore, 1990)
p. 234, fig. 3
"sip"

(Gibbon, Hardcastle,
& Moore, 1990)
p. 236, fig. 4
/s/

* = context unknown

Figure 15–18. *continued*

Chapter 16

/z/

The consonant /z/ is a voiced alveolar fricative.

Place of articulation: alveolar

Advancement: front

Voicing: voiced

Labiality: nonlabial

Sonorancy: nonsonorant (obstruent)

Continuancy: continuant

Sibilancy: sibilant

Nasality: nonnasal (oral)

STATIC IMAGES OF THE ARTICULATORY CHARACTERISTICS OF /z/

The static images of /z/ are presented via a photograph, schematic diagram, ultrasound, and electropalatograph images (Figure 16-1).

Photograph

In this photograph (Figure 16-1A), the lips are open and the teeth are shown during the production of /z/.

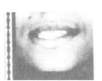

A. Photograph

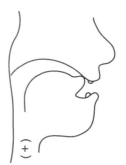

B. Schematic diagram

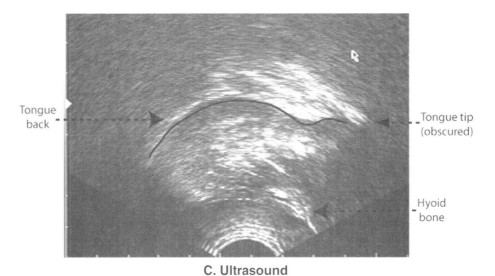

C. Ultrasound

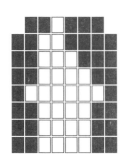

D. Electropalatograph (EPG) (single frame)

E. Electropalatograph (EPG) (cumulative frame)

Figure 16–1. Static images of the articulatory characteristics of /z/.

Schematic Diagram

The lateral view of the production of z shows the tongue approximating the front portion of the roof of the mouth (Figure 16–1B). The production of z requires a steady opening (groove) for the continuous stream of airflow. This may partially account for the designation of continuancy to the phoneme /z/. The phonemes /f, v, θ, ð/ are also continuants, requiring an opening at the point of contact in the oral cavity. The phonemes /s, z, ʃ, ʒ/ are sibilants, in addition to being continuants. Sibilants are characterized by a slightly greater opening for the emission of the airstream, resulting in greater airflow velocity and higher intensity in the very high-frequency regions. The voicing characteristic of /z/ is designated by the symbol (+) at the vocal folds.

Ultrasound

Figure 16–1C shows an ultrasound of the tongue surface during production of /z/. The tongue tip is on the right and is raised toward the alveolar ridge, with approximately 1 cm of the tongue tip being obscured from view because of the shadow of the jaw (Stone, 2005). As for /s/, the complexity of tongue positioning for the production of /z/ is shown in this image. If we follow the bright white line of the surface of the tongue from right to left shows that the tip is raised, the front is slightly lowered, the center of the tongue is slightly raised, then the back transitions from raised to lowered toward the pharynx. An air shadow can be seen above the tongue and diagonal muscle fibers can be seen below the surface of the tongue.

Electropalatograph (EPG)

The EPG image of /z/ in Figure 16–1D presents similarly to /s/ as a horseshoe shape. The tongue contacts the palate across the alveolar ridge with lateral bracing along the lateral margins of the teeth. Similar to the /s/, the EPG image of /z/ in Figure 16–1D has a groove, or inactivated electrode on the alveolar ridge. The groove is considered to be the central feature for typical /s/ and /z/ production, as it allows a corridor for the turbulent airstream to pass through creating a fricative sibilant quality.

Figure 16–1E represents the cumulation of 310 productions of /z/ by eight typical adults. As for /s/, the middle two columns of the first two rows of the cumulative frame are much lighter than for the rest of the horseshoe shape. This relates to the placement of the groove for the speakers.

McLeod, Roberts, and Sita (2006) indicated that each of 10 typical adult speakers had alveolar contact, and lateral bracing and most had a midline groove for /z/. The length and width of the groove ranged from 0 to 3 electrodes. There was a complex interaction between coarticulation with the vowel, word position, and word context (nonsense syllable and real word). For the measures alveolar palatal contact, medial groove width, and medial groove length there was significantly greater contact for /z/ compared to /s/ in word-initial position, but not in word-final position.

DYNAMIC IMAGES OF THE ARTICULATORY AND ACOUSTIC CHARACTERISTICS OF /z/

In order to obtain a comprehensive view of the production of this consonant, the dynamic aspects of the production of /z/ are shown in a filmstrip, spectrogram, and EPG images (Figure 16–2).

/z/ in Word-Initial Context: "zoom"

Filmstrip: /zum/ "zoom"

The phoneme /z/ is shown at the initial position in the word /zum/ (Figure 16–2A). These picture frames clearly demonstrate the importance of coarticulation in the understanding of phonetic events. The phoneme /z/, which would be produced with flattened lips in the context of front vowels, shows rounded lips at the very beginning, because of the influence of /u/. The voicing nature of z can be noted in the sound track beginning at frame 7. A gradual protrusion of the lips and greater lip rounding are seen in frames 10 through 14. A gradual unrounding and flattening of the lips begins about frame 15. By frame 17, the lips are flattened and closed for the production of the consonant /m/.

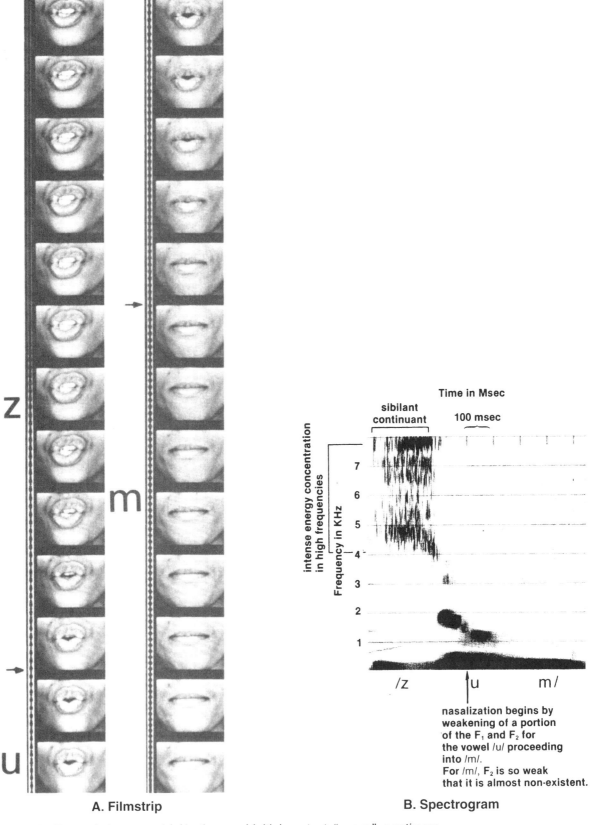

A. Filmstrip   B. Spectrogram

Figure 16–2. Dynamic images of /z/ in the word-initial context: "zoom." *continues*

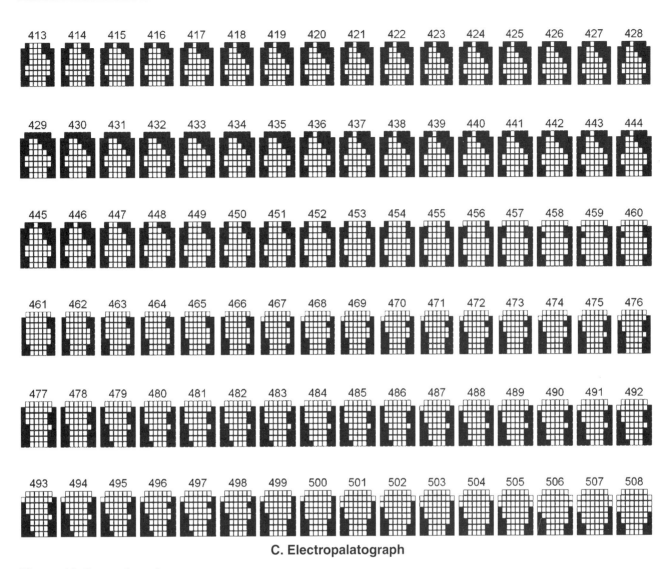

C. Electropalatograph

Figure 16–2. *continued*

Sound Spectrogram: /zum/ "zoom"

The initial consonant /z/ in the word "zoom" is a voiced sibilant produced with flattened lips (Figure 16-2B). Voicing is denoted by the presence of glottal source excitation at the base of the spectrogram, and by the rising first formant transition of the vowel /u/. The sibilancy characteristic is denoted by high-frequency, intense noise of long duration (over 200 msec). The energy for the consonant /z/ begins at 4000 Hz and ends at 8000 Hz. Because the center of energy for the /z/ consonant is high, all of the vowel formants, except for the first, show falling transitions.

Electropalatograph: /zum/ "zoom"

Figure 16-2C presents the dynamic series of EPG palates for the production of the word "zoom." The 95 EPG frames for the word "zoom" took 0.474 seconds. The EPG shape for /z/ is clearly depicted in frames 415 to 446. This shape is similar to the horseshoe shape for /t/ and /d/, but with a groove, or opening for the air to pass through causing frication. As with the phoneme /s/ (chapter 15), the groove is located at the third electrode on the first row of the palate. The coarticulatory phase between the /z/ and /u/ occurs during frames 447 to 452. The vowel /u/ (frames 453–490) has tongue/

palate contact along the lateral margins of the palate (Chapter 32). The final sound, /m/ extends from frames 491 to 505 and has limited tongue/palate contact.

/z/ in Word-Final Context: "buzz"

Filmstrip: /bʌz/ "buzz"

This series of picture frames (Figure 16–3A) displays the phoneme /z/ at the final position in the word

/bʌz/. Because of the relatively neutral nature of the mid-central vowel /ʌ/, the lip position for /z/ shows its "true" nature. The production of /b/ begins at the second frame, prior to which the lips are in the process of approximating the closure. Lip closure persists until the 10th frame. Negative voice onset time, an acoustic marker for the presence of voicing, can be seen in the sound track parallel to frames 6, 7, 8, 9, and 10. The vowel /ʌ/ is accomplished by opening the lips as shown in frames 12 through 16. The different degrees of these

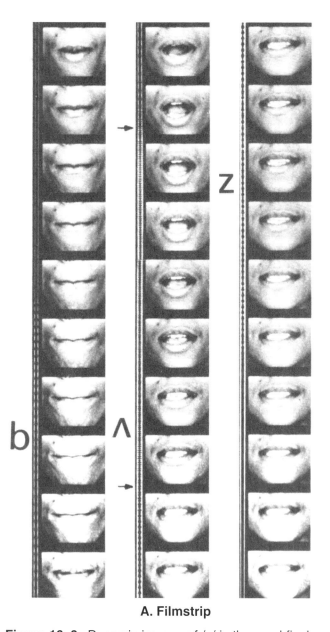

A. Filmstrip

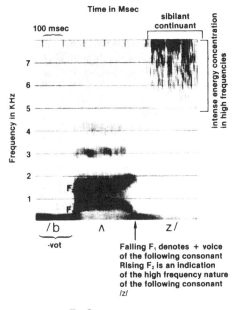

B. Spectrogram

Figure 16–3. Dynamic images of /z/ in the word-final context: "buzz." *continues*

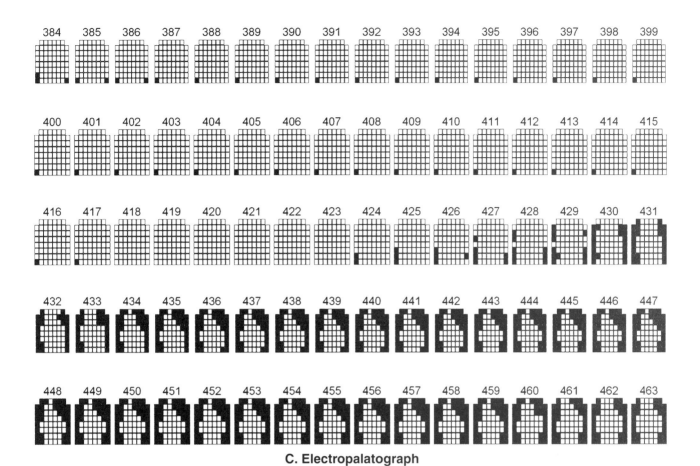

C. Electropalatograph

Figure 16–3. *continued*

openings, starting with a maximum opening in frame 12 to a minimum opening in frame 16, signify the gradual progression of articulatory efforts to approximate the tongue, jaw, and lip position for the /z/ phoneme.

Sound Spectrogram: /bʌz/ "buzz"

Figure 16-3B provides the sound spectrogram for the word "buzz." The voiced and labial components of the initial consonant are clearly denoted by the negative voice onset time and rising first and second formant transitions. The following vowel /ʌ/ has its F1 at 750 Hz, F2 at 1750 Hz, and F3 at 3000 Hz. The formants are somewhat equally spaced, demonstrating the neutrality of this vowel. The downward transition of the first formant denotes that the following consonant is voiced, whereas the upward transition of the second formant denotes that the following consonant is nonlabial-front. The voiced sibilant consonant /z/ is indicated by

long duration (approximately 250 msec), presence of high-frequency energy, and low frequency, glottal-source vibration at the baseline.

Electropalatograph: /bʌz/ "buzz"

The word "buzz" is depicted in Figure 16-3C as a series of 75 EPG frames. The /b/ extends from frames 385 to 404 and the /ʌ/ from frames 405 to 426. The juncture between the /b/ and /ʌ/ is only determined using simultaneous audio, spectrogram, waveform and EPG data (not shown in Figure 16-3C). There is limited tongue/palate contact for /b/ and /ʌ/. The transition from the vowel to the /z/ occurs in frames 427 to 433. The /z/ extends from frames 434 to 460. The groove for the /z/ is obvious as the third electrode on the first row. The air escapes through this groove causing the sibilance that is characteristic of /s/ and /z/ sounds.

INTRA- AND INTERSPEAKER VARIABILITY FOR /z/

Electropalatographic images enable consideration of intra- and interspeaker variability. First, variability between speakers of English is considered; this will be compared with German speakers' production of /z/ and finally EPG images of lateralized /z/.

Intra- and Interspeaker Variability in the Production of /z/ by Eight Typical English-Speaking Adults

Four typical adult males (M1–M4) and four typical adult females (F1–F4) produced nonsense syllables containing /t/ three times. The nonsense syllables were created with /z/ in syllable-initial and syllable-final positions in vowel contexts taken at the extremes of the vowel quadrilateral.

Maximum Contact Frames for Eight Typical English-Speaking Adults

To demonstrate both inter- and intraspeaker variability the maximum contact frame for the second production of each nonsense syllable for each speaker is provided in Figure 16–4. Most images contain a centralized groove and a horseshoe shape of tongue/palate contact where the tongue touches the alveolar ridge and the lateral margins of the palate.

Cumulative EPG Frames for Eight Typical English-Speaking Adults

Cumulative EPG patterns for /z/ were generated from maximum contact frames for each of the eight typical adults described above. Each electrode on a cumulative maximum contact display has a number, corresponding to the percentage of contact over the total number of productions. The darker the shading, the more contact.

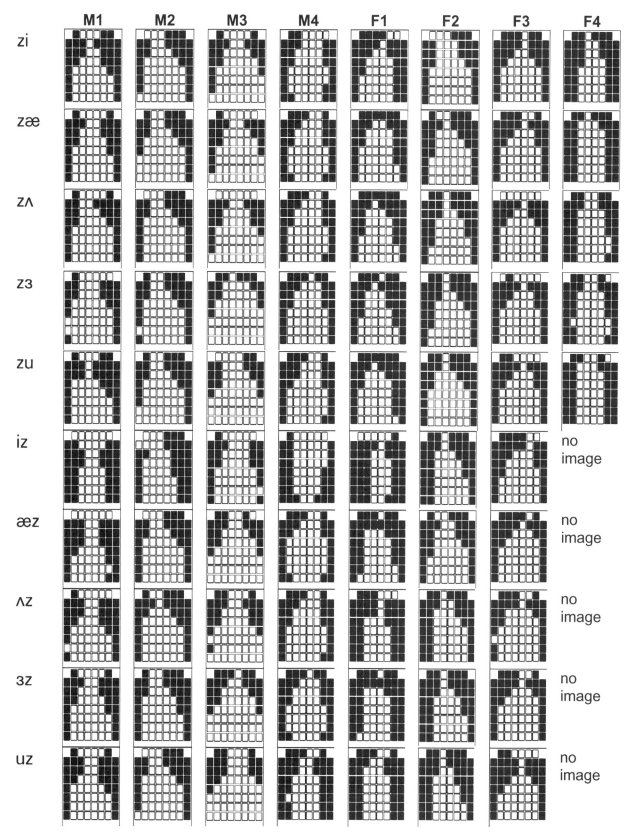

Figure 16–4. Intra- and interspeaker variability in the maximum EPG contact frame for the production of /z/ by eight typical English-speaking adults. *continues*

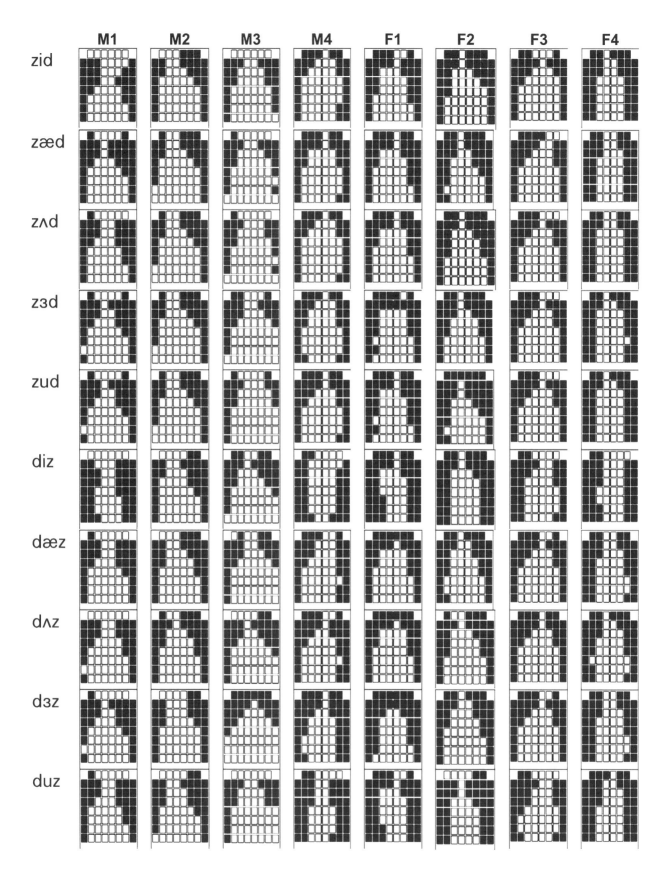

Figure 16–4. *(continues)*

In Figure 16-5 each speaker's cumulative maximum has a lighter centralized groove showing less contact in the midline on the alveolar ridge. Each speaker also has lateral bracing along the margins of the palate.

Interspeaker Variability in the Production of /z/ by Other English-Speaking Adults

English-Speaking Adults

McLeod, Roberts, and Sita (2006) considered tongue/palate contact for the production of /s/ and /z/ for 10 English speakers. Figure 16-6 demonstrates the two most common maximal contact EPG frames for the production of /z/. It can be seen that each speaker has alveolar contact, lateral bracing and most had a midline groove for both /s/ and /z/; however, there are a number of differences between speakers' images. The length and width of the groove ranged from 0 to

3 electrodes. There was significantly greater contact for /z/ compared to /s/ in word-initial position, but not in word-final position for three measures: alveolar palatal contact, medial groove width, and medial groove length.

Interspeaker Variability for /z/ in Languages Other Than English

German-Speaking Adults

Fuchs, Brunner, and Busler (2007) described the production of voicing contrasts in German fricatives. Figure 16-7 demonstrates the cumulative maximum contact EPG frame for /z/ produced by one typical adult German male (Fuchs et al., 2007). The black squares indicate that there was at least 60% contact for the electrode across the words containing /z/ in initial, medial, and final position.

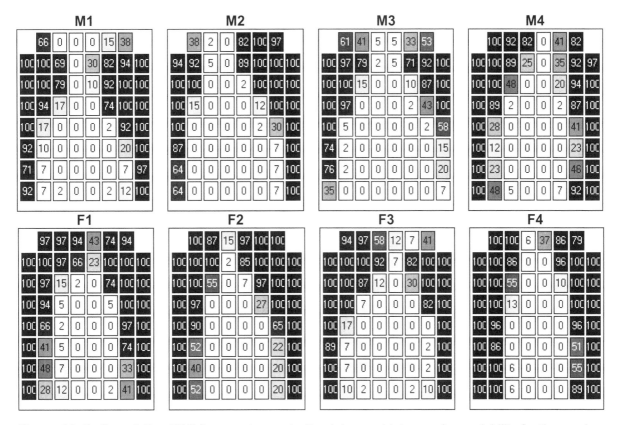

Figure 16–5. Cumulative EPG frames demonstrating intra- and interspeaker variability for the production of /z/ by eight typical English-speaking adults (adapted from McLeod et al., 2006, Figure 2, p. 57).

Speaker	P1	P2	P3	P4	P5	P6	P7	P8	P9	P10
Gender	F	F	M	M	F	M	M	F	F	M
Accent	Scottish	Canadian	Northern-Midland USA	Canadian	Australian	Scottish	Northern-Inland USA	Canadian	Canadian	Scottish
Most common /z/										
Second most common /z/										

Figure 16–6. Two most common maximum contact EPG frames for the production of /z/ by 10 typical English-speaking adults (adapted from McLeod et al., 2006, Figure 2, p. 57).

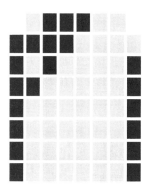

Figure 16–7. Cumulative EPG frame for the production of /z/ by one German-speaking adult (adapted from Fuchs et al., 2007, Figure 3, p. 97).

Interspeaker Variability for /z/ Speakers with Impaired Speech

Children and Adults with Lateral Lisps

Lateral productions of /s/ and /z/, are often resistant to traditional intervention (Gibbon & Hardcastle, 1987). EPG patterns for sounds heard as lateralized /s/ and /z/ are surprisingly diverse (Dent, 2001). Roberts, McLeod, and Sita (2002) collated published EPG images of pro-

ductions of /s/ and /z/ described as lateralized. These were redrawn for the purposes of the *Speech Sounds: A Pictorial Guide to Typical and Atypical Speech* (Figure 16-8) so that they were comparable with the other EPG images in the text. The main feature of the productions in Figure 16-8 is that the groove is absent. Air is therefore forced over the sides of the tongue rather than through the groove. For most of these EPG images, there is greater palatal contact than for normal productions.

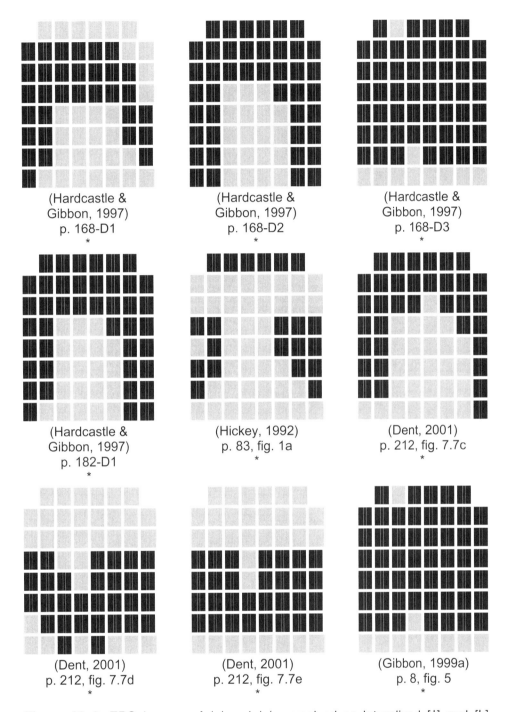

(Hardcastle & Gibbon, 1997) p. 168-D1 *

(Hardcastle & Gibbon, 1997) p. 168-D2 *

(Hardcastle & Gibbon, 1997) p. 168-D3 *

(Hardcastle & Gibbon, 1997) p. 182-D1 *

(Hickey, 1992) p. 83, fig. 1a *

(Dent, 2001) p. 212, fig. 7.7c *

(Dent, 2001) p. 212, fig. 7.7d *

(Dent, 2001) p. 212, fig. 7.7e *

(Gibbon, 1999a) p. 8, fig. 5 *

Figure 16–8. EPG images of /s/ and /z/, perceived as lateralized [ɬ] and [ɮ] (adapted from Roberts et al., 2002, Figure 5, p. 161). *continues*

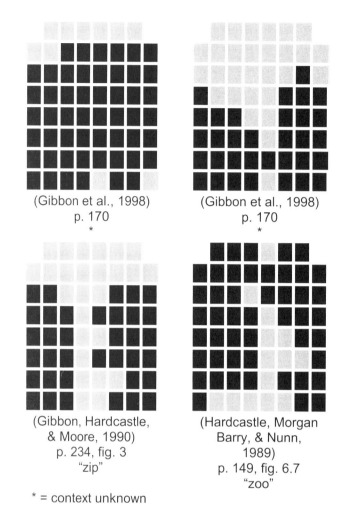

(Gibbon et al., 1998)
p. 170
*

(Gibbon et al., 1998)
p. 170
*

(Gibbon, Hardcastle,
& Moore, 1990)
p. 234, fig. 3
"zip"

(Hardcastle, Morgan
Barry, & Nunn,
1989)
p. 149, fig. 6.7
"zoo"

* = context unknown

Figure 16–8. *continued*

Chapter 17

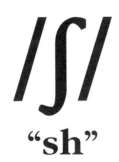

"sh"

The consonant /ʃ/ is a voiceless palatal fricative.

> Place of articulation: palatal
>
> Advancement: back
>
> Voicing: voiceless
>
> Labiality: nonlabial
>
> Sonorancy: nonsonorant (obstruent)
>
> Continuancy: continuant
>
> Sibilancy: sibilant
>
> Nasality: nonnasal (oral)

STATIC IMAGES OF THE ARTICULATORY CHARACTERISTICS OF /ʃ/

The static images of /ʃ/ are presented via a photograph, schematic diagram, ultrasound, and electropalatograph images (Figure 17–1).

Photograph

In this photograph (Figure 17–1A), the lips are rounded and the teeth are together to produce /ʃ/.

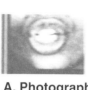

A. Photograph

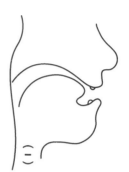

B. Schematic diagram

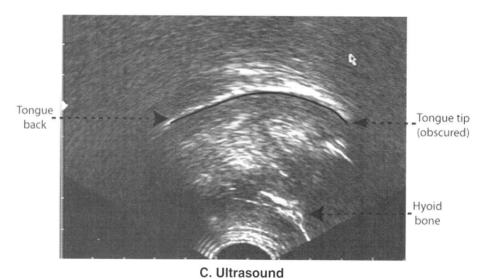

C. Ultrasound

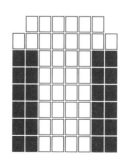

D. Electropalatograph (EPG) (single frame)

11	2	0	0	0	2		
57	55	28	0	2	17	42	42
88	83	53	0	6	46	82	84
94	92	43	1	4	37	90	96
100	98	24	0	0	15	97	100
97	77	16	0	0	4	97	99
97	70	9	0	0	10	83	99
100	71	12	0	0	16	76	99

E. Electropalatograph (EPG) (cumulative frame)

Figure 17–1. Static images of the articulatory characteristics of /ʃ/.

Schematic Diagram

The schematic diagram of the lateral view of the production of /ʃ/ in Figure 17–1B shows an opening at the point of tongue approximation at the back portion of the roof of the mouth (palatal region). The air passes through this opening. The lack of voicing of this consonant is symbolically represented at the source (the vocal folds) by a minus sign.

Ultrasound

A midsagittal ultrasound image of the tongue surface during production of /ʃ/ is shown in Figure 17–1C. The underside of the bright white line is the tongue surface. The tongue is raised compared to its resting position as described in Chapter 1; however, unlike many of the consonant sounds, the midsagittal section of the tongue in the production of /ʃ/ is flat in configuration. Stone (2005) indicates that if the ultrasound transducer is slightly off the midline, then a double image may be seen incorporating the edges of the groove. In Figure 17–1C, the sides of the tongue cannot be seen suggesting that the transducer was held correctly in the midline position (see Chapter 38 for a description of positioning of the ultrasound probe). The tongue tip is on the right of the image and is slightly obscured from view because of the shadow of the jaw (Stone, 2005). An air shadow can be seen above the tongue and diagonal muscle fibers can be seen below the surface of the tongue. The hyoid bone is seen as the bright diagonal line at the bottom right of the image.

Electropalatograph (EPG)

The EPG image of /ʃ/ (Figure 17–1D) has two rows of electrodes along the lateral margin of the palate. The central midline groove is broad, creating a corridor for the air to rush through. The cumulative EPG image (Figure 17–1E) represents multiple productions of /ʃ/ within words by eight speakers. The darker the shading the more often that part of the palate was contacted by the tongue. The numbers indicate the percentage of contact with each EPG electrode. The number 100 in the lower left square indicates that that electrode

was contacted 100% of the time by the eight speakers when producing /ʃ/. The majority of the electrodes in the two midline columns were never contacted (0%) during the production of /ʃ/ by the eight speakers.

DYNAMIC IMAGES OF THE ARTICULATORY AND ACOUSTIC CHARACTERISTICS OF /ʃ/

In order to obtain a comprehensive view of the production of this consonant, the dynamic aspects of the production of /ʃ/ are shown in a filmstrip, spectrogram, and EPG images (Figure 17–2).

/ʃ/ in the Word-Final Context: "wash"

Filmstrip: /wɔʃ/ "wash"

The filmstrip in Figure 17–2A demonstrates the phoneme /ʃ/ in the final position of the word "wash." The lips are rounded for each of the phonemes in this word. The phoneme /ʃ/ is evident in the third column of frames by the closure of the teeth simultaneously with lip rounding.

Sound Spectrogram: /wɔʃ/ "wash"

Figure 17–2b presents the sound spectrogram of the word "wash." The phoneme /w/ is presented in the initial position, followed by the vowel /ɔ/ and the consonant /ʃ/. Labiality is the only prominent feature emerging for the phoneme /w/ in this sound spectrogram. Most of the energy is vowel-like at the low frequency end of the spectrum, signaling sonorancy (at and below 500 Hz). The sonorancy feature is further indicated by a gradual rather than abrupt sloping of the rising first and second formant transitions. The vowel /ɔ/ exhibits its first formant center frequency at about 900 Hz and second formant at about 1250 Hz, with a rising second formant transition to approximate the energy spectrum of the final consonant /ʃ/. In this sound spectrogram of /ʃ/, the features continuancy and sibilancy are indicated by the long-duration, high-frequency, intense-noise spectrum. Lip rounding is indicated by a lowering of this overall spectrum to

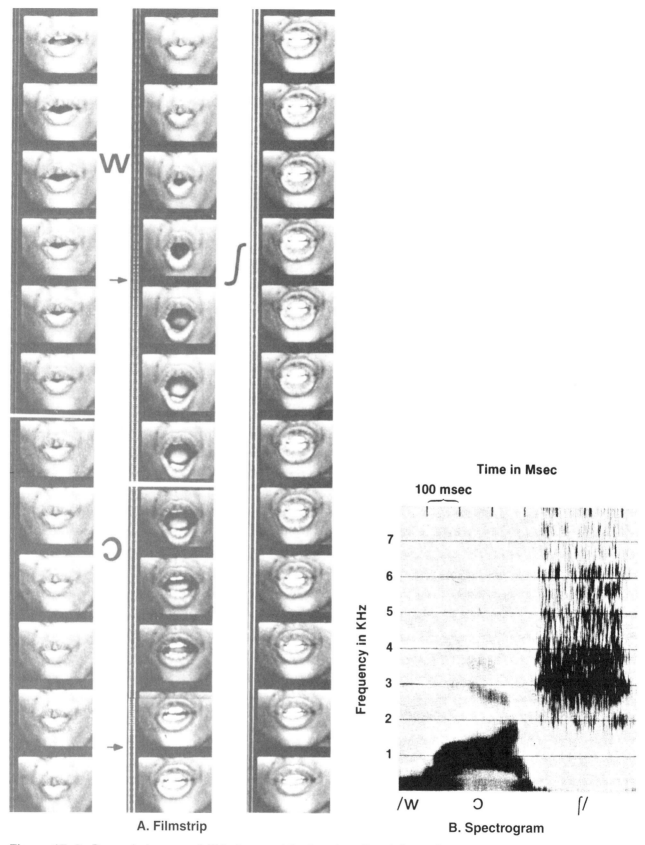

A. Filmstrip

B. Spectrogram

Figure 17–2. Dynamic images of /ʃ/ in the word-final context: "wash." *continues*

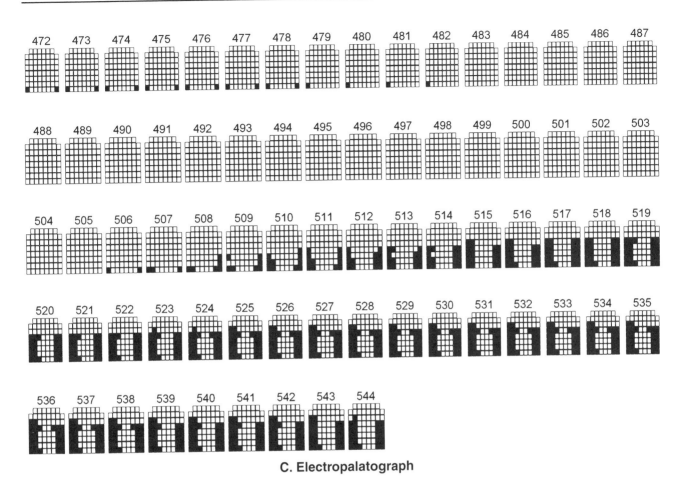

C. Electropalatograph

Figure 17–2. *continued*

exhibit most of its energy between 2500 and 4000 Hz, rather than above 4000 Hz, as can be seen for those sibilants that do not exhibit the lip rounding phenomenon (see Chapter 15, /s/).

Electropalatograph: /wɒʃ/ "wash"

Figure 17-2C contains EPG frames demonstrating tongue/palate contact for the production of /wɒʃ/[1] "wash." The /w/ sound is characterized by minimal tongue/palate contact occurring at the velar region of the palate (frames 472–482). Using the simultaneous EPG, spectrogram, waveform, and audio data, the juncture between the /w/ and /ɒ/ was identified as occur-

ring at frame 487. The transition from the vowel extending to the /ʃ/ between frames 506 to 513. The /ʃ/ sound extended from frames 514 to 544. The /ʃ/ sound is characterized by broad tongue/palate contact along the lateral margins of the palate creating a large central groove for the frication to escape.

INTRA- AND INTERSPEAKER VARIABILITY FOR /ʃ/

Electropalatographic images enable consideration of interspeaker variability. First, variability between

---

[1]/wɑʃ/ is the Australian English pronunciation of "wash."

speakers of English is considered. Then EPG images of children's productions of /ʃ/ are provided. Next, variability between the English production of /ʃ/ and the production of /ʃ/ by speakers of Polish and Norwegian is compared. Finally, variability between productions of /ʃ/ by speakers with cleft palate is presented.

Intra- and Interspeaker Variability in the Production of /ʃ/ by Eight Typical English-Speaking Adults

Four typical adult males (M1–M4) and four typical adult females (F1–F4) produced nonsense syllables containing /ʃ/ three times. The nonsense syllables were created with /ʃ/ in syllable-initial and syllable-final positions in vowel contexts taken at the extremes of the vowel quadrilateral.

Maximum Contact Frames for Eight Typical English-Speaking Adults

To demonstrate both inter- and intraspeaker variability the maximum contact frame for the second production of each nonsense syllable for each speaker is provided in Figure 17–3. The wide central groove for /ʃ/ is evident in these images.

Cumulative EPG Frames for Eight Typical English-Speaking Adults

Cumulative EPG patterns for /ʃ/ were generated from maximum contact frames for each of the eight typical adults described above. Each electrode on a cumulative maximum contact display has a number, corresponding to the percentage of contact over the 60 productions. The darker the shading, the more contact. In Figure 17–4 each speaker's cumulative maximum contact display has a wide central groove.

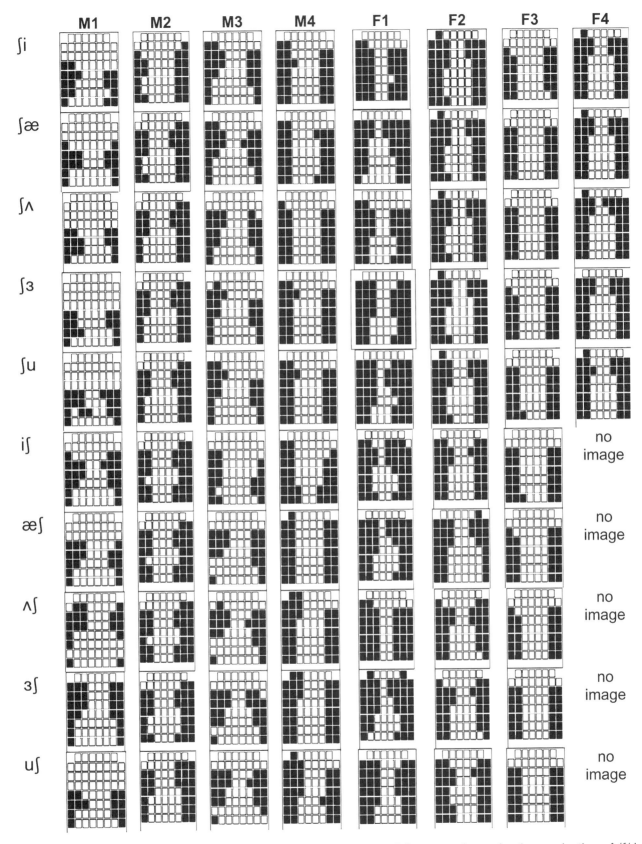

Figure 17–3. Intra- and interspeaker variability in the maximum EPG contact frame for the production of /ʃ/ by eight typical English-speaking adults. *continues*

	M1	M2	M3	M4	F1	F2	F3	F4

ʃit

ʃæt

ʃʌt

ʃɜt

ʃut

tiʃ

tæʃ

tʌʃ

tɜʃ

tuʃ

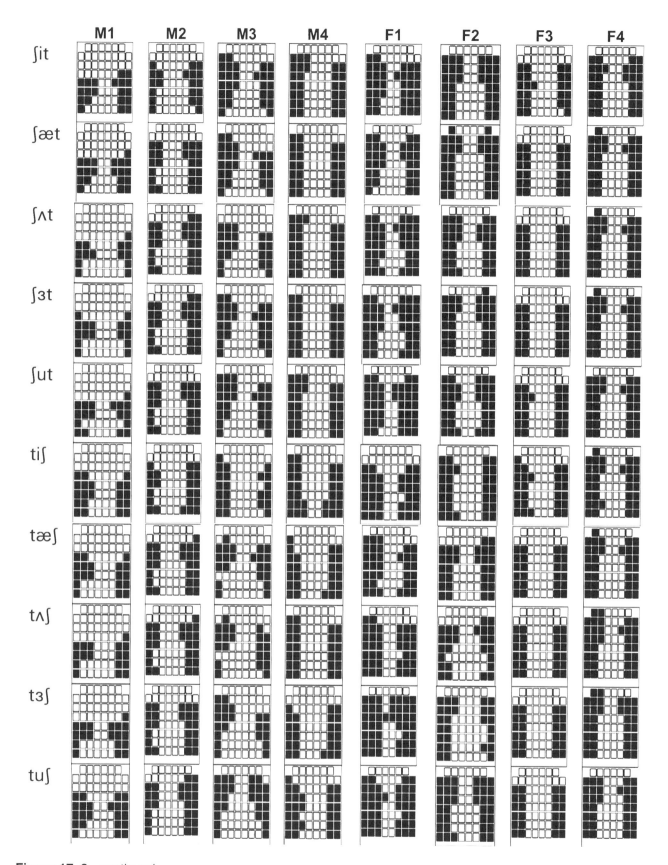

Figure 17–3. *continued*

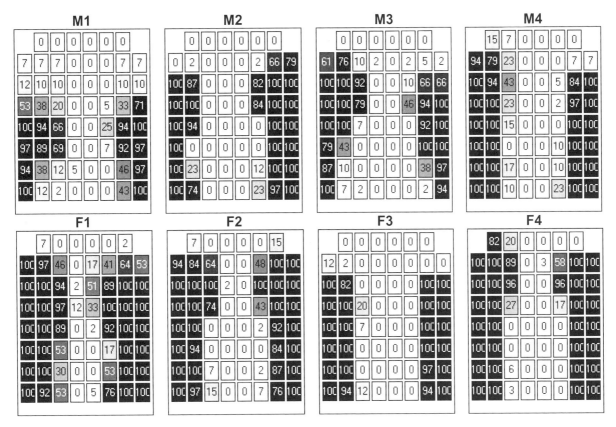

Figure 17–4. Cumulative EPG frames demonstrating intra- and inter-speaker variability for the production of /ʃ/ by eight typical English-speaking adults.

Interspeaker Variability in the Production of /ʃ/ by Other English-Speaking Adults

Scottish English-Speaking Adults

Gibbon (2004) presented EPG images of a Scottish-English adult's /ʃ/ from an unpublished honors dissertation by Shannon (2001) (as cited by Gibbon, 2004). Figure 17-5 provides the cumulative maximum contact frame for five productions of /ʃ/ across five vowel contexts by a typical adult. A black square indicates that there was at least 60% contact for that electrode across the five words containing /ʃ/. The broad midline groove is evident.

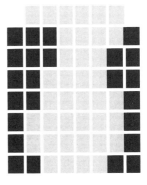

Figure 17–5. Cumulative EPG frame for the production of /ʃ/ by one typical Scottish English-speaking adult (adapted from Shannon, 2001 cited in Gibbon, 2004, Figure 10, p. 305).

Interspeaker Variability for /ʃ/ in English-Speaking Children

Scottish English-Speaking Children

Gibbon (2004) presented EPG images of Scottish-English children's productions of /ʃ/ from an unpublished honors dissertation by Shannon (2001). Figure 17–6 provides the cumulative maximum contact frame for five productions of /ʃ/ across five vowel contexts by a typical Scottish English-speaking child. A black square indicates that there was at least 60% contact for that electrode across the five words containing /ʃ/. Again, the broad midline groove is evident.

Interspeaker Variability for /ʃ/ in Languages Other Than English

Norwegian-Speaking Adults

Simonsen and Moen (2004) described the speech of seven speakers of Urban East Norwegian (three females, four males). The speakers produced real words containing /ʃ/ in the initial position. The words were produced in a carrier phrase 10 times and were randomised with productions of the other sound under examination. No systematic variation was found according to vowel context. Figure 17–7 demonstrates cumulative

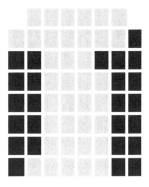

Figure 17–6. Cumulative EPG frame for the production of /ʃ/ by one typical Scottish English-speaking child (adapted from Shannon, 2001 cited in Gibbon, 2004, Figure 10, p. 305).

maximum contact EPG frames for productions of /ʃ/ for each of the seven speakers as well as a cumulative frame for all speakers combined. In Figure 17–7, a black square indicates the electrode was contacted at least 67% of the time.

Polish-Speaking Adults

Guzik and Harrington (2007) described the production of fricatives, including /ʃ/, by three typical Polish speakers in the context of a consonant cluster. Figure 17–8 presents one frame for one speaker's production of /ʃ/. The broad midline groove is again present for this speaker's production of /ʃ/.

Interspeaker Variability for /ʃ/ Speakers with Impaired Speech

Children with Cleft Palate

Gibbon (2004) presented EPG images of a Scottish-English child's productions of /ʃ/ from an unpublished honors dissertation by Shannon (2001). Figure 17–9 provides the cumulative maximum contact frame for five productions of /ʃ/ across five vowel contexts by the 7-year-old child with a cleft palate. A black square indicates that there was at least 60% contact for that electrode across the five words containing /ʃ/. Figure 17–9 illustrates that the child produced an asymmetric pattern of contact with no midline groove. Gibbon (2004) indicates that there was a high degree of variability in the production of this sound by the child with the cleft palate.

Howard (2007) described the speech of six English-speaking children aged between 9;05 and 16;03 years. Her comprehensive paper examined the interplay between articulation and prosody. Within the paper, dynamic images of the productions of words were presented. Figure 17–10 demonstrates maximum contact EPG frame for one speaker, Beth, who was 16;03 and had a history of cleft palate. The EPG frame represents the maximum contact frame for the production of the word "fish." This maximum contact frame demonstrates substantial tongue/palate contact frame across the palate and extended for 11 frames of the dynamic display.

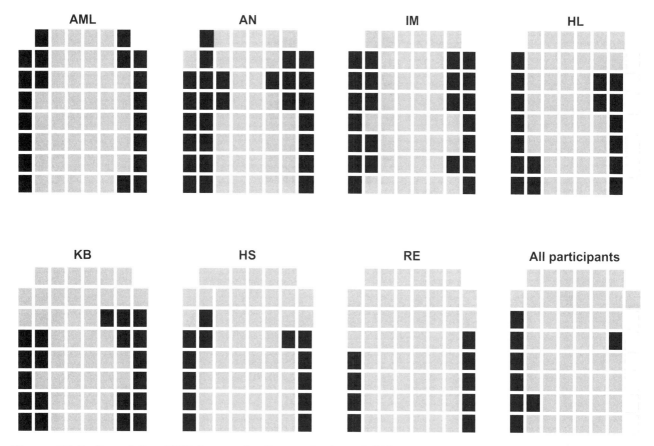

Figure 17–7. Cumulative EPG frames for the production of /ʃ/ by seven typical Norwegian-speaking adults (AML, AN, IM, HL, KB, HS, RE) (adapted from Simonsen & Moen, 2004, Figure 4, p. 601 and Figure 5, p. 611).

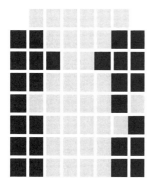

Figure 17–8. One EPG frame at the midpoint of production of /ʃ/ produced by one Polish-speaking adult (adapted from Guzik & Harrington, 2007, Figure 1, p. 111).

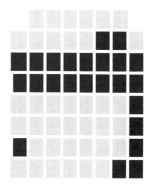

Figure 17–9. A cumulative EPG frame for the production of /ʃ/ by one Scottish English-speaking child with a cleft palate (adapted from Shannon, 2001 cited in Gibbon, 2004, Figure 10, p. 305).

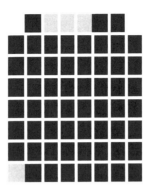

Figure 17–10. Maximum contact EPG frame for the production of /ʃ/ in the word "fish" by an English-speaking adolescent with cleft palate (adapted from Howard, 2007, Figure 1, p. 24).

Chapter 18

/ʒ/

"zh"

The consonant /ʒ/ is a voiced palatal fricative.

Place of articulation: palatal

Advancement: back

Voicing: voiced

Labiality: nonlabial

Sonorancy: nonsonorant (obstruent)

Continuancy: continuant

Sibilancy: sibilant

Nasality: nonnasal (oral)

STATIC IMAGES OF THE ARTICULATORY CHARACTERISTICS OF /ʒ/

The static images of /ʒ/ are presented via a photograph, schematic diagram, ultrasound, and electropalatograph images (Figure 18-1).

Photograph

The photograph in Figure 18-1A shows lip rounding with the teeth visible in order to produce /ʒ/.

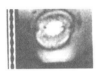

A. Photograph

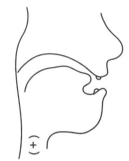

B. Schematic diagram

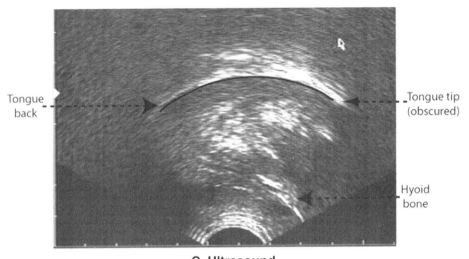

C. Ultrasound

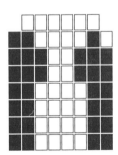

D. Electropalatograph (EPG) (single frame)

15	3	0	0	1	6		
62	55	34	4	2	27	44	42
86	86	54	3	9	53	82	85
92	92	55	2	4	47	92	95
99	99	25	2	0	17	99	100
99	83	18	0	0	5	95	99
98	71	14	2	0	9	83	99
100	63	12	0	0	11	75	99

E. Electropalatograph (EPG) (cumulative frame)

Figure 18–1. Static images of the articulatory characteristics of /ʒ/.

Schematic Diagram

The lateral view of the production of /ʒ/ in this schematic diagram (Figure 18-1B) can be compared with the frontal view in the filmstrip (Figure 18-2A). Because of the continuancy rather than the stop characteristic of /ʒ/, there is an opening at the point of tongue approximation at the back portion of the roof of the mouth. The voicing characteristic of /ʒ/ is indicated by a plus sign (+) in the vicinity of the vocal folds.

Ultrasound

The bright white line in Figure 18-1C is a midsagittal image immediately above the tongue surface during production /ʒ/. As for the production of /ʃ/, the tongue is raised compared to its resting position; however, unlike many of the consonant sounds, the midsagittal section of the tongue in the production of /ʃ/ is flat in configuration. The tongue tip is on the right of the image and is slightly obscured from view because of the shadow of the jaw (Stone, 2005). In Figure 18-1C, the sides of the tongue cannot be seen suggesting that the transducer was held in the midline position. Stone (2005) indicates that if the ultrasound transducer is slightly off the midline, then a double image may be seen incorporating the edges of the groove. An air shadow can be seen above the tongue and diagonal muscle fibers can be seen below the surface of the tongue. The hyoid bone is seen as the bright diagonal line at the bottom right of the image.

Electropalatograph (EPG)

The EPG image of /ʒ/ (Figure 18-1D) has two rows of electrodes along the lateral margin of the palate. The central midline groove is broad, creating a corridor for the air to rush through.

The cumulative EPG image (Figure 18-1E) represents multiple productions of /ʒ/ within words by eight speakers. The darker the shading the more often that part of the palate was contacted by the tongue. The numbers indicate the percentage of contact with each EPG electrode. The number 100 in the lower left square indicates that that electrode was contacted 100% of the time by the eight speakers when producing /ʒ/. The two midline columns are rarely contacted, as a result of the broad midline grooving of the tongue.

DYNAMIC IMAGES OF THE ARTICULATORY AND ACOUSTIC CHARACTERISTICS OF /ʒ/

In order to obtain a comprehensive view of the production of this consonant, the dynamic aspects of the production of /ʒ/ are shown in a filmstrip, spectrogram, and EPG images (Figures 18-2).

/ʒ/ in the Within-Word Context: "measure"

Filmstrip: /ˈmɛʒɚ/ "measure"

The phoneme /ʒ/ is shown in the medial position in the word /ˈmɛʒɚ/ (Figure 18-2A). Labiality can be clearly viewed in the first three frames. The next four frames show the lips in an open position, which is characteristic of the vowel /ɛ/. Ordinarily the vowel /ɛ/ is less open and less rounded than as shown in frames 6 and 7. The difference is attributable to its presence in the context of /ʒ/ followed by /ɚ/. Both of these sounds involve lip rounding.

Sound Spectrogram: /ˈmɛʒɚ/ "measure"

The consonant phoneme /ʒ/ is presented (Figure 18-2B) in the medial position, where it is phonemic in most English dialects. Voicing is clearly indicated by the continuation of the glottic pulsation across this consonant, which started for the phoneme /m/ at the initial position and continued through the vowel /ɛ/ to the final vowel /ɚ/. Because of the nasalization of the vowel /ɛ/, there exists a weakening, as indicated by the lighter shade of F1. The sibilancy and continuancy nature of /ʒ/ is manifested in the presence of a noisy spectrum of energy for approximately 150 msec. Because of lip rounding in the production of /ʒ/, as can be seen in the filmstrip in this module (in frames 15 through 16), there is a lowering of the energy spectrum for this sibilant as compared to /s/ and /z/.

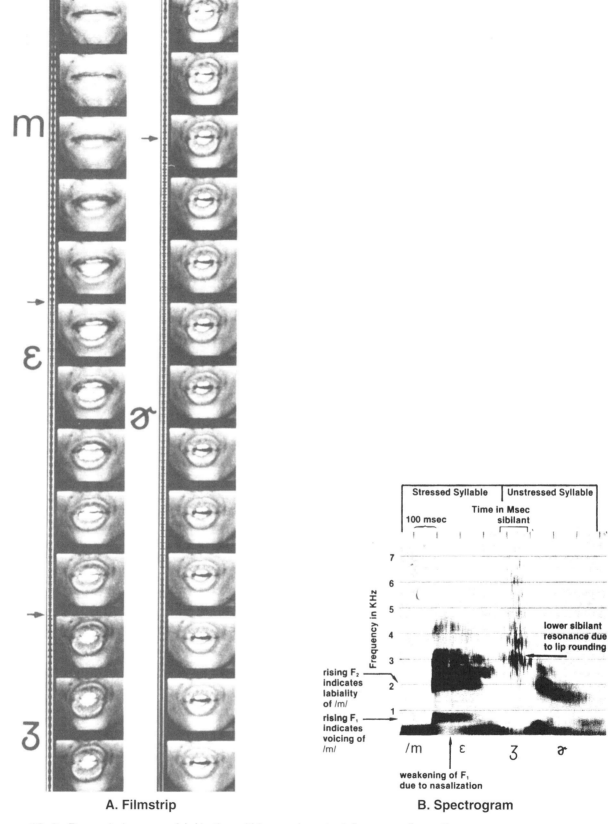

A. Filmstrip

B. Spectrogram

Figure 18–2. Dynamic images of /ʒ/ in the within-word context: "measure." *continues*

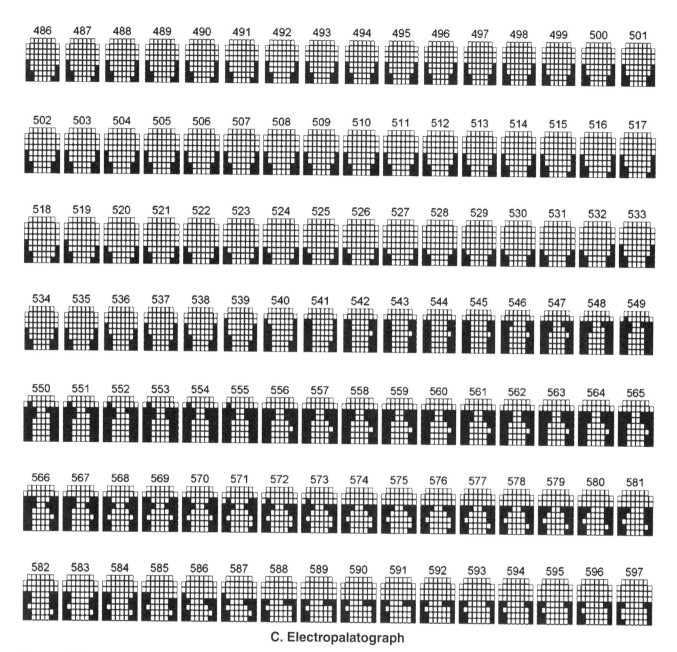

C. Electropalatograph

Figure 18–2. *continued*

Most of the energy for this sibilant is between 2500 and 4500 Hz. The following vowel shows a falling F2 transition, a short duration, and a low level of energy as compared to the vowel of the first syllable. This is primarily the result of the unstressed nature of this syllable in this word.

Electropalatograph: /ˈmɛʒə/ "measure"

Figure 18-2C provides 112 consecutive EPG frames for the production of /ˈmɛʒə/[1] "measure." The initial phoneme /m/ extends from frames 486 to 521 and is characterized by limited tongue/contact along the

___

[1] /ˈmɛʒə/ is the Australian English pronunciation of "measure."

posterior lateral margins of the palate. The vowel /ɛ/ extends from 522 to 541 and looks similar to the /m/. The juncture between /m/ and /ɛ/ was identified using simultaneous EPG, spectrogram, waveform and audio data (not shown in Figure 18–2C). The consonant /ʒ/ extends from frames 542 to 567 and is characterized by broad contact along the lateral margins of the palate in order to create the central groove for the frication. There is a long period of transition from /ʒ/ to the final vowel. The final vowel /ə/ extends from 574 to 596.

INTRA- AND INTERSPEAKER VARIABILITY FOR /ʒ/

Electropalatographic images enable consideration of interspeaker variability.

Intra- and Interspeaker Variability in the Production of /ʒ/ by Eight Typical English-Speaking Adults

Four typical adult males (M1–M4) and four typical adult females (F1–F4) produced nonsense syllables containing /ʒ/ three times. The nonsense syllables were created with /ʒ/ in syllable-initial and syllable-final positions in vowel contexts taken at the extremes of the vowel quadrilateral.

Maximum Contact Frames for Eight Typical English-Speaking Adults

To demonstrate both inter- and intraspeaker variability the maximum contact frame for the second production of each nonsense syllable for each speaker is provided in Figure 18–3. The width of the groove varies between 1 and 3 electrodes; however, most are 2 to 3 electrodes wide. Compared with groove for /z/, the groove for /ʒ/ is produced more posteriorly and there is wider lateral bracing.

Cumulative EPG Frames for Eight Typical English-Speaking Adults

Cumulative EPG patterns for /ʒ/ were generated from maximum contact frames for each of the eight typical adults described above. Each electrode on a cumulative maximum contact display has a number, corresponding to the percentage of contact over the 60 productions. The darker the shading, the more contact. In Figure 18–4 each speaker's cumulative maximum contact display has a broad midline groove with lateral bracing. M1's cumulative frame shows a slightly retracted tongue placement compared with the other speakers.

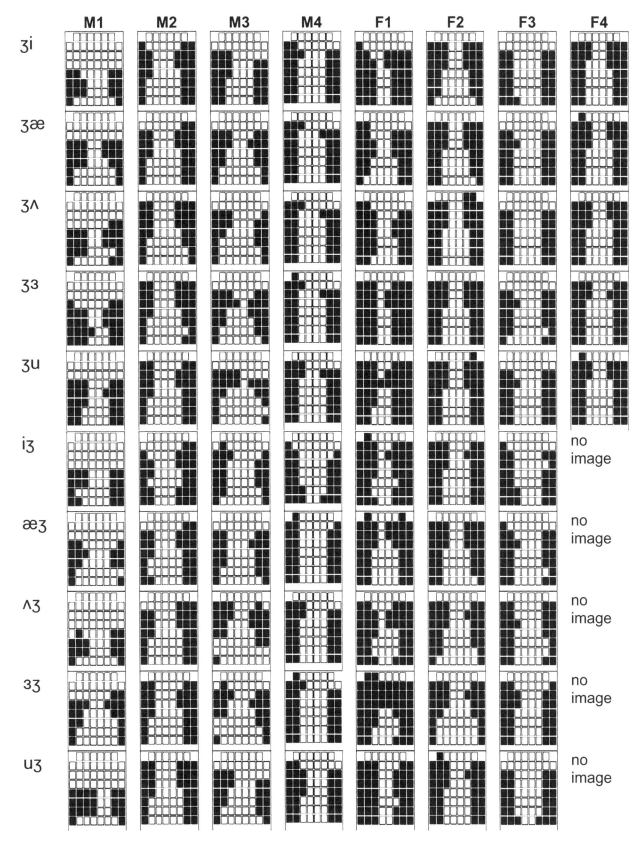

Figure 18–3. Intra- and interspeaker variability in the maximum EPG contact frame for the production of /ʒ/ by eight typical English-speaking adults. *continues*

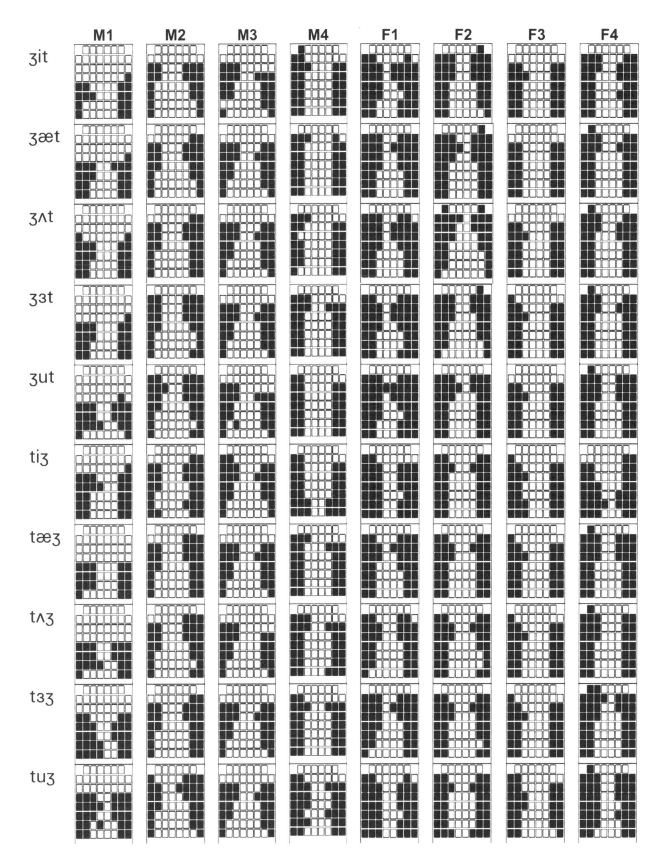

Figure 18–3. *continues*

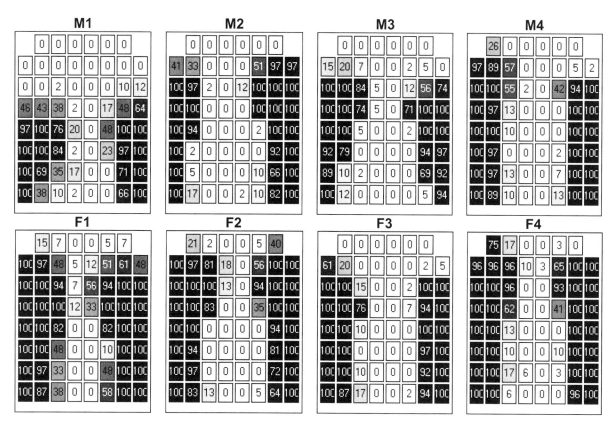

Figure 18–4. Cumulative EPG frames demonstrating intra- and interspeaker variability for the production of /ʒ/ by eight typical English-speaking adults.

Chapter 19

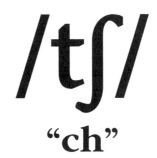

"ch"

The consonant /tʃ/ is a voiceless palatal affricate.

> Place of articulation: palatal
>
> Advancement: back
>
> Voicing: voiceless
>
> Labiality: nonlabial
>
> Sonorancy: nonsonorant (obstruent)
>
> Continuancy: noncontinuant (stop)
>
> Sibilancy: sibilant
>
> Nasality: nonnasal (oral)

STATIC IMAGES OF THE ARTICULATORY CHARACTERISTICS OF /tʃ/

The static images of /tʃ/ are presented via a photograph, schematic diagram, ultrasound, and electropalatograph images (Figure 19-1).

Photograph

In this photograph (Figure 19-1A), the image of /tʃ/ is taken from within spontaneous speech and is marked by considerable lip rounding due to the coarticulatory influence of the rounded vowel.

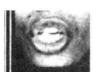

A. Photograph

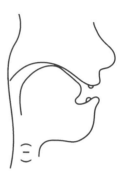

B. Schematic diagram

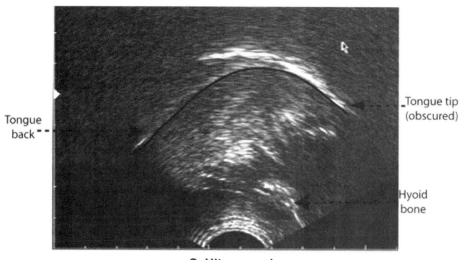

C. Ultrasound

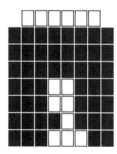

D. Electropalatograph (EPG) (single frame)

Figure 19–1. Static images of the articulatory characteristics of /tʃ/.

Schematic Diagram

Only the stop aspect of this phoneme is shown in the lateral view of the production of /tʃ/ (Figure 19-1B). After blocking the airstream at the point of contact, the high-velocity airstream is emitted, resulting in a high-frequency, intense noise for a considerable period of time. The phoneme /tʃ/ is voiceless, as indicated by the minus sign at the vocal fold region.

Ultrasound

The bright white line on the ultrasound image in Figure 19-1C represents the air above the tongue surface during the occlusion phase for the production of /tʃ/. The tongue tip is on the right and is slightly lowered so that the tongue blade touches the alveolar ridge. Approximately 1 cm of the tongue tip is obscured from view because of the acoustic shadow of the jaw (Stone, 2005). The electropalatographic image in Figure 19-1D shows that the first row of electrodes was not contacted at this point in the production of /tʃ/. In the ultrasound, the back of the tongue is also raised in the oral cavity. The double line at the highest point of the tongue could be created by the body of air ready to produce the release phase for /tʃ/. The white line of the hyoid bone can be seen in the lower right side of the image.

Electropalatograph (EPG)

The EPG image of /tʃ/ (Figure 19-1D) shows that the majority of the palate is contacted by the tongue during the occlusion phase. This large amount of tongue/palate contact is similar to the voiced cognate /dʒ/ in Figure 20-1D. In this static image for the production of /tʃ/, there is no contact on the first row of electrodes on the alveolar ridge. Bernhardt et al. (2005) indicated that speakers move their tongues posteriorly to a postalveolar position during production of /tʃ/.

Liker, Gibbon, Wrench, and Horga (2007) compared EPG data of production of /tʃ/ and /t/ for seven British English speakers. They found the production of /tʃ/:

- had more posterior tongue placement than /t/ (significant difference for all speakers)
- had greater amount of tongue/palate contact than /t/ (significant difference for five speakers)
- had a longer occlusion phase than /t/ (significant difference for six speakers). The occlusion phase ranged from 60 to 100 msec. Liker et al. report that this finding is consistent with other studies (i.e., Crystal & House, 1982; Umeda, 1977)
- had greater variability in the *closure* phase for /tʃ/ than /t/ (present in five speakers; significant for three speakers), but that tongue placement was stable for the *occlusion* phase for both /t/ and /tʃ/.

DYNAMIC IMAGES OF THE ARTICULATORY AND ACOUSTIC CHARACTERISTICS OF /tʃ/

To obtain a comprehensive view of the production of this consonant, the dynamic aspects of the production of /tʃ/ are shown in a filmstrip, spectrogram, and EPG images (Figure 19-2).

/tʃ/ in Word-Initial and Word-Final Contexts: "church"

Filmstrip: /tʃɝtʃ/ "church"

The phoneme /tʃ/ is at the initial and final positions (Figure 19-2A) of the word "church." The phoneme /tʃ/ is marked by considerable lip rounding. The first 13 frames show the lip rounding that occurs before the emission of the acoustic energy. Because the following vowel is /ɝ/, the rounding persists through the vowel. The boundary between the rounded /tʃ/ and the rounded /ɝ/ is exhibited by the mouth opening for the /ɝ/ phoneme, as seen in frames 17 through 26. After frame 27, the teeth contact, the lips remain rounded, and the final consonant /tʃ/ is produced.

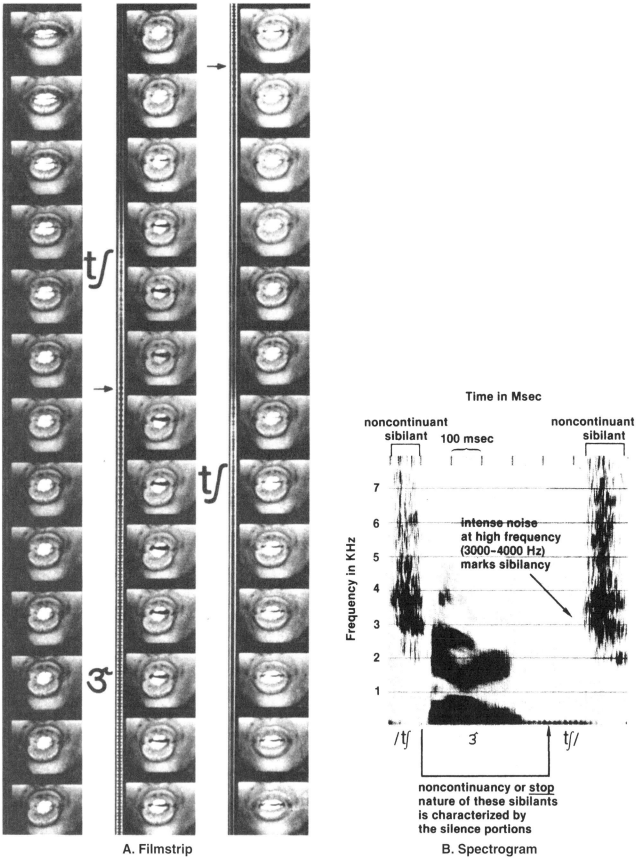

A. Filmstrip

B. Spectrogram

Figure 19–2. Dynamic images of /tʃ/ in word-initial and word-final contexts: "church." *continues*

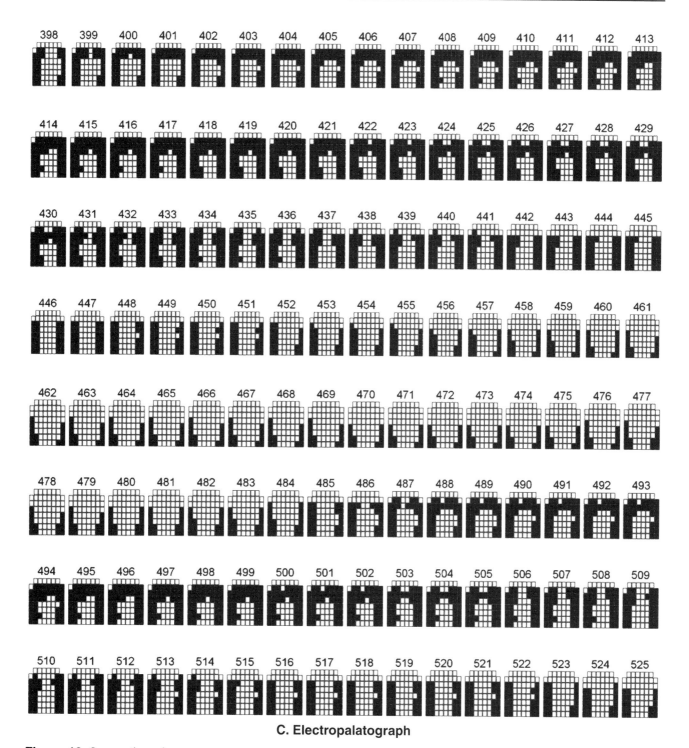

C. Electropalatograph

Figure 19–2. *continued*

Sound Spectrogram: /tʃɝtʃ/ "church"

The sound spectrogram (Figure 19-2B) shows that the initial consonant is a voiceless sibilant with the presence of lip rounding. The sibilancy of the consonant /tʃ/ is denoted by a durational characteristic of approximately 125 msec. The energy concentration is between 2600 and 4000 Hz. The transitions for all of the vowel formants are falling. The final consonant, again, is a voiceless sibilant with lip rounding. There exists a total silence for approximately 200 msec at the termination of the vowel /ɝ/ and the beginning of the presence of energy representing the phoneme /tʃ/. This silence reaffirms our classification of /tʃ/ into the category of stops.

Electropalatograph: /tʃɝtʃ/ "church"

Figure 19-2C presents the word /tʃɝtʃ/[1] "church" in 128 EPG frames. The initial /tʃ/ extends from 400 to 455. The occlusion phase of the /tʃ/ extends from 400 to 430 and the friction phase extends from 431 to 455. The vowel /ɜ/ extends from 456 to 487 (identified by using simultaneous spectrogram and audio data, not shown in Figure 19-2C). The final /tʃ/ extends from 488 to 523. The occlusion phase of the /tʃ/ extends from 488 to 505 and the friction phase extends from 506 to 523.

/tʃ/ in the Within-Word Context: "searching"

Filmstrip: /ˈsɝtʃɪŋ/ "searching"

The phoneme /tʃ/ is presented in the medial position in the word /ˈsɝtʃɪŋ/. This filmstrip (Figure 19-3A) demonstrates the strong influence of neighboring sounds on each other. In addition, it can be seen here that the production of speech is a dynamic event. The very first frame shows rounding of the lips, which is atypical for the production of /s/. This rounding persists throughout the production of /s/. The influence of lip rounding caused by /ɝ/ and /tʃ/ can be viewed in both the backward and forward coarticulators. The example of backward coarticulation is the rounding of /s/, and the example of forward coarticulation is the rounding of /ɪ/ and /ŋ/.

Sound Spectrogram: /ˈsɝtʃɪŋ/ "searching"

Figure 19-3B contains the sound spectrogram of the word "searching." The initial consonant is the voiceless sibilant /s/. Sibilancy is indicated by a high-frequency component starting at 4000 Hz and ending at 8000 Hz,

coupled with a long duration of approximately 200 msec. All four formants of the following vowel /ɝ/ show a falling transition. The absence of voicing is clearly indicated by the lack of any negative voice onset time markings and the lack of a rising transition of the first formant of the vowel. The vowel /ɝ/ shows its first formant at approximately 400 Hz and its second formant at 1800 Hz. Following the vowel /ɝ/, the stop characteristic of /tʃ/ is denoted by a silence of approximately 150 msec. This silence is then followed by a sibilancy-type noise, with most of its energy concentrated between 3000 and 4000 Hz. The relatively lower energy for the sibilant /tʃ/, as compared to the sibilant /s/, which appears in the initial position, is attributed to the phenomenon of lip rounding. The four sibilants that involve lip rounding are /ʃ/, /ʒ/, /tʃ/, and /dʒ/, and the remaining two, which do not involve lip rounding, are /s/ and /z/. The former contain energy in the lower frequencies (between 3000 and 4000 Hz), as compared to the latter, whose energy is concentrated higher than 4000 Hz.

Electropalatograph: /ˈsɝtʃɪŋ/ "searching"

Figure 19-3C contains 135 EPG frames for the word /ˈsɝtʃɪŋ/[2] "searching." The word extends over 0.669 seconds and was produced within a sentence context. The /s/ extends from 455 to 487, the vowel /ɜ/ extends from 498 to 512, the affricate /tʃ/ extends from 520 to 547, the vowel /ɪ/ extends from 554 to 567 (identified using simultaneous EPG, audio, spectrogram, and waveform data not shown in Figure 19-3C) and the velar nasal /ŋ/ extends from 568 to 583. The frames that are unaccounted for are periods of transition (coarticulation) between the sounds. The EPG frames for the affricate /tʃ/ show the occlusion phase from frames 520 to 537 and the friction phase from frames 538 to 547.

INTRA- AND INTERSPEAKER VARIABILITY IN THE PRODUCTION OF /tʃ/

To date there is limited research on the production of affricates.

---

[1]/tʃɝtʃ/ is the Australian English pronunciation of "church."
[2]/ˈsɝtʃɪŋ/ is the Australian English pronunciation of "searching."

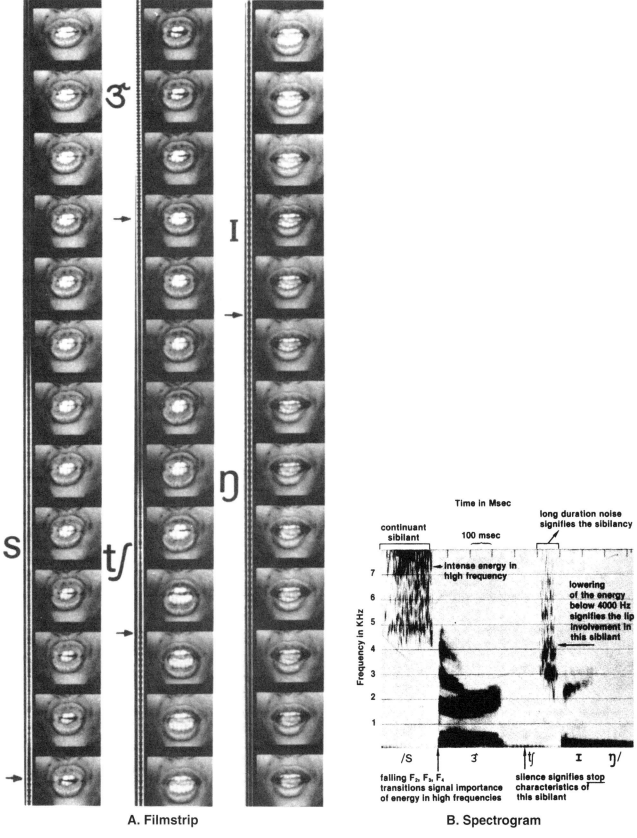

A. Filmstrip

B. Spectrogram

Figure 19–3. Dynamic images of /tʃ/ in the within-word context: "searching." *continues*

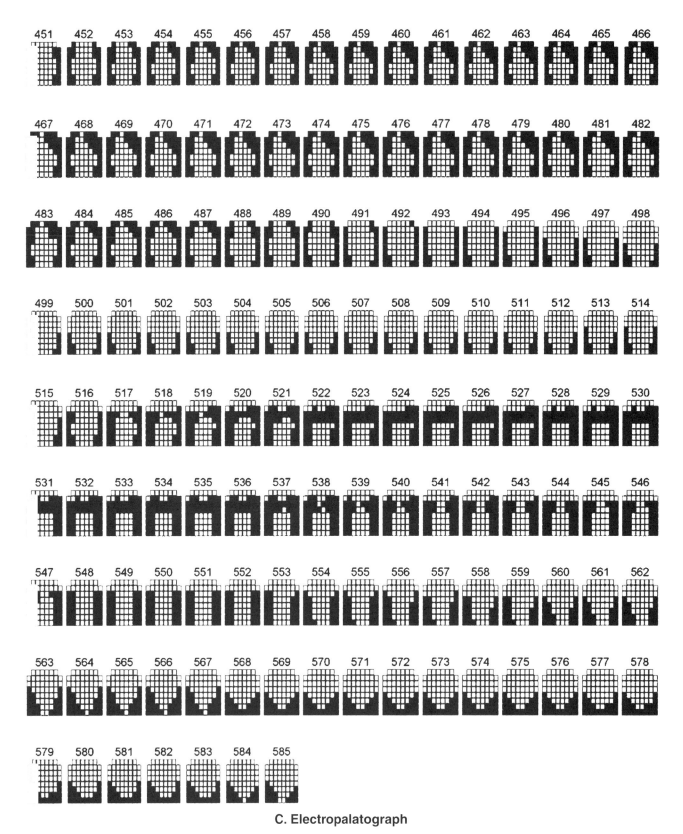

C. Electropalatograph

Figure 19–3. *continued*

220

Interspeaker Variability in the Production of /tʃ/ by English-Speaking Adults

British English-Speaking Adults

Liker et al. (2007) created cumulative maximum contact EPG frames for the *occlusion phase* of /tʃ/ in order to compare /t/ with /tʃ/. Seven British English speakers, four females and three males, produced /tʃ/ in VCV sequences in differing combinations with the vowels /a, i, u/. Thus, they produced 630 tokens of /tʃ/. Similar to these speakers' productions of /t/, each speaker's cumulative maximum contact display is a horseshoe shape. The production was more posterior than for /t/: none of these speakers had contact on the first row of the palate (Figure 19–4).

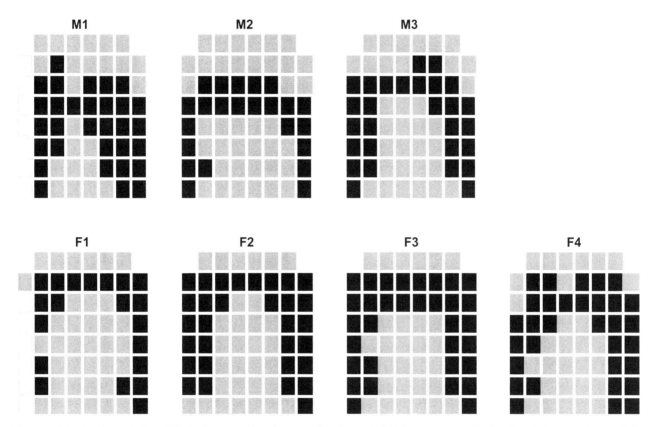

Figure 19–4. Cumulative EPG frames for the production of /tʃ/ by seven British English-speaking adults (adapted from Liker et al., 2007, Appendix, p. 108).

Chapter 20

/dʒ/

"j"

The consonant /dʒ/ is a voiced palatal affricate.

Place of articulation: palatal

Advancement: back

Voicing: voiced

Labiality: nonlabial

Sonorancy: nonsonorant (obstruent)

Continuancy: noncontinuant (stop)

Sibilancy: sibilant

Nasality: nonnasal (oral)

STATIC IMAGES OF THE ARTICULATORY CHARACTERISTICS OF /dʒ/

The static images of /dʒ/ are presented via a photograph, schematic diagram, ultrasound, and electropalatograph images (Figure 20–1).

Photograph

Figure 20-1A is a photograph of the production of /dʒ/. The lips are rounded and forward and the teeth are together.

A. Photograph

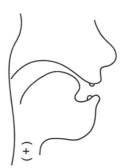

B. Schematic diagram

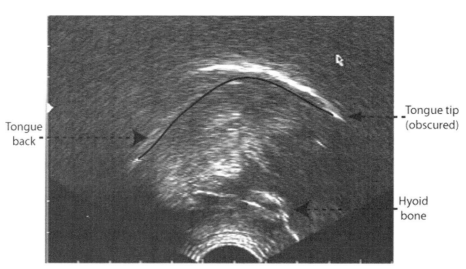

C. Ultrasound

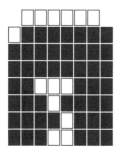

D. Electropalatograph (EPG) (single frame)

Figure 20–1. Static images of the articulatory characteristics of /dʒ/.

Schematic Diagram

Only the stop aspect of this phoneme is shown in the lateral view of the production of /dʒ/ in Figure 20–1B. After blocking the airstream at the point of contact, the high-velocity airstream is emitted, resulting in a high frequency, intense noise for a considerable period of time. The phoneme /dʒ/ is a voiced consonant, as indicated by the plus sign at the vocal fold region.

Ultrasound

Figure 20–1C shows the tongue surface during the occlusion phase for the production of /dʒ/. The bright white line is the air directly above the tongue surface. The tongue tip is on the right and is slightly lowered so that the tongue blade touches the alveolar ridge. In the simultaneous electropalatographic image shown in Figure 20–1D, the first row of electrodes was not contacted at this point in the production of /dʒ/, adding support to the notion that the tongue blade was touching the alveolar ridge. Additionally, approximately 1 cm of the tongue tip is obscured from view because of the acoustic shadow of the jaw (Stone, 2005). In the ultrasound, the back of the tongue is also raised in the oral cavity. The double image at the highest point of the tongue could be created by the air ready to produce the release phase for /dʒ/. The white line of the hyoid bone can be seen in the lower right side of the image and the diagonal lines under the tongue surface indicate the sound waves bouncing off the muscle fibers and fatty tissue in the tongue.

Electropalatograph (EPG)

The occlusion phase of the /dʒ/ is presented in Figure 20–1D. The tongue touches all but the central portion of the palate as it stops the airflow before it is released.

DYNAMIC IMAGES OF THE ARTICULATORY AND ACOUSTIC CHARACTERISTICS OF /dʒ/

To obtain a comprehensive view of the production of this consonant, the dynamic aspects of the production of /dʒ/ are shown in a filmstrip, spectrogram, and EPG images (Figure 20–2).

/dʒ/ in Word-Initial and Word-Final Contexts: "judge"

Filmstrip: /dʒʌdʒ/ "judge"

The /dʒ/ phoneme is presented at the initial and final positions (Figure 20–2A) with the vowel /ʌ/ in the medial position in the word /dʒʌdʒ/. Like /tʃ/, the phoneme /dʒ/ influences the production of the mid-central vowel /ʌ/. The voicing aspect of /dʒ/ can be seen in the sound track parallel to frames 8 and 9. The transition to the vowel /ʌ/ can be seen in frame 10. During the production of both the initial and final /dʒ/, the lips form the shape of a round tunnel through which the acoustic energy is emitted. The nature of this energy is high-frequency, intense noise accompanied by low frequency glottal pulses.

Sound Spectrogram: /dʒʌdʒ/ "judge"

The initial consonant /dʒ/ is a voiced sibilant (Figure 20–2B), in which voicing is indicated by the rising first formant of the medial vowel /ʌ/ and sibilancy is indicated by the high-frequency noise spectrum (ranging from 3000 Hz to 8000 Hz). The initial consonant /dʒ/ is followed by a neutral vowel /ʌ/, with formant frequencies at 600, 1750, and 3000 Hz. Because of the strong sibilant energy in the high-frequency domain of the initial consonant, both the second and third formants for the vowel show a downward transition.

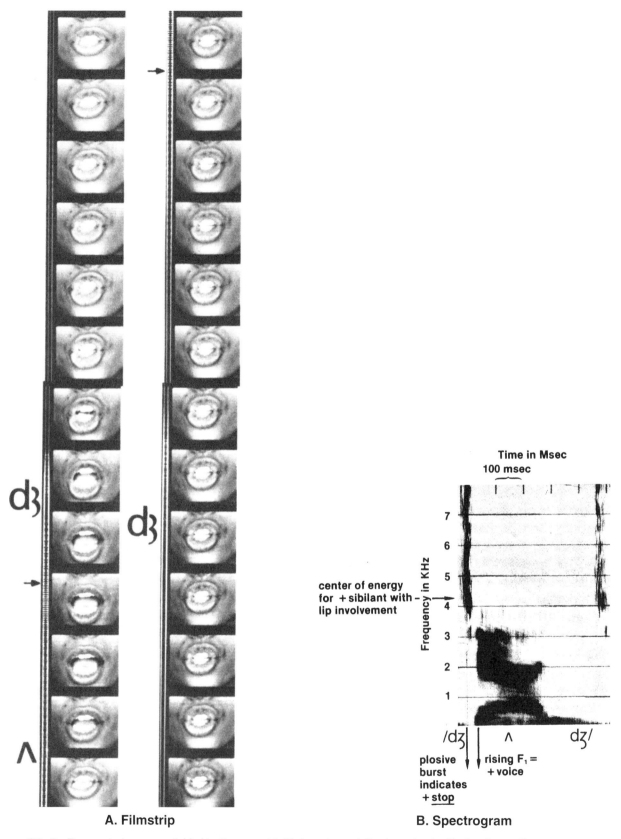

A. Filmstrip

B. Spectrogram

center of energy
for + sibilant with –
lip involvement

plosive
burst
indicates
+ <u>stop</u>

rising F₁ =
+ voice

Time in Msec
100 msec

Frequency in KHz

/dʒ   ʌ   dʒ/

Figure 20–2. Dynamic images of /dʒ/ in the word-initial and word-final contexts: "judge." *continues*

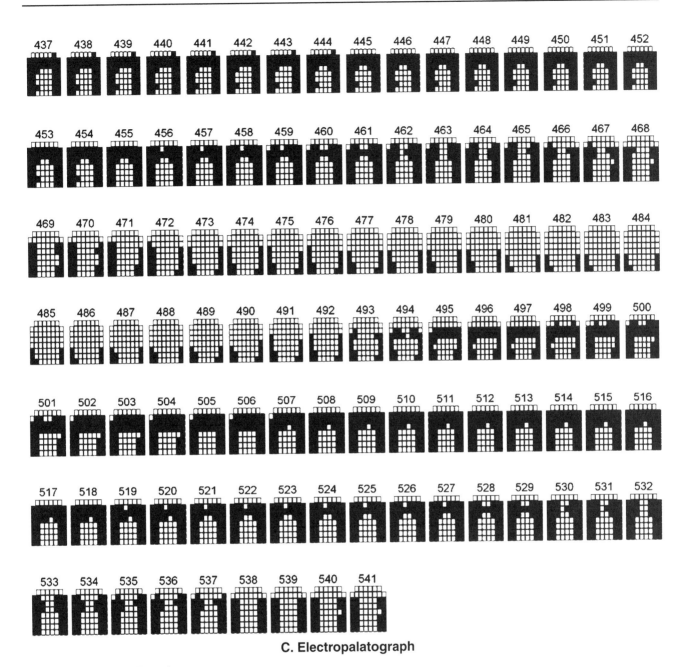

C. Electropalatograph

Figure 20–2. *continued*

The final consonant /dʒ/ is, again, a voiced sibilant, in which voicing is indicated by a falling F1, and the high-frequency spectrum of energy is indicated by a rising F2.

Electropalatograph: /dʒʌdʒ/ "judge"

Figure 20-2C presents the word "judge" in 101 EPG frames. The word-initial /dʒ/ extends from 437 to 470. The occlusion phase of the /dʒ/ extends from 437 to 461 and the friction phase extends from 462 to 470. The vowel /ʌ/ extends from 471 to 492 (identified by using simultaneous spectrogram and audio data, not shown in Figure 20-2C). The word-final /dʒ/ extends from 495 to 537. The occlusion phase of the /dʒ/ extends from 495 to 529 and the friction phase extends from 530 to 537.

Chapter 21

/h/

The consonant /h/ is a voiceless glottal fricative.

Place of articulation: glottal

Advancement: back

Voicing: voiceless

Labiality: nonlabial

Sonorancy: nonsonorant (obstruent)

Continuancy: continuant

Sibilancy: nonsibilant

Nasality: nonnasal (oral)

STATIC IMAGES OF THE ARTICULATORY CHARACTERISTICS OF /h/

The static images of /h/ are presented via a photograph, schematic diagram, ultrasound, and electropalatograph images (Figure 21-1).

Photograph

In this photograph (Figure 21-1A), the mouth is open allowing unobstructed airstream to produce /h/.

A. Photograph

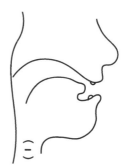

B. Schematic diagram

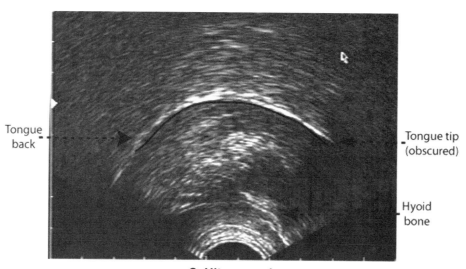

Tongue back

Tongue tip (obscured)

Hyoid bone

C. Ultrasound

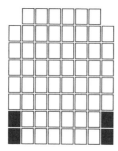

D. Electropalatograph (EPG) (single frame)

Figure 21–1. Static images of the articulatory characteristics of /h/.

Schematic Diagram

In the lateral view (Figure 21–B) of the production of the consonant /h/, the tongue maintains a neutral position ensuring no stoppage of the airstream in the oral cavity. The lack of voicing of this consonant is symbolically represented at the source (the vocal folds) by a minus sign.

Ultrasound

The ultrasound image of /h/ is depicted in Figure 21–1C. The tongue is in a neutral position in the mouth, resting on the floor of the mouth. This image can be compared with the image in Chapter 1 of the tongue at rest in the mouth. If the mouth is open farther, there will be no contact.

Electropalatograph (EPG)

The EPG image of /h/ (Figure 21–1D) demonstrates limited contact between the tongue and the palate during the production of this sound.

DYNAMIC IMAGES OF THE ARTICULATORY AND ACOUSTIC CHARACTERISTICS OF /h/

To obtain a comprehensive view of the production of this consonant, the dynamic aspects of the production of /h/ are shown in a filmstrip, spectrogram, and EPG images (Figure 21–2).

/h/ in Word-Initial Context: "have"

Filmstrip: /hæv/ "have"

The filmstrip (Figure 21–2A) shows the continuants /h/ and /v/ at the initial and final positions, respectively, in the word /hæv/. The vowel /æ/ is in the medial position. In the production of this word, the articulatory gestures associated with the vowel /æ/ predominate throughout the filmstrip. Jaw excursion and unrounded lips are characteristic of this vowel. The phoneme /h/ is considered to be vocalic because it does not require closure, as for stop consonants, or stricture, as for continuant consonants. Because of its vocalic nature, its production has been assimilated with the following vowel /æ/. The voiceless characteristic of /h/ can be verified in the filmstrip by examining the sound track. A very high-frequency, low-amplitude energy appears at frame 8. The transition to the vowel begins by frame 12.

Sound Spectrogram: /hæv/ "have"

The phoneme /h/ is presented in initial position in the word "have." There is no trace of any high-frequency acoustic energy present at this initial position on the sound spectrogram in Figure 21–2B.

Electropalatograph: /hæv/ "have"

Figure 21–2C presents tongue/palate contact for the word "have." Throughout this word the EPG frames have limited tongue/palate contact along the posterior lateral margins. Simultaneous audio, EPG, and waveform data are required to determine the boundaries of the consonants and vowels. The /h/ extends from 558 to 569, the /æ/ from 570 to 599 and the /v/ from 600 to 621, detectable only by the activation of one and two electrodes respectively.

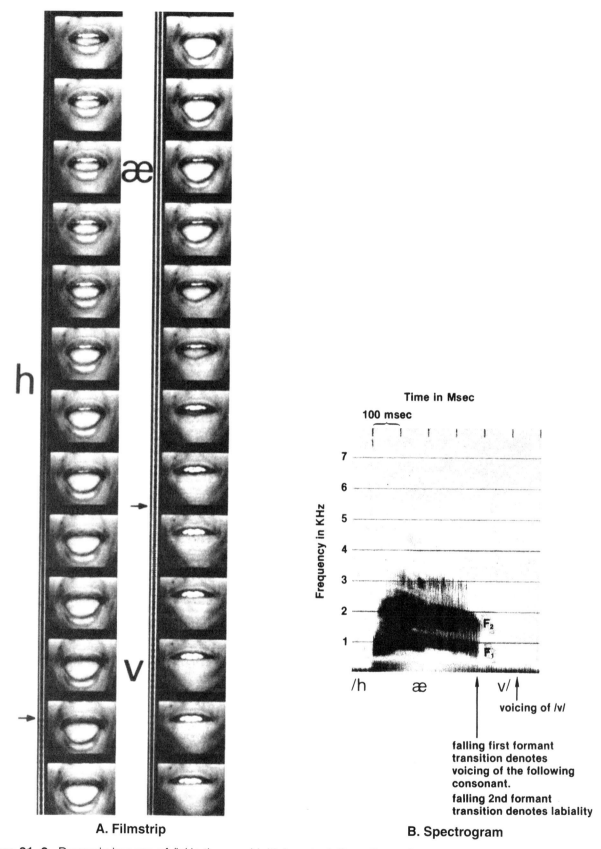

A. Filmstrip

B. Spectrogram

Figure 21–2. Dynamic images of /h/ in the word-initial context: "have." *continues*

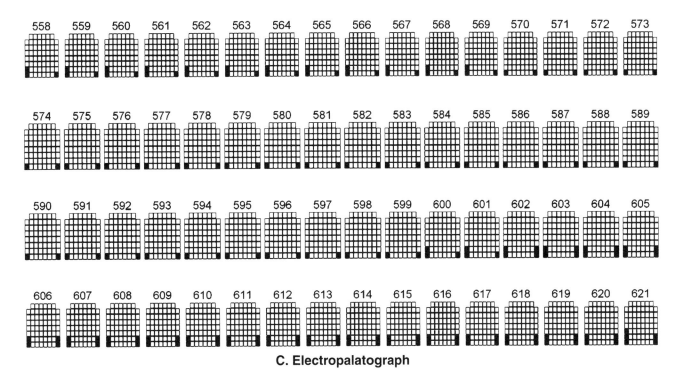

C. Electropalatograph

Figure 21–2. *continued*

Chapter 22

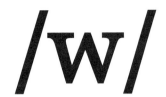

The consonant /w/ is a voiced labiovelar approximant.

Place of articulation: labiovelar

Advancement: back

Voicing: voiced

Labiality: labial

Sonorancy: sonorant

Continuancy: —

Sibilancy: nonsibilant

Nasality: nonnasal (oral)

STATIC IMAGES OF THE ARTICULATORY CHARACTERISTICS OF /w/

The static images of /w/ are presented via a photograph, schematic diagram, ultrasound, and electropalatograph images (Figure 22–1).

Photograph

In this photograph (Figure 22–1A), the lips are rounded to produce /w/.

A. Photograph

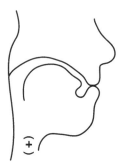

B. Schematic diagram

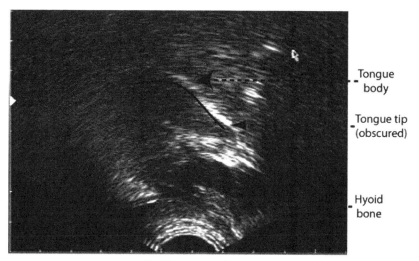

Tongue body

Tongue tip (obscured)

Hyoid bone

C. Ultrasound

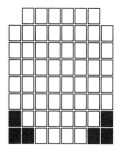

D. Electropalatograph (EPG) (single frame)

Figure 22–1. Static images of the articulatory characteristics of /w/.

Schematic Diagram

The lateral view of the production of /w/ in this schematic diagram (Figure 22-1B) can be compared with the frontal view shown in the filmstrip. The lips are open and protruded in the production of /w/. The tongue is raised toward the velum. The symbol (+) at the vocal folds indicates their involvement in the production of the phoneme /w/.

Ultrasound

The ultrasound image of /w/ in Figure 22-1C demonstrates why this sound is called a labio*velar* approximant. The tongue is arched similarly to the tongue shape for the other velar sounds, /k, g, ŋ/. The tongue tip is down (right of the image) and the back of the tongue is high and back in the mouth. The tongue surface is not as clearly seen in this image. This lack of clarity is a feature of other ultrasound images where the tongue is steeply sloping such as in velars and high vowels (Stone, 2005).

Electropalatograph (EPG)

The EPG image of /w/ in Figure 22-1D also demonstrates why this sound is called a labio*velar* approximant. There is tongue/palate contact along the posterior (velar) corners of the palate. The extent of tongue/palate contact for /w/ is influenced by the surrounding vowels.

DYNAMIC IMAGES OF THE ARTICULATORY AND ACOUSTIC CHARACTERISTICS OF /w/

To obtain a comprehensive view of the production of this consonant, the dynamic aspects of the production of /w/ are shown in a filmstrip, spectrogram, and EPG images (Figure 22-2).

[1]/wɒʃ/ is the Australian English pronunciation of "wash."

/w/ in Word-Initial Context: "wash"

Filmstrip: /wɔʃ/ "wash"

The phoneme /w/ is presented at the initial position (Figure 22-2A) in the word /wɔʃ/. Labiality can be clearly viewed in the filmstrip. Labiality is seen in the rounding and approximation of the lower and upper lips. One of the differences between /b/ and /w/, both labials, is that /b/ requires that the lips be completely closed, whereas in /w/ they remain open. The advantage of the filmstrip is that we can view the complete process of lip approximation. The protrusion of the lips starts in frame 1 and continues through frame 14, with no two frames showing the same protrusion/opening ratio.

Sound Spectrogram: /wɔʃ/ "wash"

The phoneme /w/ is presented (Figure 22-2B) in the initial position, followed by the vowel /ɔ/ and the consonant /ʃ/ in the word "wash." Labiality is the only prominent feature emerging for the phoneme /w/ in this sound spectrogram. Most of the energy is vowel-like at the low frequency end of the spectrum, signaling sonorancy (at and below 500 Hz). The sonorancy feature is further indicated by a gradual rather than abrupt sloping of the rising first and second formant transitions. The vowel /ɔ/ exhibits its first formant center frequency at about 900 Hz and second formant at about 1250 Hz, with a rising second formant transition to approximate the energy spectrum of the final consonant /ʃ/ In this sound spectrogram of /ʃ/, the features continuancy and sibilancy are indicated by the long-duration, high-frequency, intense-noise spectrum. Lip rounding is indicated by a lowering of this overall spectrum to exhibit most of its energy between 2500 and 4000 Hz, rather than above 4000 Hz, as can be seen for those sibilants that do not exhibit the lip rounding phenomenon (such as /s/).

Electropalatograph: /wɒʃ/ "wash"

Figure 22-2C contains EPG frames demonstrating tongue/palate contact for the production of /wɒʃ/[1] "wash." The /w/ sound is characterized by minimal

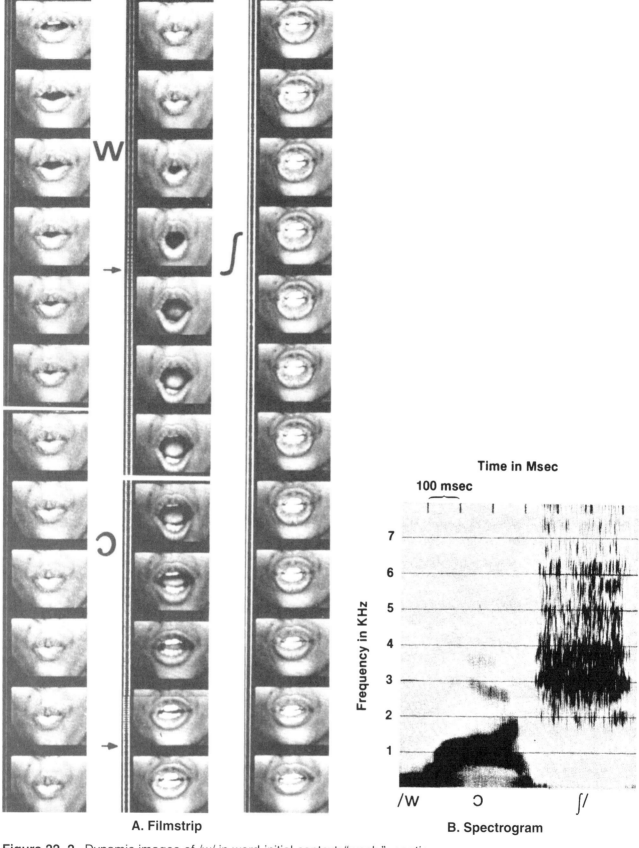

A. Filmstrip

B. Spectrogram

Figure 22–2. Dynamic images of /w/ in word-initial context: "wash." *continues*

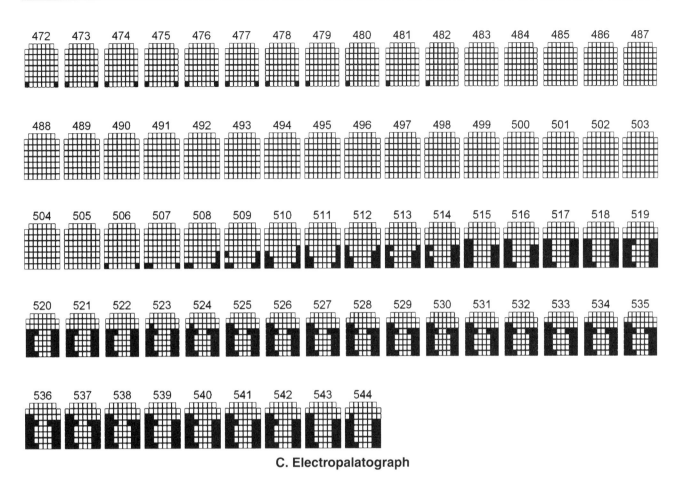

C. Electropalatograph

Figure 22–2. *continued*

tongue/palate contact occurring at the velar region of the palate (frames 472–482). Using the simultaneous EPG, spectrogram, waveform and audio data, the juncture between the /w/ and /ɒ/ was identified as occurring at frame 487. The transition from the vowel extending to the /ʃ/ between frames 506 to 513. The /ʃ/ sound extended from frames 514 to 544. The /ʃ/ sound is characterized by broad tongue/palate contact along the lateral margins of the palate creating a large central groove for the frication to escape.

Chapter 23

/1/

The consonant /l/ is a voiced alveolar lateral approximant.

Place of articulation: alveolar

Advancement: front

Voicing: voiced

Labiality: nonlabial

Sonorancy: sonorant

Continuancy: —

Sibilancy: nonsibilant

Nasality: nonnasal (oral)

The speech sound /l/ has been classified as dark or clear /l/. The term light /l/ is also used for clear /l/. Different types of /l/ predominate in different languages:

◆ Dark [l]: allophones of English, Portuguese, Catalan (Valencià), Russian
◆ Clear [l]: Spanish, Catalan (Mallorquí, Eastern Catalan), Italian, French, German, Greek

There are a number of articulatory and acoustic properties distinguishing dark from clear /l/ (Recasens, 2004). Clear [l] only involves activation of the tongue tip on the alveolar ridge. Dark /l/ involves activation of the tongue tip as well as retraction of the postdorsum region of the tongue. Dark /l/ is often described as velarized or pharyngealized due to this post-dorsal velar or pharyngeal constriction. Additionally, on a sound spectrogram F2 is lower and F1 is raised for a dark /l/ compared with a clear /l/ (Recasens, 2004).

For English, many papers report lighter /l/ in word-initial positions and darker /l/ in word-final positions during the production of isolated words. However, Oxley, Buckingham, Roussel, and Daniloff (2006) recommend consideration of prosodic word boundaries when describing /l/. They found that word-initial /l/ was darkened in "front vowel prosodic word boundaries" (p. 109) and word-final /l/ was darkened within prosodic word boundaries.

STATIC IMAGES OF THE ARTICULATORY CHARACTERISTICS OF /l/

The static images of /l/ are presented via a photograph, schematic diagram, ultrasound, and electropalatograph images (Figure 23–1).

Photograph

In this photograph (Figure 23–1A), the mouth is open and the tongue can be seen touching the alveolar ridge to create closure of the airstream to produce /l/.

Schematic Diagram

The lateral view of the phoneme /l/ (Figure 23–1B) shows the tip of the tongue contacting the hard palate behind the upper incisors. During the production of /l/, the velum is raised, thus closing the velopharyngeal port. In addition, it should be noted that the direction of the airflow through the oral cavity for /l/ differs in manner from that of all other phonemes of English. In the case of /l/, the airflow passes laterally through the mouth rather than centrally; it is directed on either side of the tongue. The vocal folds vibrate in the production of this phoneme as noted by the plus symbol (+).

Ultrasound

A midsagittal ultrasound image of the tongue surface during production /l/ is shown in Figure 23–1C. Underneath the bright white line is the tongue surface. The tongue tip is on the right of the image, with approximately 1 cm of the tip being obscured by the acoustic shadow of the jaw (Stone, 2005). The raising of the tongue tip and tongue back with the lowering of the tongue center is clear in this image. This retraction of the postdorsum region of the tongue is typical in productions of dark /l/ for languages such as English. An air shadow can be seen above the tongue and diagonal muscle fibers can be seen below the surface of the tongue. The hyoid bone is seen as the bright diagonal line at the lower right of the image.

Electropalatograph (EPG)

The EPG image of /l/ (Figure 23–1D) presents primarily as having tongue contact along the alveolar ridge. This contact is narrower than for the alveolar stops /t, d/ (Dagenais, Lorendo, & McCutcheon, 1994). There is minimal amount of contact along the left lateral margin of the palate, which may be a result of a coarticulatory gesture as the image was created during spontaneous speech.

The cumulative EPG image (Figure 23–1E) represents multiple productions of words containing /l/ by eight speakers. The darker the shading the more often that part of the palate was contacted by the tongue.

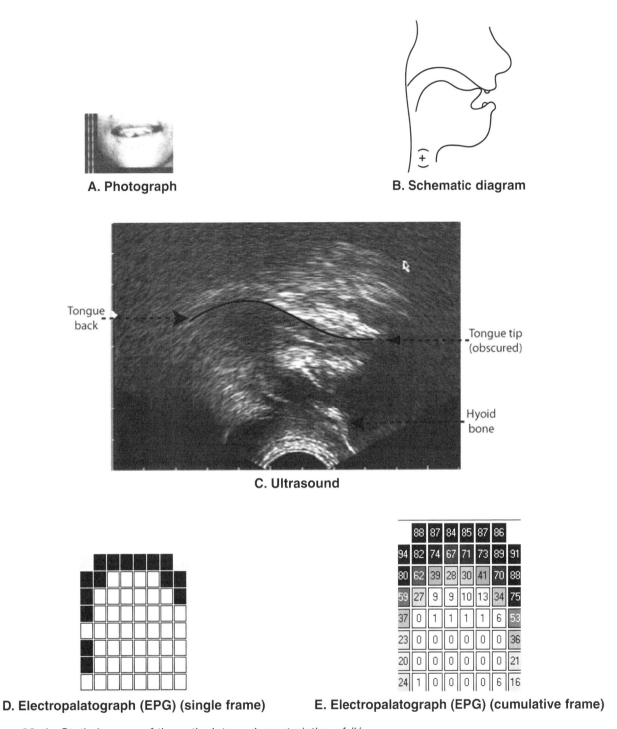

A. Photograph

B. Schematic diagram

C. Ultrasound

D. Electropalatograph (EPG) (single frame)

E. Electropalatograph (EPG) (cumulative frame)

Figure 23–1. Static images of the articulatory characteristics of /l/.

The numbers indicate the percentage of contact with each EPG electrode. The number 24 in the lower left square indicates that that electrode was contacted 24% of the time by the eight speakers over the words when producing /l/. It can be seen that the speakers' tongues predominantly touched the alveolar ridge during production of /l/. However, there was contact along the lateral margins of the palate some of the time.

DYNAMIC IMAGES OF THE ARTICULATORY AND ACOUSTIC CHARACTERISTICS OF /l/

To obtain a comprehensive view of the production of this consonant, the dynamic aspects of the production of /l/ are shown in a filmstrip, spectrogram and EPG images for the words "lily" (Figure 23–2) and "veal" (Figure 23–3).

/l/ in Word-Initial and Within-Word Contexts: "lily"

Filmstrip: /ˈlɪlɪ/ "lily"

The phoneme /l/ is shown (Figure 23–2A) at the initial and medial positions in the word /ˈlɪlɪ/. The frontal view of tongue contact for the phoneme /l/ is like the tongue contact shown for the phoneme /n/ in the word /nʌn/ (see Figure 9–2). However, as can be seen by comparing the electropalatographic images, during the production of /l/ the tongue does not extend along the lateral margins of the palate as it does for /n/. The influence of the vowel /ɪ/ on the consonant /l/ can be seen in both the initial and final positions. The lips are flattened and widespread throughout the production of the word /ˈlɪlɪ/.

Sound Spectrogram: /ˈlɪlɪ/ "lily"

On the temporal continuum, it can be seen from the sound spectrogram (Figure 23–2B) that the phoneme boundary showing /l/+/ɪ/+/l/+/ɪ/ is difficult to determine. The phoneme /l/, being a sonorant consonant, behaves like a vowel, showing a clear F1 and F2 at about 300 Hz and 1500 Hz, respectively. The second formant of the consonant /l/ slopes upward to make a smooth transition into the second formant of the vowel /ɪ/ at 2000 Hz. The /l/ in the medial position is shorter in duration, but has approximately the same F1 and F2 values as the initial /l/. The final vowel /ɪ/ has been pronounced more like the vowel /i/, showing a higher F2 value (about 2500 Hz), and a sharper transition from /l/ to /ɪ/ or /i/. Because neither a voiceless nor obstruent consonant was involved in this word, it can be noted that a continuous pulsation of the vocal folds has been maintained from beginning to end.

Electropalatograph: /ˈlili/ "lily"

Figure 23–2C presents tongue/palate contact for the word /ˈlɪli/[1] "lily." The 93 EPG frames took approximately 0.477 seconds to produce. Closure for the initial /l/ extends from frames 476 to 504, the vowel /ɪ/ extends from 507 to 526 and the medial /l/ extends from 527 to 542, and the final /i/ from 543 to 569. The /l/ sound is produced with tongue contact along the alveolar ridge as well as along the anterior lateral margins of the palate. There is more anterior tongue/palate contact for the /l/ produced at the beginning of the word than for the /l/ within the word "lily." Prevocalic /l/ is typically found farther forward in the mouth than postvocalic /l/ (Shriberg & Kent, 2003).

---

[1]/ˈlɪli/ is the Australian English pronunciation of "lily."

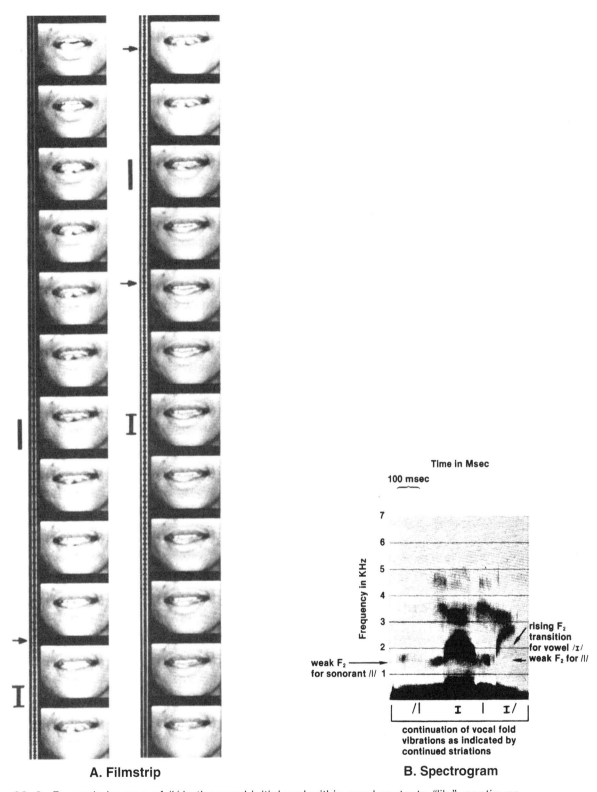

A. Filmstrip

B. Spectrogram

Figure 23–2. Dynamic images of /l/ in the word-initial and within-word contexts: "lily." *continues*

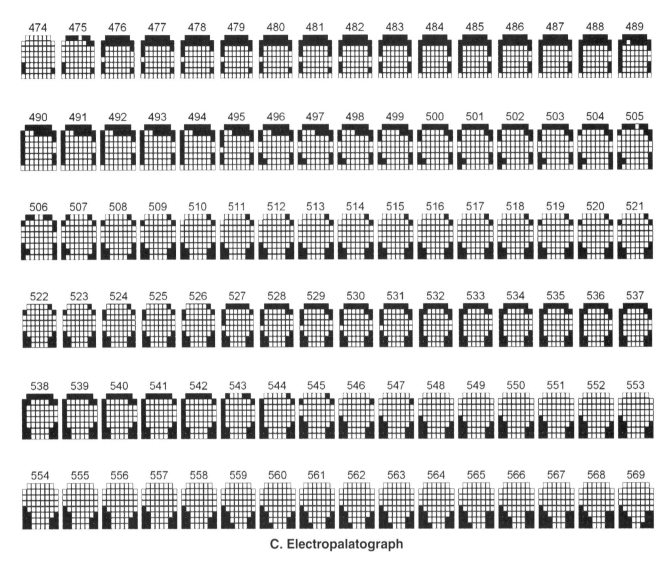

C. Electropalatograph

Figure 23–2. *continued*

/l/ in Word-Final Context: "veal"

Filmstrip: /vil/ "veal"

The criterion phoneme /l/ is at the final position of the word /vil/ "veal." The first six frames (Figure 23–3A) show the lips before the labiodental closure for /v/. Frames 7 through 15 show the state of labiodental contact necessary for the production of English consonants /f/ and /v/. Frame 16 shows the beginning sign of lip opening for the vowel /i/. Frames 17 through 23 show the tongue at the front-high position for the production of the vowel /i/. Frame 24 shows the upward movement of the tongue tip for the production of the final consonant /l/. The last two frames show the tongue touching the alveolar ridge area.

Sound Spectrogram: /vil/ "veal"

This is a good example of transitions from voiced labial fricative /v/ to the high vowel /i/ ending into a low frequency sonorant /l/. As is marked on this spectrogram (Figure 23–3B), labiality is represented by the presence of low frequency energy at approximately 1250 Hz.

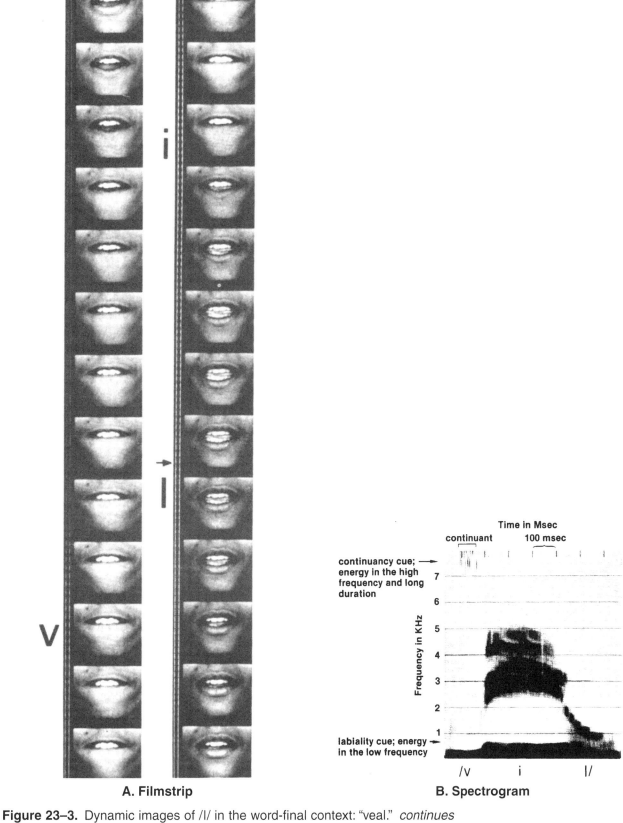

A. Filmstrip

B. Spectrogram

Figure 23–3. Dynamic images of /l/ in the word-final context: "veal." *continues*

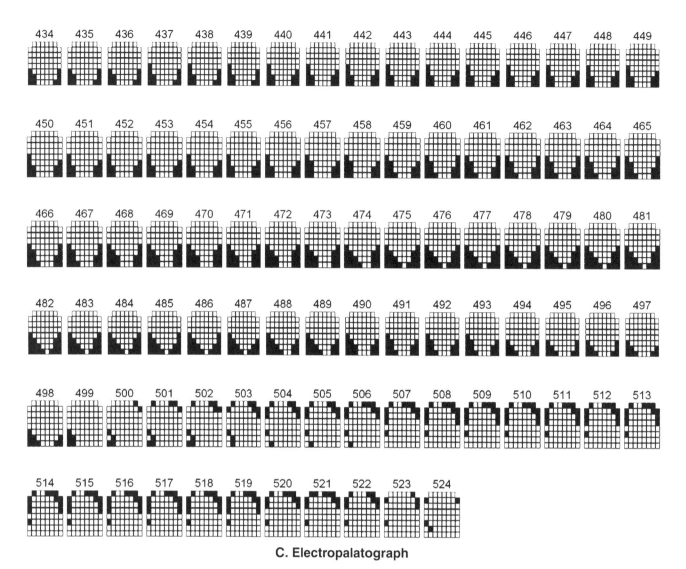

C. Electropalatograph

Figure 23–3. *continued*

The transition from this low frequency domain into the high formant frequencies of vowel /i/ is sharp—almost 90 degrees. The center frequency for the second formant is approximately 2250 Hz and third formant 3250 Hz. As is well known for the vowel /i/, the distance between first and second formant frequencies is substantially greater than the almost nonexistant distance between the frequencies of the second and third formant. /l/ is a vowel-like sonorant consonant with low frequency energy. Thus, the second and third formants of vowel /i/ by necessity make abrupt tran-sitions—almost at 90 degrees again—to the second formant of the vowel-like consonant /l/. In this spectrogram, /l/ behaves like a vowel with clear indication of a formantlike structure because it is influenced by the coarticulation effect of the vowel /i/.

Electropalatograph: /vil/ "veal"

Figure 23-3C presents tongue/palate contact for the word "veal" in the phase "I see a veal again." The 89 EPG frames took 0.452 seconds to produce. The initial

/v/ extends from frames 434 to 458, the vowel /i/ extends from 459 to 493 and the final /l/ extends from 507 to 521. The simultaneous sound spectrogram and waveform (not shown in Figure 23–3C) were used to identify the boundaries between /v/ and /i/ as there was no detectable difference at this point on the EPG palate trace. The EPG frames 493 to 506 represent a period of coarticulatory transition between the vowel and the /l/. The word-final /l/ predominantly has contact with the tongue along the alveolar ridge and there also may be some contact with the front teeth.

INTRA- AND INTERSPEAKER VARIABILITY FOR /l/

Electropalatographic images enable consideration of interspeaker variability. Variability productions of /l/ by typical speakers of English, typical speakers of languages other than English, and between speakers with differing types of speech impairment are considered.

Intra- and Interspeaker Variability in the Production of /l/ by Eight Typical English-Speaking Adults

Four typical adult males (M1–M4) and four typical adult females (F1–F4) produced nonsense syllables containing /l/ three times. The nonsense syllables were created with /l/ in syllable-initial and syllable-final positions in vowel contexts taken at the extremes of the vowel quadrilateral. In order to demonstrate both inter- and intraspeaker variability the maximum contact frame for the second production of each nonsense syllable for each speaker is provided in Figure 23–4. The influence of word position is very evident in the production of /l/ with more tongue/palate contact for word-initial than word-final sounds.

Some speakers of Australian English vowelize /l/ to /ʊ/ in word-final position (Horvath, 1985). M4, who was described as having broad Australian accent may have produced the vowel /ʊ/ instead of /l/ in words such as "deal" /dil/. This could explain why M4's productions of some words only had contact with the back of the palate.

Cumulative EPG patterns for /l/ were generated from maximum contact frames for each of the eight typical adults described above. Each electrode on a cumulative maximum contact display has a number, corresponding to the percentage of contact over many productions. The darker the shading, the more contact. Figure 23–5 shows that each speaker's cumulative maximum contact display is centred around the alveolar ridge. Speaker M3 had no contact on the posterior three rows of the palate. Speakers M2 and M3 had limited contact at the posterior lateral margins of the palate. In contrast, speakers M4 and F4 had extensive contact along the lateral margins of the palate during production of exactly the same words containing /l/.

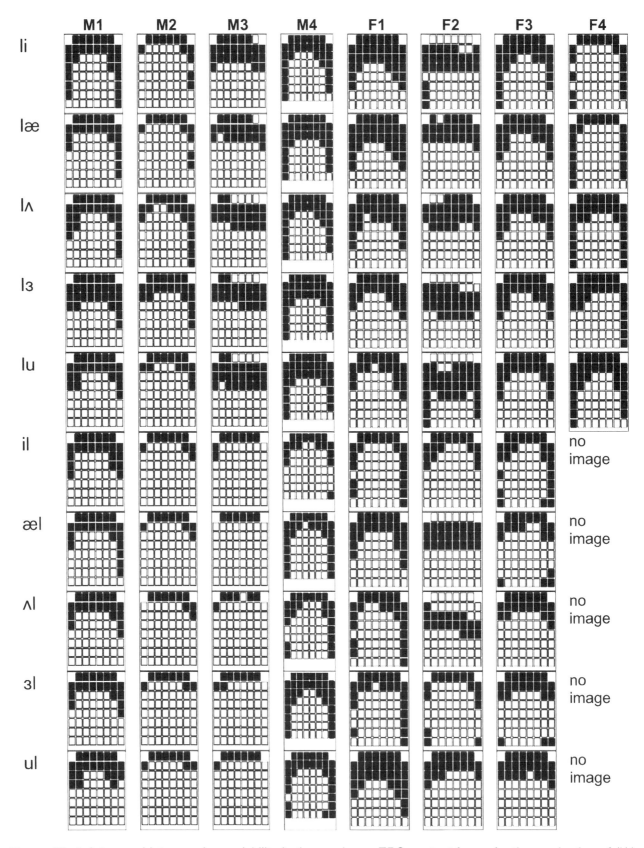

Figure 23–4. Intra- and interspeaker variability in the maximum EPG contact frame for the production of /l/ by eight typical English-speaking adults. *continues*

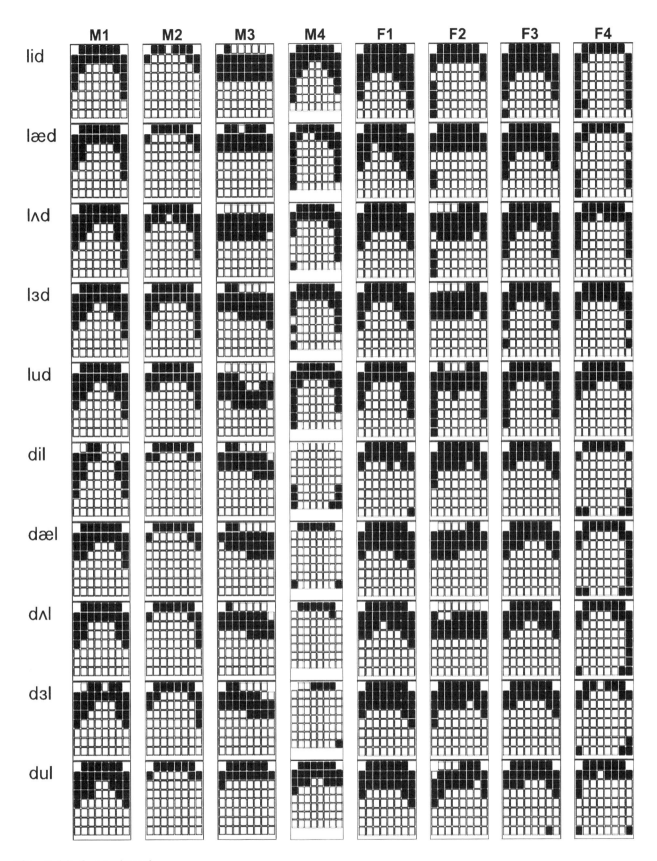

Figure 23–4. *continued*

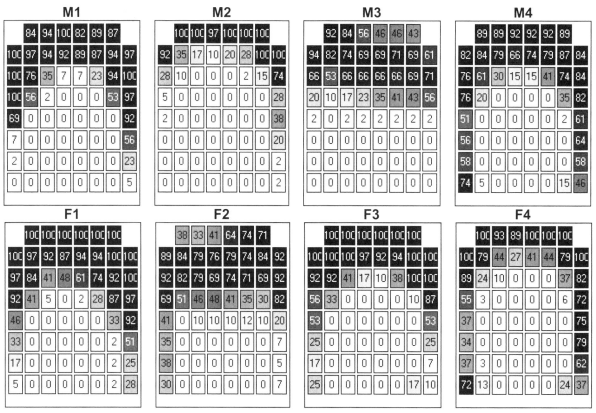

Note. F3 had one electrode in the third row that incorrectly recorded activation

Figure 23–5. Cumulative EPG frames demonstrating intra- and interspeaker variability for the production of /l/ by eight typical English-speaking adults.

Interspeaker Variability in the Production of /l/ by Other English-Speaking Adults

Australian English-Speaking Adults

McAuliffe, Ward, and Murdoch (2006a) described the speech of fifteen typical Australian-English speaking people in order to provide a comparison with the speech of people with Parkinson's disease. The typical speakers were divided into two groups. The seven aged controls were males and were aged between 50 and 79 years (mean = 67.71). Seven of the young controls were female and the eighth was male. The young control group was aged between 23 to 31 years (mean = 25.63). Figure 23-6 demonstrates two cumulative maximum contact EPG frames for productions of /l/ in the contexts /li/ and /la/. The participants were asked to produce these words in a sentence " I saw a _____ today" 10 times. In Figure 23-6, a black square indicates that that electrode was contacted at least 67% of the time. McAuliffe et al. found that there was no significant difference in the amount of tongue/palate contact between the aged and young control groups for the production of /l/.

Cheng, Murdoch, Goozée, and Scott (2007) conducted a study to describe typical speech production for 12 Australian English-speaking adults. The six male and six female adult participants, aged between 23 and 38 years, produced /l/ in CV and CVC words that were embedded within a phrase. Each phrase was produced five times, resulting in 10 productions of /l/ per speaker. Figure 23-7 provides a cumulative maximum contact frame for the production of /l/ by the adults. In Figure 23-7, a black square indicates that

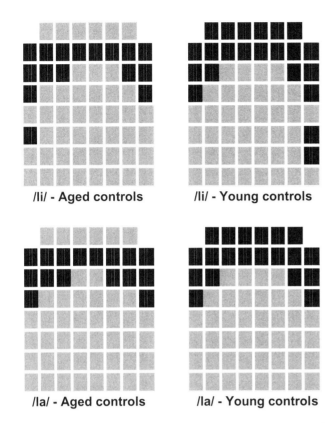

/li/ - Aged controls   /li/ - Young controls

/la/ - Aged controls   /la/ - Young controls

Figure 23–6. Cumulative maximum contact EPG frames for the production of /l/ by 15 typical Australian English-speaking adults (adapted from McAuliffe et al., 2006, Figure 1, p. 8).

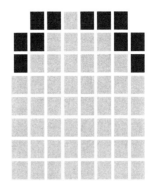

Figure 23–7. Cumulative maximum contact EPG frames for the production of /l/ by 12 typical Australian English-speaking adults (adapted from Cheng et al., 2007, Figure 1, p. 380).

that electrode was contacted at least 67% of the time. Although it appears that there may be a central groove in this image, the unshaded electrode on the first row was contacted by the participants 58% of the time.

Interspeaker Variability in the Production of /l/ by English-Speaking Children

Australian English-Speaking Children

Cheng et al. (2007) also described typical speech production for 36 children. There were six males and six females in each of the following age groups: 6 to 7 years, 8 to 11 years, and 12 to 17 years. Like the adults, the children produced /l/ in CV and CVC words that were embedded within a phrase. Each phrase was produced

five times, resulting in 10 productions of /l/ per speaker. Figure 23-8 provides a cumulative maximum contact frame for the production of /l/ by the children. In Figure 23-8, a black square indicates that that electrode was contacted at least 67% of the time. Cheng et al. described the maturation of the speech motor system as nonlinear and nonuniform.

Interspeaker Variability in the Production of /l/ by Adults Who Speak Languages Other Than English

Catalan-Speaking Adults

Recasens (2004) described the production of /l/ by 15 speakers of Catalan. There were five speakers for each of the following Catalan dialects: Mallorquí, Eastern Catalan, and Valencià. Recasans described the first two dialects as having a clear /l/; that is, "more [i] - like" and the third dialect as having a dark /l/; that is "more [u]-like" (Recasans, 2004, p. 593). Each speaker produced /l/ in meaningful words containing /ili/ and /ala/. Each word was produced seven times by each speaker. The cumulative EPG frames for each speaker for the seven words that contained /ili/ is shown in Figure 23-9. A black square indicates that that electrode was contacted at least 80% of the time (most other images in *Speech Sounds: A Pictorial Guide to*

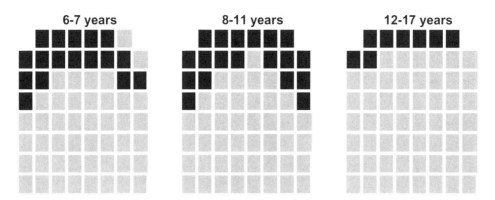

Figure 23–8. Cumulative maximum contact EPG frames for the production of /l/ by 36 typical Australian English-speaking children (adapted from Cheng et al., 2007, Figure 1, p. 380).

Typical and Atypical Speech use 67% contact). Comparing the images across the three dialects, reveals that the speakers of Mallorquí and Eastern Catalan (dark /l/) had less palatal contact across the four last rows of the palate than the speakers of Valencià (clear /l/) with the exception of speaker AR.

German-Speaking Adults

Recasens (2004) also described the production of /l/ by four speakers of German. Like Valèncian Catalan (above), Recasans described German as having a "dark [l]"; that is "more [u]-like" (Recasans, 2004, p. 593). Each speaker produced /l/ seven times in meaningful words containing /ili/ and /ala/. The cumulative EPG frames for each speaker for the seven words that contained /ili/ is shown in Figure 23–10. A black square indicates that that electrode was contacted at least 80% of the time. The German speakers had similar contact to the Valencià dialect (above), confirming its status as clear [l]. The German speakers generally had more contact across the palatal region (last four rows of the EPG) than for the speakers of English and the two Catalan dialects as described above, differentiating it from these dark [l] languages.

Greek-Speaking Adults

Nicolaidis (2004) described the speech of one typical Modern Standard Greek-speaking adult in order to provide comparative data for the speech of four Greek-speaking people with hearing impairment. Figure 23–11 demonstrates two cumulative maximum contact EPG frames for productions of /l/ in the contexts /ala/ and /ili/. The female participant was asked to produce these phoneme combinations ten times in a dysyllabic word of the form /pVlV/ within a carrier phrase. In Figure 23–11, a black square indicates that that electrode was contacted at least 60% of the time. This Greek speaker had more tongue/palate contact, particularly with the posterior region of the palate compared with the cumulative palates produced by English-speaking adults shown above again suggesting the status of Greek as using clear /l/.

Interspeaker Variability for /l/ Speakers with Impaired Speech

Adults with Parkinson's Disease

McAuliffe et al. (2006a) described the speech of nine people diagnosed with Parkinson's disease. Figure 23–12 demonstrates two cumulative maximum contact EPG frames for productions of /l/ in the contexts /li/ and /la/. The participants were asked to produce these words in a sentence " I saw a _____ today" 10 times. In Figure 23–12, a black square indicates that that electrode was contacted at least 67% of the time. McAuliffe et al. indicated that the people with Parkinson's disease had "reductions in the amplitude of lingual movement, or articulatory undershoot" (p. 16).

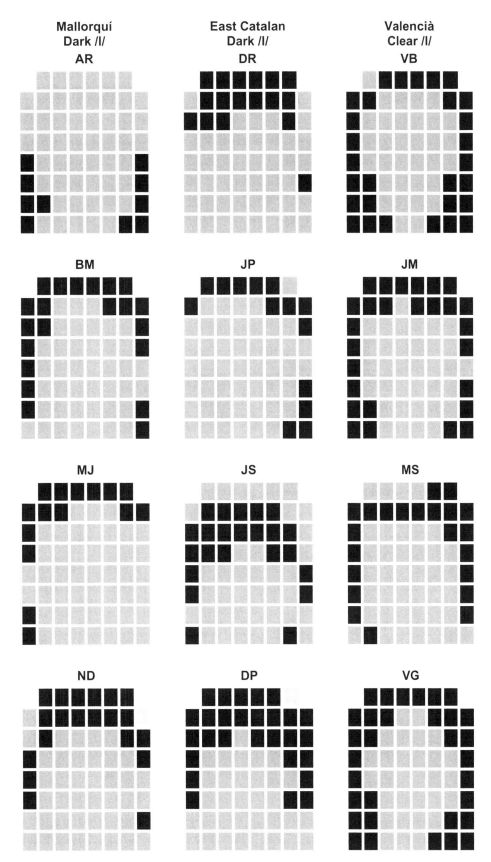

Figure 23–9. Cumulative maximum contact EPG frames for the production of /l/ by 15 Catalan-speaking adults from 3 different dialects (adapted from Recasens, 2004, Figure 1, p. 598). *continues*

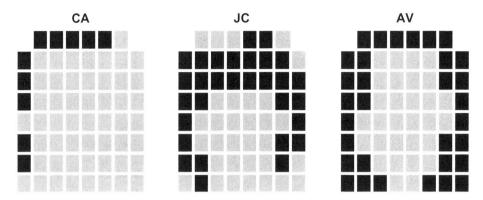

Figure 23–9. *continued*

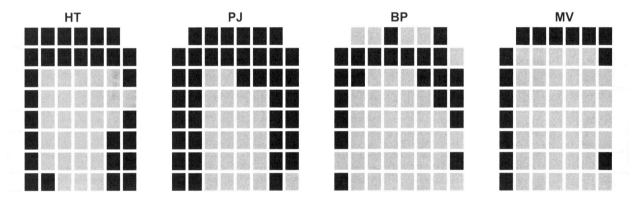

Figure 23–10. Cumulative maximum contact EPG frames for the production of /l/ by four typical German-speaking adults (HT, PJ, BP, MV) (adapted from Recasens, 2004, Figure 1, p. 598).

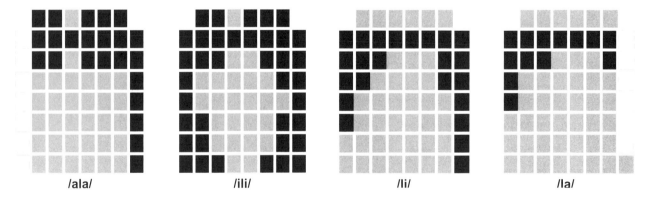

/ala/ /ili/ /li/ /la/

Figure 23–11. Cumulative maximum contact EPG frames for the production of /l/ by one typical Greek-speaking adult (adapted from Nicolaidis, 2004, Figure 1, p. 8).

Figure 23–12. Cumulative maximum contact EPG frames for the production of /l/ by nine English-speaking adults with Parkinson's disease (adapted from McAuliffe et al., 2006, Figure 1, p. 8).

Adults with Hearing Impairment

Nicolaidis (2004) described the speech of four adults (three females and one male) with hearing impairment aged between 23 to 26 years. Each spoke typical Modern Standard Greek. Each of the four people produced /l/ in the contexts /ala/ and /ili/ within the word form /pVlV/ within a carrier phrase. Each word was produced 10 times. Figure 23-13 demonstrates two cumulative maximum contact EPG frames for each speaker (HI1-HI4) for productions of /l/ in the two contexts /ala/ and /ili/. In Figure 23-13, a black square indicates that that electrode was contacted at least 60% of the time. The vowel context heavily influenced the amount of tongue/palate contact for /l/,

particularly for speakers HI2 and HI3. In fact, there was limited contact for these speakers in the context of /ili/, which is not typical of for people without speech impairment.

Children with Speech Impairment

Howard (2007) described the speech of six English-speaking children with speech impairment aged between 9;05 and 16;03 years. Her comprehensive paper examined the interplay between articulation and prosody. Within the paper, dynamic images of the prductions of words were presented. Figure 23-14 demonstrates maximum contact EPG frames for three speakers' productions of words containing /l/. Tara

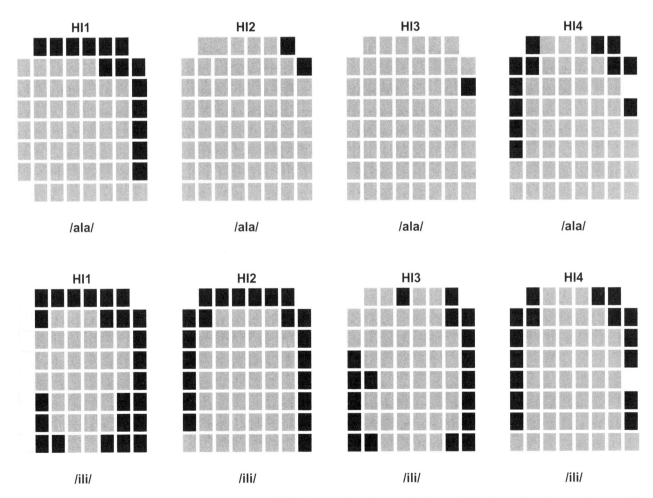

Figure 23–13. Cumulative maximum contact EPG frames for the production of /l/ by four Greek-speaking adults with hearing impairment (adapted from Nicolaidis, 2004, Figure 1, p. 8).

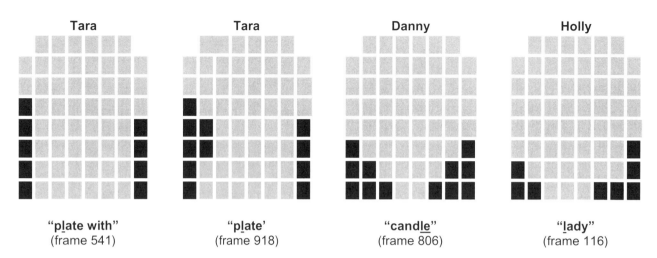

Figure 23–14. Maximum contact EPG frames during the production of words containing /l/ produced by three English-speaking children with speech impairment (adapted from Howard, 2007, Figure 2, p. 25, Figure 4, p. 27, Figure 8, p. 30).

(aged 14;3) was a bilingual English-Punjabi speaker who had a deflected nasal septum and her uvula attached at the left side at birth. Luke (aged 10;0) had no associated medical conditions. Holly (aged 9;06) had Worster-Drought syndrome. Each produced /l/ with velar tongue/palate contact as evident in Figure 23-14. Velar contact is not typical for the production of /l/. Typical productions have alveolar contact.

Chapter 24

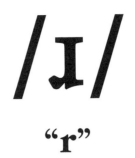

"r"

The consonant /ɹ/ is a voiced alveolar approximant.

Place of articulation: alveolar

Advancement: front

Voicing: voiced

Labiality: labial

Sonorancy: sonorant

Continuancy: —

Sibilancy: nonsibilant

Nasality: nonnasal (oral)

The articulation of /ɹ/ is probably the most variable of consonants (Shriberg & Kent, 2003), with the two major articulations being described as retroflexed (tongue tip up and slightly back) or bunched (either in the middle or front of the mouth). Lip rounding also is present in some speakers' articulations of /ɹ/ (Shriberg & Kent, 2003).

In order to avoid confusion between the trilled /r/ found in languages such as Spanish, and the voiced alveolar approximant found in languages such as English, the IPA symbol /ɹ/ is used within this text. However, readers may be interested to note that Ladefoged (2001, p. 176) states "When you are not trying to make such precise distinctions [between trilled and alveolar r], the IPA recommends that you use the simplest possible phonetic symbol, which in this case is r, even for transcribing a BBC English pronunciation. Then at the end of the transcript, you should simply say r = ɹ."

STATIC IMAGES OF THE ARTICULATORY CHARACTERISTICS OF /ɹ/

The static images of /ɹ/ are presented via a photograph, schematic diagram, ultrasound, and electropalatograph images (Figure 24–1).

Photograph

In this photograph (Figure 24–1A), the lips and teeth are slightly open. The lips are not rounded.

Schematic Diagram

In the lateral view of the production of the consonant /ɹ/ (Figure 24–1B), the tongue does not contact the middle of the palate. This schematic view does not demonstrate the contact along the posterior lateral margins of the palate. The voicing of this consonant is symbolically represented at the source (the vocal folds) by a plus sign.

Ultrasound

The bright white line on the ultrasound image in Figure 24–1C shows the air above the tongue surface during production of /ɹ/. The tongue tip is on the right and is raised toward the alveolar ridge. Approximately 1 cm of the tongue tip is obscured from view because of the acoustic shadow of the jaw (Stone, 2005). The bunched nature of this production of /ɹ/ is suggested by this image with the back of the tongue moved forward in the oral cavity. Diagonal muscle fibers can be seen below the surface of the tongue and an air shadow can be seen above the tongue.

Electropalatograph (EPG)

There is limited tongue/palate contact in the EPG image of /ɹ/ displayed in Figure 24–1D. The tongue is contacted along the posterior lateral margins of the palate. The speaker did not use retroflexed /ɹ/ as she spoke Australian English. However, an EPG display from a speaker of American English should be similar. Dagenais, Lorendo, and McCutcheon (1994, p. 235) described the production of /ɹ/ by speakers of American English in the following way: "Contact patterns for /r/ showed linguapalatal contact along the posterior regions of the alveolar process."

The cumulative frame in Figure 24–1E was also created by eight speakers of Australian English. Again, contact is concentrated at the posterior lateral margins of the palate.

DYNAMIC IMAGES OF THE ARTICULATORY AND ACOUSTIC CHARACTERISTICS OF /ɹ/

To obtain a comprehensive view of the production of this consonant, the dynamic aspects of the production of /ɹ/ are shown in EPG images (Figure 24–2).

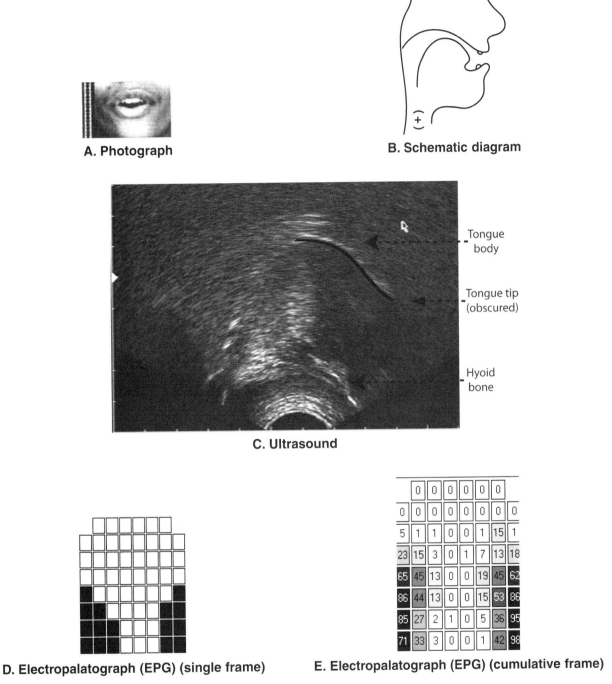

A. Photograph

B. Schematic diagram

Tongue body

Tongue tip (obscured)

Hyoid bone

C. Ultrasound

D. Electropalatograph (EPG) (single frame)

E. Electropalatograph (EPG) (cumulative frame)

Figure 24–1. Static images of the articulatory characteristics of /ɹ/.

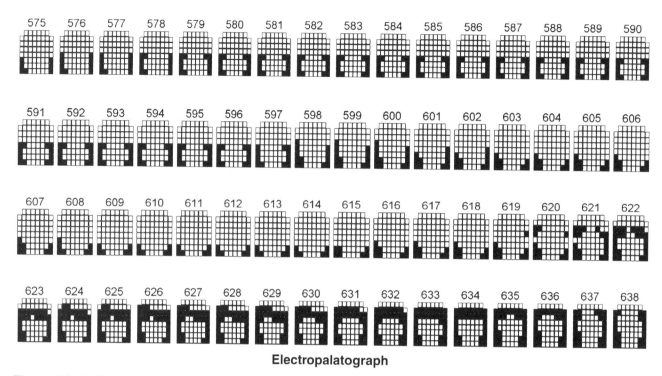

Electropalatograph

Figure 24–2. Dynamic images of /ɹ/ in the word-initial context: "round."

/ɹ/ in the Word-Initial Context: "round"

Electropalatograph: /ɹaʊnd/ "round"

Figure 24-2 presents 56 EPG frames for the production of "round." The initial /ɹ/ extends from frames 579 to 597. The /ɹ/ is characterized by contact along the posterior lateral margins of the palate. The diphthong extends from 598 to 623 with evidence of coarticulation at the points of juncture. The final consonant cluster /nd/ extends from frames 623 to 636.

INTRA- AND INTERSPEAKER VARIABILITY FOR /ɹ/

Variability between images created by speakers of Australian and American English is considered.

Intra- and Interspeaker Variability in the Production of /ɹ/ by Eight Typical English-Speaking Adults

Eight typical Australian adults, four males (M1–M4) and four females (F1–F4) produced nonsense syllables containing /ɹ/ three times in syllable-initial positions in five vowel contexts. Syllable-final /ɹ/ does not occur in Australian English, so was not sampled.

Maximum Contact Frames for Eight Typical English-Speaking Adults

In order to demonstrate both inter- and intraspeaker variability the maximum contact frame for the second production of each nonsense syllable for each speaker is provided in Figure 24-3. In almost each case few electrodes are contacted. Contact occurs at the lateral margins towards the palatal and velar sections of the

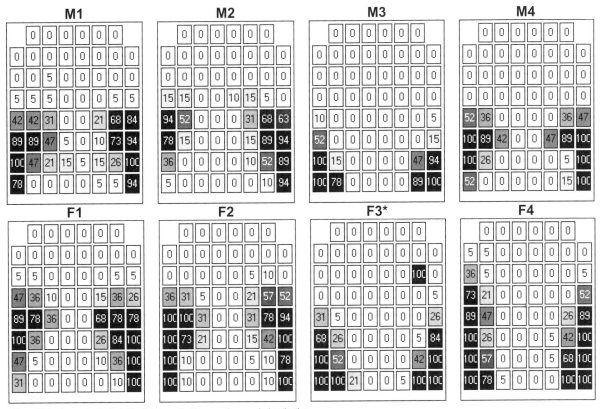

*Note: F3 had one electrode in the third row that incorrectly recorded activation.

Figure 24–3. Intra- and interspeaker variability in the maximum EPG contact frame for the production of /ɹ/ by eight typical English-speaking adults.

palate. There was never contact on the two alveolar rows of the palate; this was true for all speakers and all words. For some speakers, such as M3 and M4, contact only occurred in the posterior half of the palate.

Cumulative EPG Frames for Eight Typical English-Speaking Adults

Cumulative EPG patterns for /ɹ/ were generated from 20 maximum contact frames for each of the eight typical Australian English adults described above. Each electrode on a cumulative maximum contact display has a number, corresponding to the percentage of contact over the 20 productions. The darker the shading, the more contact. In Figure 24-4 each speaker's cumulative maximum contact display shows concentration along the posterior margins of the palate.

Interspeaker Variability in the Production of /ɹ/ by Other English-Speaking Adults

American English

Dagenais Lorendo, et al. (1994) described the production of /ɹ/ produced by American speakers using the 96 electrode palatometer. They indicated "The anterior limit of this contact appeared to be strongly context dependent . . . the length of contacts on both right and left sides are the smallest in the /a/ context. The lengths of contact are similar for the /i/ and /u/ contexts" (p. 235). This description is comparable to the Australian English examples shown above.

Schmidt (2007) also described an EPG image of the production of /ɹ/ by one speaker of American English (Figure 24-5) in the following way: "Note the

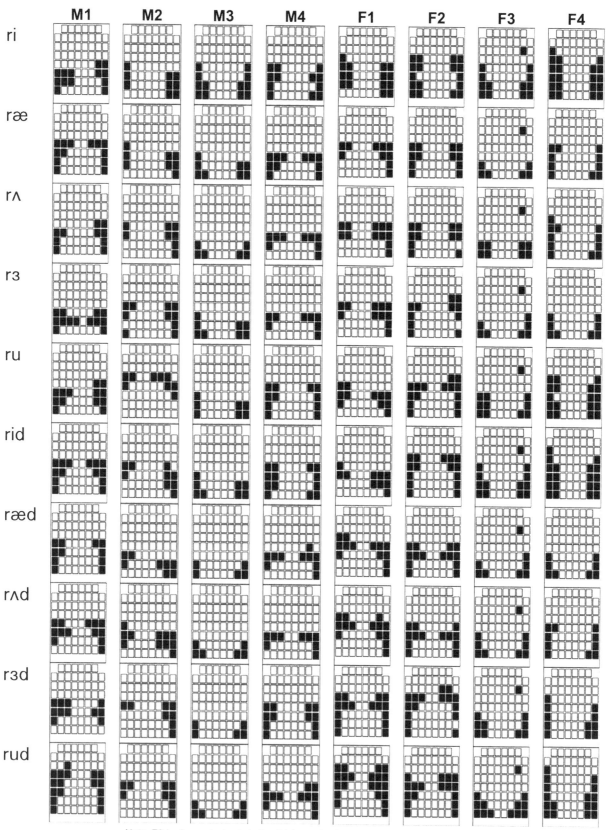

Note. F3 had one electrode in the third row that incorrectly recorded activation

Figure 24–4. Cumulative EPG frames demonstrating intra- and interspeaker variability for the production of /ɹ/ by eight typical English-speaking adults.

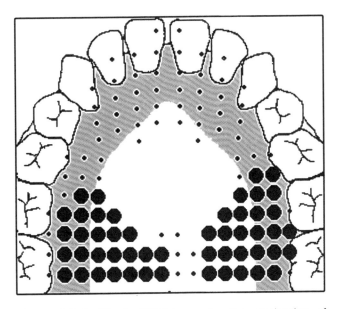

Figure 24–5. Single EPG frame for the production of /ɹ/ by one American English-speaking adult using the Logometrix system (reprinted with permission from Schmidt, 2007, Figure 5, p. 77).

broad lateral tongue contact along the posterior hard palate and the lack of contact centrally." (p. 77). Figure 24-5 captures the production of /ur/ at the point of maximum contact by a typical speaker of American English. The Reading WIN/EPG system used in *Speech Sounds: A Pictorial Guide to Typical and Atypical Speech* was not used by Schmidt; her image is from a Logometrix EPG system.

Chapter 25

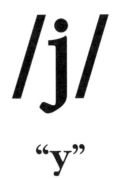

"y"

The consonant /j/ is a voiced palatal approximant.

Place of articulation: palatal

Advancement: back

Voicing: voiced

Labiality: nonlabial

Sonorancy: sonorant

Continuancy: —

Sibilancy: nonsibilant

Nasality: nonnasal (oral)

STATIC IMAGES OF THE ARTICULATORY CHARACTERISTICS OF /j/

The static images of /j/ are presented via a photograph, schematic diagram, ultrasound, and electropalatograph images (Figure 25–1).

Photograph

In this photograph (Figure 25-1A), the mouth is open and the tongue is slightly visible.

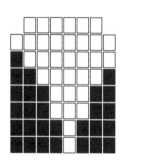

A. Photograph

B. Schematic diagram

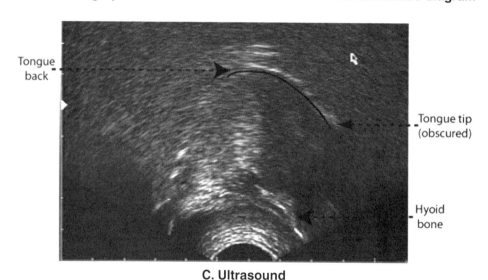

C. Ultrasound

D. Electropalatograph (EPG) (single frame)

E. Electropalatograph (EPG) (cumulative frame)

Figure 25–1. Static images of the articulatory characteristics of /j/.

Schematic Diagram

In the lateral view of the production of the consonant /j/ (Figure 25–1b), the tongue contacts the palatal region. The voicing of this consonant is symbolically represented at the source (the vocal folds) by a plus sign.

Ultrasound

Figure 25–1C presents a midsagittal ultrasound image of the tongue surface during production /j/. The white line above the tongue's surface is faint in this image. The tongue is high in the oral cavity and the tip is located toward the right of the image.

Electropalatograph (EPG)

The EPG image of /j/ (Figure 25–1D) has slightly more contact than for the vowel /i/ (Chapter 26). The EPG image of /j/ is characterized by broad contact along the lateral and velar margins of the palate, with absence of contact along the midline. The cumulative image in Figure 25–1E represents contact during multiple productions of words commencing with /j/ by eight typical speakers. The darker the shading the more often that part of the palate was contacted by the tongue. This cumulative image has a similar contact to Figure 25–1D.

INTRA- AND INTERSPEAKER VARIABILITY FOR /j/

Electropalatographic images enable consideration of intra- and interspeaker variability.

Intra- and Interspeaker Variability in the Production of /j/ by Eight Typical English-Speaking Adults

Four typical adult males (M1–M4) and four typical adult females (F1–F4) produced nonsense syllables containing /j/ three times. The nonsense syllables were created with /j/ in syllable-initial positions in vowel contexts taken at the extremes of the vowel quadrilateral.

Maximum Contact Frames for Eight Typical English-Speaking Adults

To demonstrate both inter- and intraspeaker variability in the production of /j/ the maximum contact frame for the second production of each nonsense syllable for each of the eight speakers is provided in Figure 25–2. For almost every production the speakers have broad contact along the lateral and velar margins of the palate with a midline gap.

Cumulative EPG Frames for Eight Typical English-Speaking Adults

Cumulative EPG patterns for /j/ were generated from maximum contact frames for each of the eight typical adults described above. Each electrode on a cumulative maximum contact display has a number, corresponding to the percentage of contact over the multiple productions (Figure 25–3). The darker the shading, the more contact. In Figure 25–3 each speaker's cumulative maximum contact display is focused around the lateral and velar regions of the palate. M2's contacts were more asymmetric than productions by the other speakers; however, he still had lateral contact along both sides of the palate.

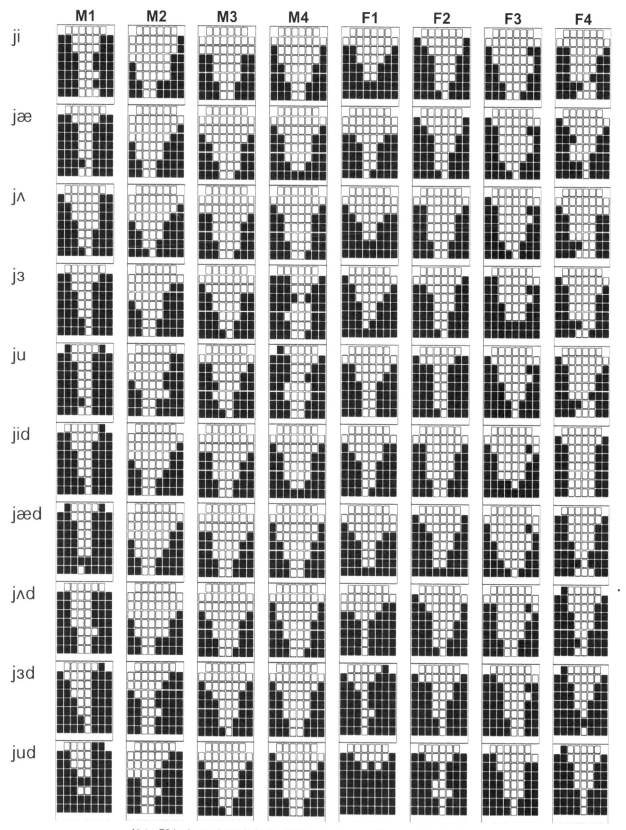

Note. F3 had one electrode in the third row that incorrectly recorded activation

Figure 25–2. Intra- and interspeaker variability in the maximum EPG contact frame for the production of /j/ by eight typical English-speaking adults.

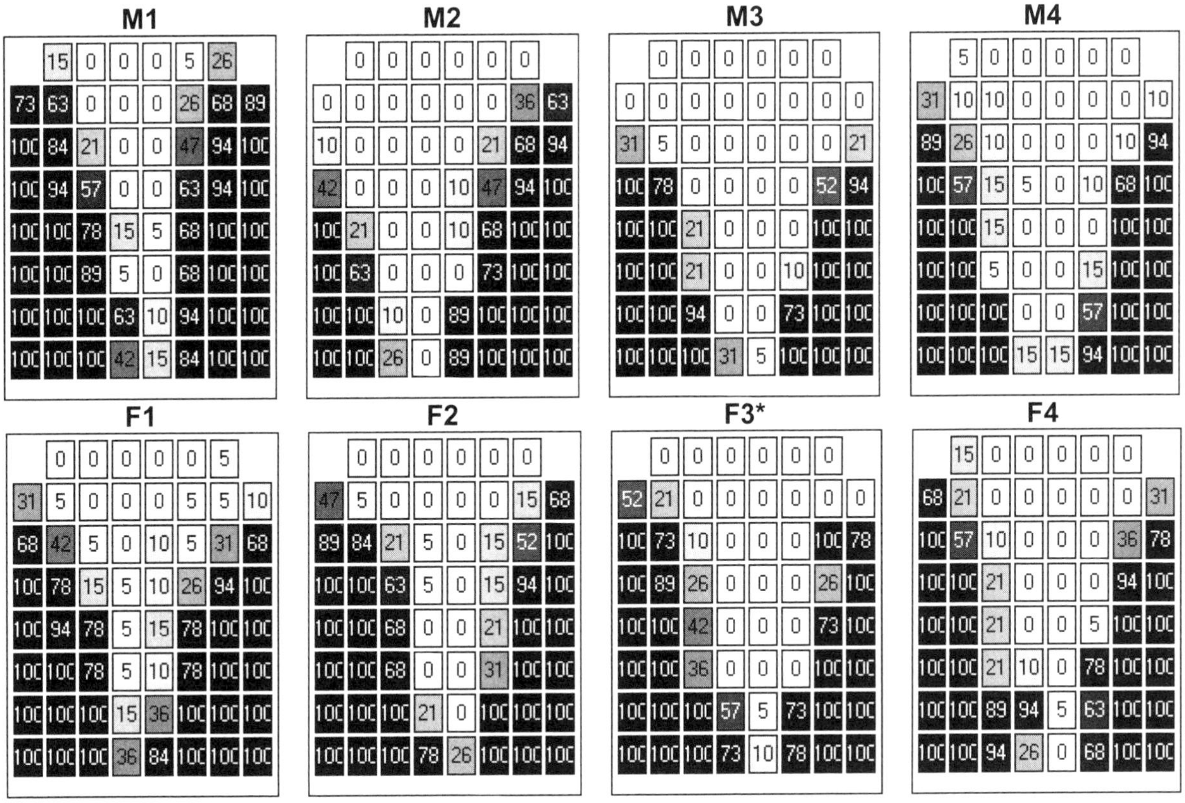

*One electrode on the third row of F3's EPG palate incorrectly intermittently recorded contact.

Figure 25–3. Cumulative EPG frames demonstrating intra- and interspeaker variability for the production of /j/ by eight typical English-speaking adults.

Chapter 26

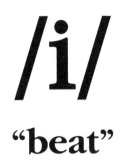

"beat"

The vowel /i/ is described as high, front, tense, and unrounded.

Advancement: front

Height: high

Tenseness: tense

Roundness: unrounded

STATIC IMAGES OF /i/

Figure 26-1 presents static images of the articulatory and acoustic characteristics of /i/.

Photograph

The photograph of /i/ in Figure 26-1A has been taken from the continuous production of the sustained vowel /i/ to show the most open state of this vowel.

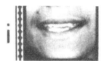

A. Photograph

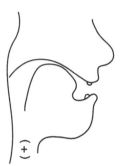

B. Schematic diagram

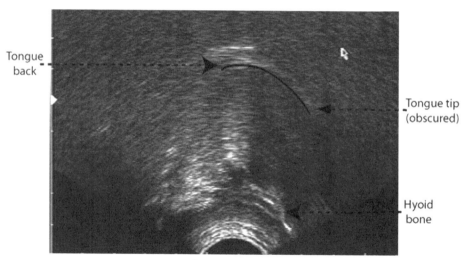

C. Ultrasound

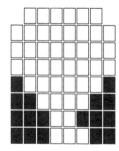

D. Electropalatograph (EPG) (single frame)

Figure 26–1. Static images of the articulatory characteristics of /i/.

The photograph demonstrates that the lip position for the vowel /i/ is the least round, widest, and least open of all the vowels of English. Typically, the teeth are visible in the production of /i/.

Schematic Diagram

The schematic drawing of the vowel /i/ tongue position (Figure 26–1B) is shown to assume a very high-front tongue position within the oral cavity. The vocal folds are the source for the production of vowel speech sounds. Therefore, all vowel diagrams will have the symbol (+) in the vicinity of the vocal folds to denote vocal fold vibration.

Ultrasound

Figure 26–1C shows the tongue in an ultrasound image during production of the vowel /i/. The surface of the tongue is difficult to see during production of sounds that have steeply sloping tongue shapes such as the high vowels and velars (Stone, 2005). The bulk of the tongue can be seen as an inverted U shape in the middle of the image and the tip is pointing toward the floor of the mouth at the right of the image. The diagonal lines below the surface of the tongue are the muscle fibers.

Electropalatograph (EPG)

Tongue/palate contact is indicated by the dark shading (Figure 26–1D). Contact is extended along the lower back quadrants (margins) of the palate during production of /i/. The vowels /i/ and /ɪ/ (Chapter 27) have the greatest amount of tongue/palate contact for any English vowel owing to their high front status. For example, Stone, Faber, Raphael, and Shawker (1992), reported greater tongue/palate contact occurred for consonants preceding /i/ than for those preceding /ɛ/, /ɑ/ or /o/. Similarly, Gibbon, Smeaton-Ewins, and Crampin (2005) indicated that /i/ had the most contact, followed by /ʉ/, /ɑ/, /o/ and finally, /ɔ/ with the least.

DYNAMIC IMAGES OF /i/

In order to obtain a comprehensive view of the production of this vowel, the dynamic aspects of the production of /i/ are shown in a filmstrip, spectrogram, and EPG frames (Figure 26–2).

/i/ in Within-Word Context: "beat"

Filmstrip: /bit/ "beat"

The criterion phoneme /i/ is at the medial position of the word /bit/ "beat." The lip closure for the initial phoneme /b/ can be seen in the first five frames (Figure 26–2A). In frame 6, the lips begin to relax for the opening into the vowel. The lip position for the vowel /i/ is the least round, widest, and least open of all of the vowels of English. That /i/ is a tense vowel is well represented in the production of the preceding consonant /b/. A comparison of Chapters 26 and 27 reveals that the lip closure for /b/ in the context of the tense vowel /i/ is more intense than the lip closure for /b/ in the context of the lax vowel /ɪ/.

Sound Spectrogram: /bit/ "beat"

Here (Figure 26–2B) the vowel /i/ is presented in the medial position in the word /bit/ "beat." The first formant is centered at approximately 250 Hz, the second formant at approximately 2750 Hz. The stressed nature of this vowel in English is revealed by its long duration. The duration of the vowel in this example is 300 msec. The rising transition of the second formant signals the low-frequency characteristic of the preceding consonant, which in this case is a labial consonant. It can be seen from comparing this vowel /i/ to the vowel /ɪ/ in Chapter 27 that a wider gap exists between the F1 and F2 for the vowel /i/ than for the vowel /ɪ/ and, importantly, the vowel /i/ has a considerably longer duration than the vowel /ɪ/.

Electropalatograph: /bit/ "beat"

The dynamic series of EPG palates for the production of the word "beat" is presented in Figure 26–2C.

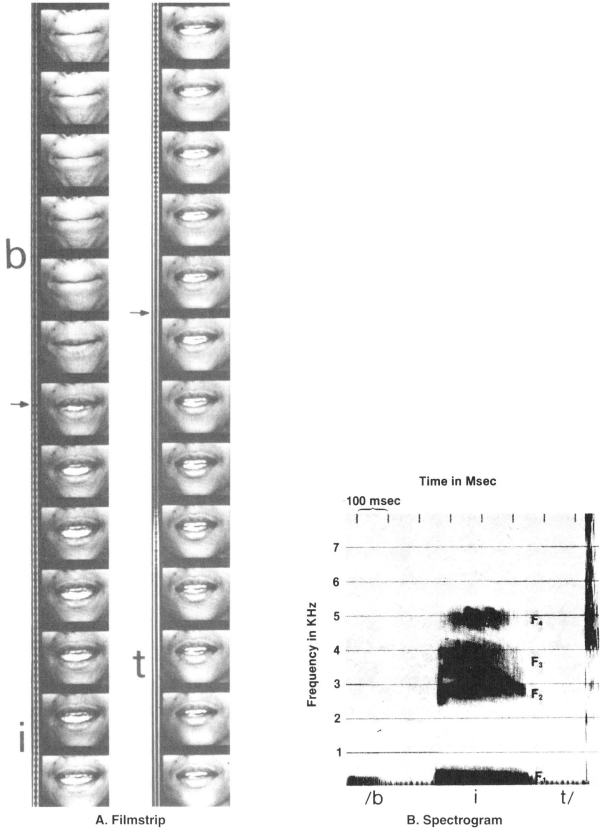

A. Filmstrip

B. Spectrogram

Figure 26–2. Dynamic images of /i/ in the within-word context: "beat." *continues*

276

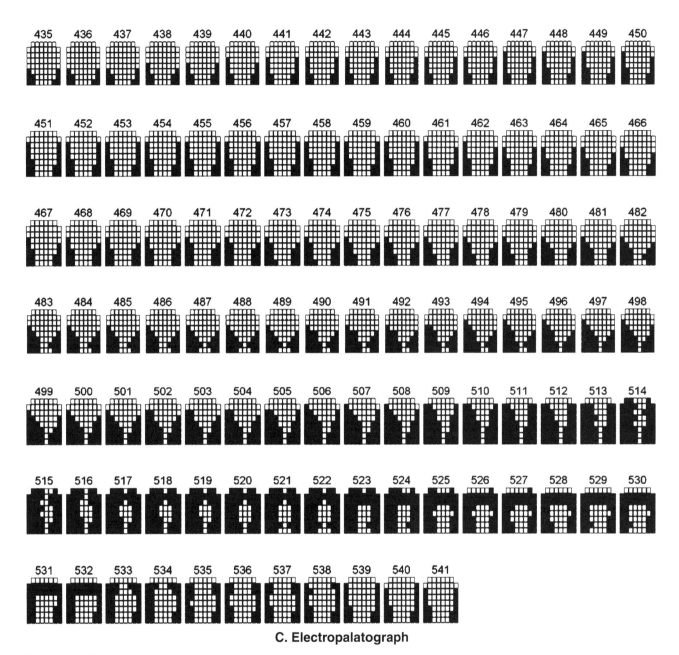

C. Electropalatograph

Figure 26–2. *continued*

The word "beat" was extracted from the sentence "I see a beat again." The /b/ extends from 435 to 469. The vowel /i/ extends from frames 470 to 516 and has more than anticipated tongue/palate contact, particularly due to the coarticulatory influence of the /t/. The juncture between the /b/ and /i/ was determined by using simultaneous EPG, sound spectrogram, wave-

form and audio data (not shown in Figure 26-2C). The horseshoe shape for the final /t/ is depicted in frames 517 to 532. Again, there is more tongue/palate contact in this production of /t/ than is typically found (see Chapter 4). However, this production of the word "beat" was judged as typical by a speech-language pathologist.

INTERSPEAKER VARIABILITY IN THE PRODUCTION OF /i/

Electropalatography enables consideration of inter-speaker variability between speakers of English and by speakers with speech impairment.

Scottish English-Speaking Adults

Gibbon, Smeaton-Ewins, and Crampin (2005) described the speech of five typical Scottish-English speaking people to provide a comparison with the speech of 18 children with cleft palate. The participants were asked to produce four designated words containing five different vowels. Figure 26–3 demonstrates the cumulative maximum contact EPG frames for four productions of /i/ spoken by the five adults. In Figure 26–3, a black square indicates that that electrode was

contacted at least 67% of the time. As mentioned above, /i/ had more contact than the four other vowels that were studied.

Scottish English-Speaking Children with Repaired Cleft Lip and Palate

Gibbon et al. (2005) described the speech of 18 Scottish-English-speaking children with repaired cleft lip and palate. The children produced four designated words containing five different vowels. Figure 26–4 demonstrates the cumulative maximum contact EPG frames for four productions of /i/ spoken by one child (participant 3) who had a unilateral cleft lip and palate. In Figure 26–4, a black square indicates that that electrode was contacted at least 67% of the time. Participant 3 produced the other vowels with tongue/palate contact that was similar to the adult target; however, /i/ had more tongue/palate contact than was typical.

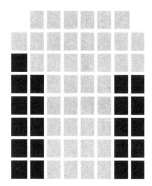

Figure 26–3. Cumulative EPG frame for the production of /i/ by five English-speaking adults (adapted from Gibbon et al., 2005, Figure 3, p. 188).

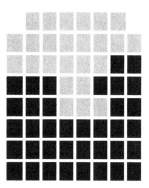

Figure 26–4. Cumulative EPG frame for the production of /i/ by one Scottish English-speaking child with a repaired unilateral cleft lip and palate (adapted from Gibbon et al., 2005, Figure 4, p. 189).

Chapter 27

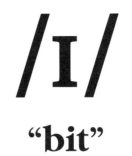

"bit"

The vowel /ɪ/ is described as high, front, lax, and unrounded.

Advancement: front

Height: high

Tenseness: lax

Roundness: unrounded

STATIC IMAGES OF /ɪ/

Figure 27-1 presents static images of the articulatory and acoustic characteristics of /ɪ/.

Photograph

In this photograph (Figure 27-1A) the lips are open, a characteristic of the vowel /ɪ/. The lips are slightly more open and slightly more rounded for the vowel /ɪ/ than for the vowel /i/.

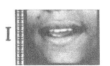

A. Photograph

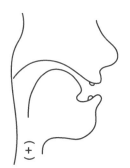

B. Schematic diagram

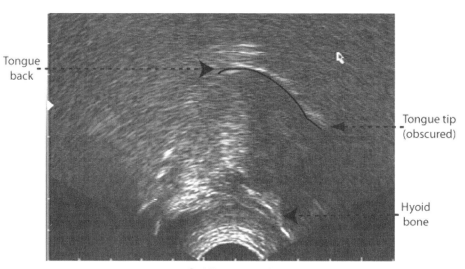

Tongue back

Tongue tip (obscured)

Hyoid bone

C. Ultrasound

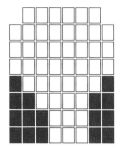

D. Electropalatograph (EPG) (single frame)

Figure 27–1. Static images of the articulatory characteristics of /ɪ/.

Schematic Diagram

The lateral view of the tongue position for the vowel /ɪ/ is shown in Figure 27–1B. The tongue assumes a high-front position for the production of the vowel /ɪ/. In both the height and front aspects, the vowel /ɪ/ assumes a less high and slightly less front position than the vowel /i/ (Chapter 26).

Ultrasound

Figure 27–1C shows the surface of the tongue displayed via ultrasound during production of the vowel /ɪ/. Stone (2005) suggests that the surface of the tongue is difficult to see during production of sounds that have steeply sloping tongue shapes such as the high vowels and velars. In Figure 27–1C, the bulk of the tongue is an inverted U shape in the middle of the image and the tip is pointing toward the floor of the mouth at the right of the image. The diagonal lines below the surface of the tongue are the muscle fibers. The hyoid bone is the bright diagonal line in the lower right part of the image.

Electropalatograph (EPG)

Along with the vowel /i/ (Chapter 26), the vowel /ɪ/ has the greatest amount of tongue/palate contact for any English vowel owing to its high front status. Tongue/palate contact is indicated by the dark shading. Contact is extended along the lower back quadrants (margins) of the palate during production of /i/.

DYNAMIC IMAGES OF /ɪ/

In order to obtain a comprehensive view of the production of this vowel, the dynamic aspects of the production of /ɪ/ are shown in Figure 27–2 using a filmstrip, spectrogram, and EPG frames.

/ɪ/ in the Within-Word Context: "bit"

Filmstrip: /bɪt/ "bit"

The criterion vowel /ɪ/ is displayed in the filmstrip (Figure 27–2A) in the context of the consonants /b/ in the initial and /t/ in the final position. The 10th frame shows the beginning of lip opening for the production of the vowel /ɪ/. Frames 11 through 14 demonstrate the open status of the lips, which is characteristic of this vowel. The lips are slightly more open and slightly more rounded for the vowel /ɪ/ than for the vowel /i/ (Chapter 26).

Sound Spectrogram: /bɪt/ "bit"

The vowel /ɪ/ is presented in the medial position in this spectrogram (Figure 27–2B). This is primarily an unstressed vowel in English, which is indicated by the fairly short duration (about 100 msec). The first formant for this vowel is centered at approximately 375 Hz, the second at approximately 2200 Hz. The effect of the preceding and following consonants on this vowel is clear in the lack of any steady-state portion. The beginning portion of this vowel shows a rising transition for all formants—for F1, because of the voicing nature of the preceding consonant, and for F2, because of the labiality of the preceding consonant.

Electropalatograph: /bɪt/ "bit"

The dynamic series of EPG palates for the production of the word "bit" is presented in Figure 27–2C. The word "bit" was extracted from the sentence "I see a bit again." The /b/ extends from 433 to 468. The vowel /ɪ/ extends from frames 469 to 488 and consists of tongue contact concentrated towards the posterior lateral margins of the palate. The juncture between the /b/ and /ɪ/ was determined by using simultaneous EPG, sound spectrogram, waveform, and audio data (not shown in Figure 27–2C). The horseshoe shape for the final /t/ is depicted in frames 489 to 518. The final frames (459-462) correspond with the burst of frication following the /t/.

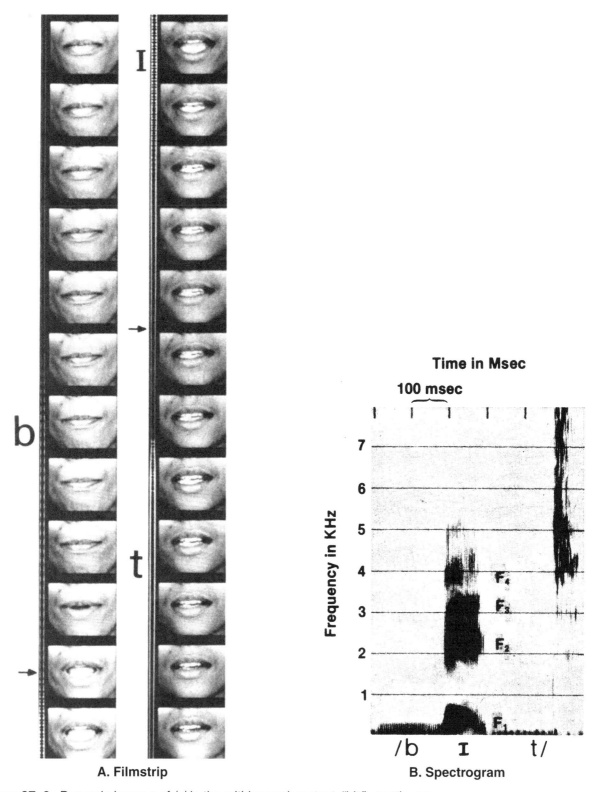

A. Filmstrip

B. Spectrogram

Figure 27–2. Dynamic images of /ɪ/ in the within-word context: "bit." *continues*

C. Electropalatograph

Figure 27–2. *continued*

INTERSPEAKER VARIABILITY IN THE PRODUCTION OF /ɪ/

Electropalatography enables consideration of interspeaker variability between speakers of English and speakers with speech impairment.

Scottish English-Speaking Adults

Gibbon, Smeaton-Ewins, and Crampin (2005) described the speech of five typical Scottish-English speaking adults to provide a comparison with the speech of 18 children with cleft palate. The participants were asked to produce four designated words containing five different vowels. Figure 27–3 demonstrates the cumulative maximum contact EPG frames for four productions of /ɪ/ spoken by the five adults. A black square indicates that that electrode was contacted at least 67% of the time.

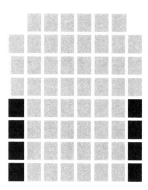

Figure 27–3. Cumulative EPG frame for the production of /ɪ/ by five English-speaking adults (adapted from Gibbon et al., 2005, Figure 3, p. 188).

Chapter 28

/ɛ/

"bed"

The vowel /ɛ/ is described as lower-mid, front, lax, and unrounded.

Advancement: front

Height: lower-mid

Tenseness: lax

Roundness: unrounded

STATIC IMAGES OF /ɛ/

Photograph

In this photograph (Figure 28–1A), the lips are spread and separated to produce the vowel /ɛ/.

Schematic Diagram

The tongue position for the vowel /ɛ/ is shown in this diagram (Figure 28–1B) without any coarticulatory influences. This is a front-mid vowel; the body of the tongue elevates to a mid-position in the front area of the oral cavity.

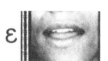

A. Photograph

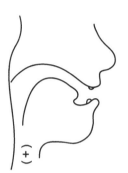

B. Schematic diagram

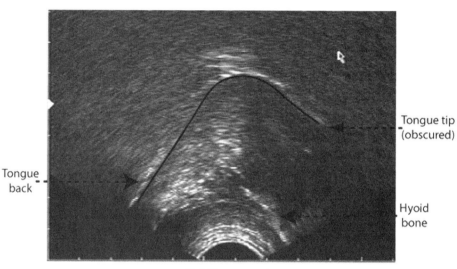

C. Ultrasound

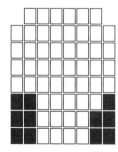

D. Electropalatograph (EPG) (single frame)

Figure 28–1. Static images of the articulatory characteristics of /ɛ/.

Ultrasound

The bright white line on the ultrasound image in Figure 28-1C highlights the tongue surface during production of /ɛ/. The tongue tip is on the right and is directed toward the floor of the mouth. The center of the tongue is raised in the oral cavity. An air shadow can be seen above the tongue and diagonal muscle fibers can be seen below the surface of the tongue.

Electropalatograph (EPG)

The EPG image (Figure 28-1D) presents tongue/palate contact along the lateral margins of the teeth during the production of /ɛ/.

DYNAMIC IMAGES OF /ɛ/

To obtain a comprehensive view of the production of this vowel, Figure 28-2 presents dynamic images of the articulatory and acoustic characteristics of /ɛ/ via a filmstrip, spectrogram, and EPG frames.

/ɛ/ in the Within-Word Context: "bed"

Filmstrip: /bɛd/ "bed"

The vowel /ɛ/ is shown in the context of the consonants /b/ and /d/ (Figure 28-2A). The lips begin to separate in the eighth frame, with the distance between the upper and lower lips being approximately 3 mm. This opening increases in the subsequent frames. The 9th, 10th, and 11th frames show openings of 4½, 5, and 5 mm, respectively. Beginning at the 12th frame, the distance between the upper and lower lips decreases. The distances in the 12th, 13th, and 14th frames are 4½, 4, and 3½ mm, respectively. A comparison of the lip movements involved in the production of this vowel with that of the vowel /i/ (Chapter 27) clearly shows greater lip opening for the vowel /ɛ/ than for /i/.

Sound Spectrogram: /bɛd/ "bed"

The vowel /ɛ/ appears in the word "bed" in the medial position (Figure 28-2B). The first formant of this vowel is approximated at 675 Hz and the second formant at 2,150 Hz. This is a stressed vowel in the English language and, consequently, its duration is long (approximately 280 msec). As can be predicted, the vowel formants are influenced by both the initial and final consonants. Because of the labial nature of the initial consonant, the F2 shows a rising transition, whereas, because of the front nature of the final consonant, the F2 shows a rising transition to the final consonant. The distance between F1 and F2 is relatively smaller for /ɛ/ than for the vowels /i/ (Chapter 26) or /i/ (Chapter 27).

Electropalatograph: /bɛd/ "bed"

The dynamic series of EPG palates for the production of the word "bed" is presented in Figure 28-2C. The word "bed" was extracted from the sentence "I see a bed again." The /b/ extends from 465 to 495. The vowel /ɛ/ extends from frames 496 to 519 and has limited tongue/palate contact, concentrated toward the velar region of the palate. The juncture between the /b/ and /ɛ/ was determined by using simultaneous EPG, sound spectrogram, waveform, and audio data (not shown in Figure 28-2C). The horseshoe shape for the final /d/ is depicted in frames 520 to 536.

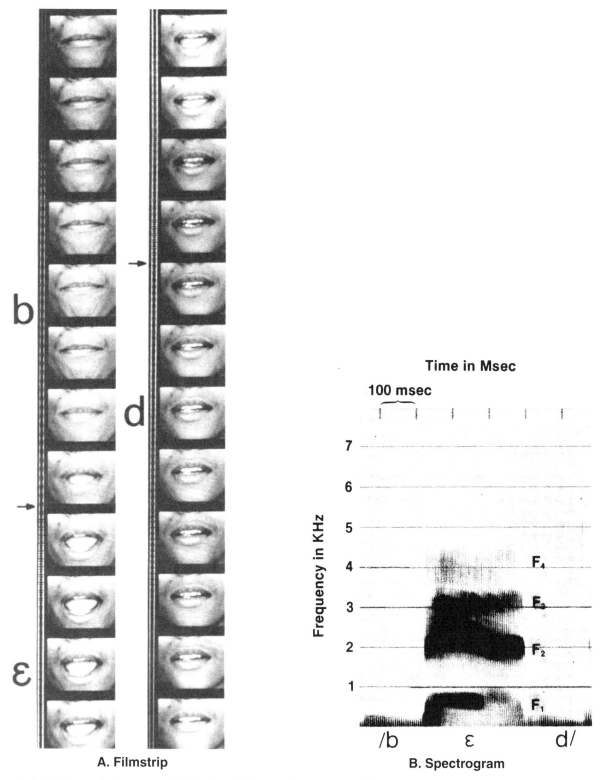

A. Filmstrip

B. Spectrogram

Figure 28–2. Dynamic images of /ɛ/ in the within-word context: "bed." *continues*

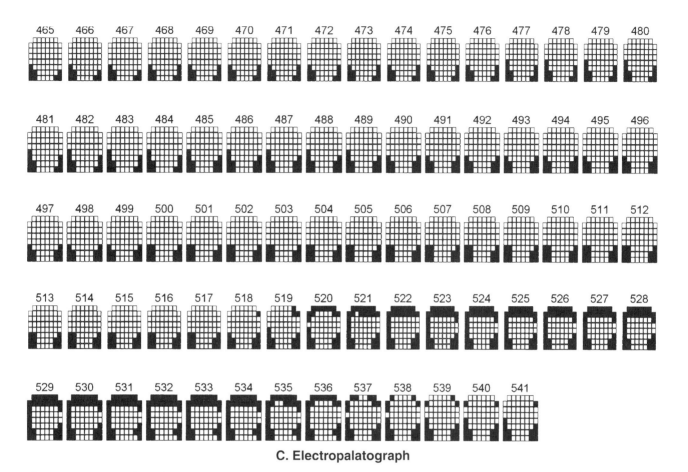

C. Electropalatograph

Figure 28–2. *continued*

Chapter 29

/æ/

"cat"

The vowel /æ/ is described as low, front, neutral and unrounded.

Advancement: front
Height: low
Tenseness: neutral
Roundness: unrounded

STATIC IMAGES OF /æ/

Figure 29-1 presents static images of the articulatory and acoustic characteristics of /æ/.

Photograph

This photograph (Figure 29-1A) has been taken from the sustained isolated production of the vowel /æ/. This frame presents the most open lip position for this vowel.

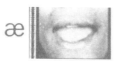

A. Photograph

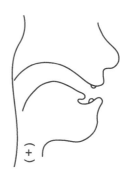

B. Schematic diagram

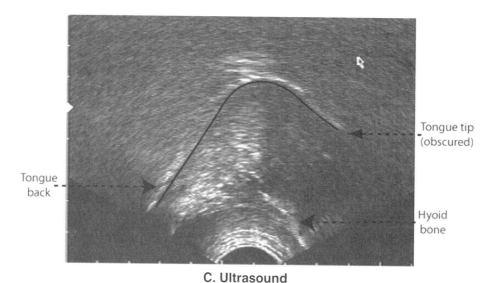

Tongue tip (obscured)

Tongue back

Hyoid bone

C. Ultrasound

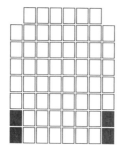

D. Electropalatograph (EPG) (single frame)

Figure 29–1. Static images of the articulatory characteristics of /æ/.

Schematic Diagram

The schematic diagram (Figure 29–1B) representing the tongue position for the vowel /æ/ shows a front-low tongue position. The voicing, typical of all vowels is symbolically represented at the source (the vocal folds) by a plus (+) sign.

Ultrasound

The ultrasound image for /ɛ/ in Chapter 28, is similar to the ultrasound image in Figure 29–1C for /æ/. The surface of the tongue corresponds to the lower edge of the bright white line. The tongue tip is on the right and is directed toward the floor of the mouth. The center of the tongue is raised in the oral cavity. An air shadow can be seen above the tongue and diagonal muscle fibers can be seen below the surface of the tongue.

Electropalatograph (EPG)

There is limited tongue/palate contact in the EPG image (Figure 29–1D) of /æ/. The tongue only contacts the palate near the back teeth (molars). The limited contact is because /æ/ is produced a low vowel.

DYNAMIC IMAGES OF /æ/

To obtain a comprehensive view of the production of this vowel, the dynamic of the articulatory and acoustic characteristics of /æ/ are shown in Figure 29–2 via a filmstrip, spectrogram, and EPG frames.

/æ/ in Within-Word Context: "cat"

Filmstrip: /kæt/ "cat"

The criterion phoneme /æ/ is at the medial position of the word /kæt/ "cat." In the first frame, the influence of the vowel on the initial consonant /k/ can be clearly seen (Figure 29–2A). Although the audible sound tracing for /k/ cannot be seen until frame 4 or 5, the production of the vowel /æ/ is initiated in the beginning

frames. The tongue turns downward in concert with the lowering of the mandible. In addition to the greater excursion of the mandible and spreading of the lips, there is also considerably greater distance between the upper and lower lips in the production of this vowel. The lips open to 5 mm in the sixth frame, with an increase in opening in the subsequent three frames. The distance between the upper and lower lips in frames 7 through 9 is 5½, 6, and 6½ mm, respectively. In frame 9, a complete vowel /æ/ position has been assumed by the lips, tongue, and mandible. The mouth is wide open, the tongue is low, and there is a lack of noticeable rounding. In frames 9 through 13, the opening remains at a steady 6½ mm. This open position results in the steady-state vowel formants. The lips begin to close in the 15th frame, which shows an opening of 5½ mm.

Sound Spectrogram: /kæt/ "cat"

The vowel /æ/ is presented in the medial position (Figure 29–2B) in the word "cat." This is a stressed vowel in English, as indicated by the long duration of approximately 175 msec. The first formant of this vowel is at about 1100 Hz, the second formant is at about 1900 Hz. The second formant shows a greater concentration of energy than the first. Ordinarily the F2 of this vowel is lower than that shown in this spectrogram. The higher energy concentration in this case may be attributed to the coarticulatory effect of the high frequency noise of the initial consonant /k/ at about 3000 Hz and the final consonant /t/ at about 4000 Hz.

Electropalatograph: /kæt/ "cat"

The dynamic series of EPG palates for the production of the word "cat" is presented in Figure 29–2C. The word "cat" was extracted from the sentence "I see a cat again." The closure phase for the /k/ extends from 471 to 487. The vowel /æ/ extends from frames 489 to 530 and has limited tongue/palate contact, concentrated towards the velar region of the palate. The steady state of the vowel is from frames 505 to 521 where the surrounding consonants do not provide coarticulatory influence over the vowel. The horseshoe shape for the final /t/ is depicted in frames 531 to 548. The final frames (549–562) correspond with the burst of frication following the /t/.

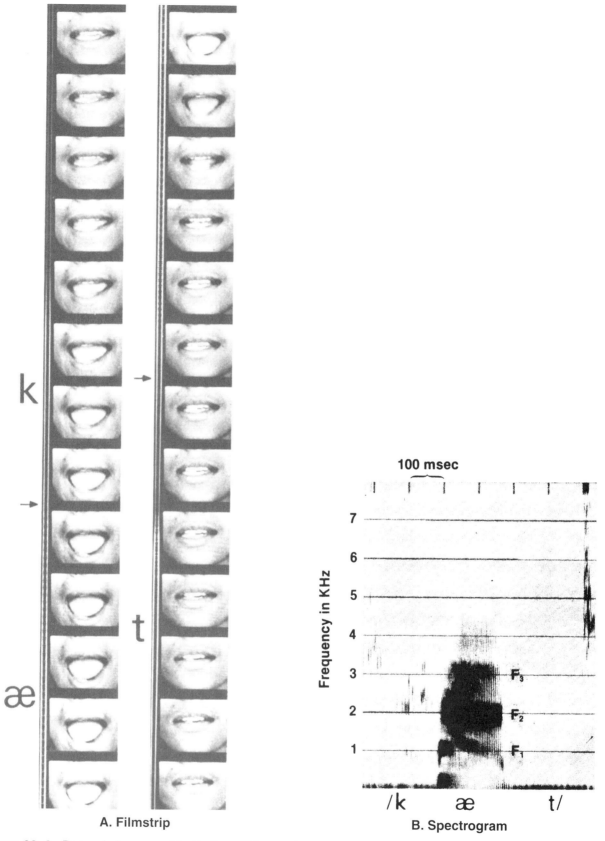

A. Filmstrip

B. Spectrogram

Figure 29–2. Dynamic images of /æ/ in the within-word context: "cat." *continues*

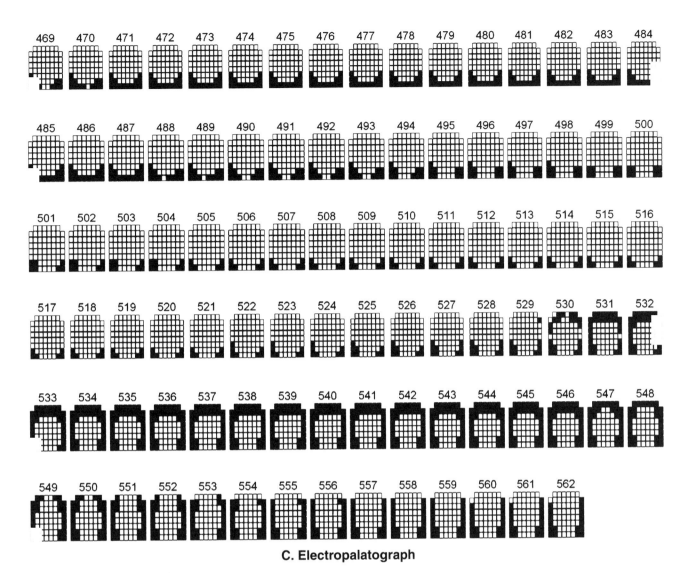

C. Electropalatograph

Figure 29–2. *continued*

Chapter 30

/ɑ/

"father"

The vowel /ɑ/ is described as low, back and unrounded.

Advancement: back

Height: low

Tenseness: neutral

Roundness: unrounded

STATIC IMAGES OF /ɑ/

Figure 30-1 presents static images of the articulatory and acoustic characteristics of /ɑ/.

Photograph

The photograph (Figure 30-1A) has been taken from the production of the vowel /ɑ/ in "father". This frame represents the most open lip position for this vowel.

A. Photograph

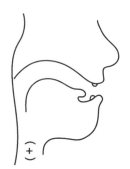

B. Schematic diagram

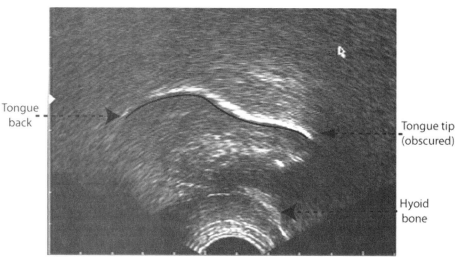

C. Ultrasound

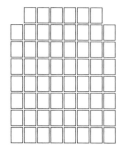

D. Electropalatograph (EPG) (single frame)

Figure 30–1. Static images of the articulatory characteristics of /ɑ/.

Schematic Diagram

The schematic diagram (Figure 30–1B) shows a central-low tongue position for the vowel /ɑ/.

Ultrasound

Figure 30–1C is an ultrasound image of the production of the vowel /ɑ/. The bright white line shows the air reflecting on the tongue surface. The tongue is low in the oral cavity compared with vowels such as /i/ (Chapter 26) and /ɪ/ (Chapter 27). The tongue tip is on the right and is directed toward the floor of the mouth.

Electropalatograph (EPG)

The vowel /ɑ/ is a low back vowel, thus the lowering of the jaw moves the tongue away from the palate. Typically, the tongue does not contact the palate during the production of /ɑ/, as indicated by the absence of activated electrodes on the EPG frame (Figure 30–1D).

DYNAMIC IMAGES OF /ɑ/

To obtain a comprehensive view of the production of this vowel, dynamic images of the articulatory and acoustic characteristics of /ɑ/ are shown via a filmstrip, spectrogram, and EPG frames (Figure 30–2).

/ɑ/ in the Within-Word Context: /ˈfɑðɚ/ "father"

Filmstrip: /ˈfɑðɚ/ "father"

The criterion vowel /ɑ/ is at the medial position of the word /ˈfɑðɚ/ "father." In addition, the vowel /ɑ/ can be viewed at the final position of this word. The acoustic energy for the vowel /ɑ/ following the consonant /f/ begins at the first frame of the second strip of film (Figure 30–2A). The two frames preceding this full

opening show the state of the articulatory transition between the consonant /f/ and the vowel /ɑ/. The vowel is maintained through the first seven frames of the second filmstrip. This vowel differs from the vowels in the previous chapters in two important ways: the lips are more open and more rounded. Although the extent of lip opening for the vowels /æ/ and /ɑ/ may be the same, the major difference is in the rounding of the vowel /ɑ/ as compared to the flattening of vowel /æ/. A measurement of the lip opening for the vowel /ɑ/ in frames 12 through 18 shows 5, 5, 5½, 6, 6, 5½, and 4½ mm, respectively. The final eight frames of the third filmstrip show the lip position for the vowel /ɑ/. For the vowel /ɑ/, the lips are fairly open and the tongue is low and somewhat in the central region. For the vowel /ɚ/, the lips are less open. The degree of lip rounding for both of these vowels is approximately the same.

Sound Spectrogram: /ˈfɑðɚ/ "father"

The vowel /ɑ/ is presented in a bisyllabic word, "father." The vowel /ɑ/ is stressed in English and, hence, is a long-duration vowel. Here (Figure 30–2B) it is approximately 350 msec in duration. The first formant is at about 850 Hz; the second formant at about 1250 Hz. The lack of a rising transition for the F1 signals the devoicing nature of the preceding consonant /f/, whereas the falling transitions for the second, third, and fourth formants indicate the presence of high-frequency energy. However, the only cue indicating the presence of the initial consonant /f/ in the production of this word is in the transition of vowel formants. No clear trace of any energy representing the phoneme /f/ can be seen in the utterance. It may be noted that the transition cues signaling the features of the initial consonant, for example, voicelessness and continuancy, have been considered adequate for the perception of the consonant. Following the vowel /ɑ/ is the consonant /ð/. The voicing nature of this consonant is clearly indicated by the presence of glottal vibration for approximately 140 msec. The rising transition of F1 for the vowel /ɚ/ indicates the voicing nature of the preceding consonant /ð/. The falling transitions of the second and third formants indicate the high frequency elements of the consonant /ð/.

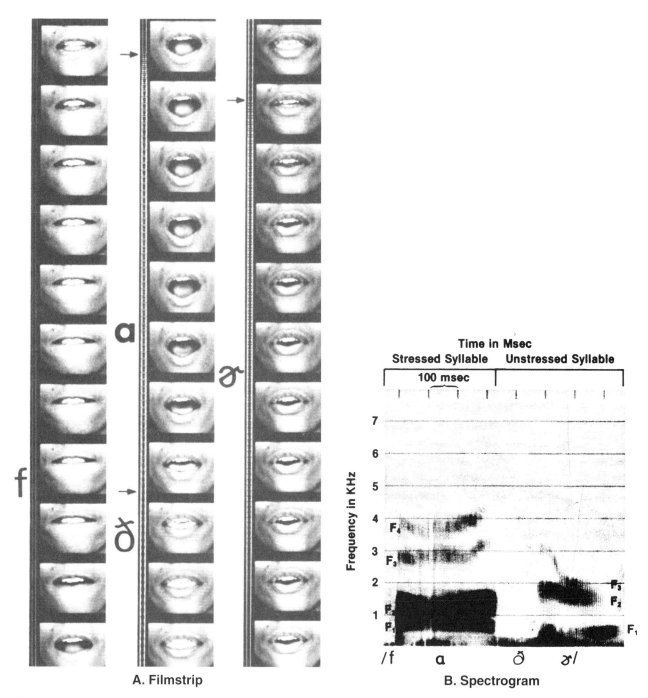

Figure 30–2. Dynamic images of /ɑ/ in the within-word context: "father." *continues*

Electropalatograph: /ˈfaðə/ "father"

The dynamic series of EPG palates for the production of the word /ˈfaðə/[1] "father" is presented in Figure 30-2C.

The word "father" was extracted from the sentence "I see a father again" and contains limited tongue/palate contact. The juncture between each of the sounds was determined by using simultaneous EPG, sound

---

[1]/ˈfaðə/ is the Australian English pronunciation of "father."

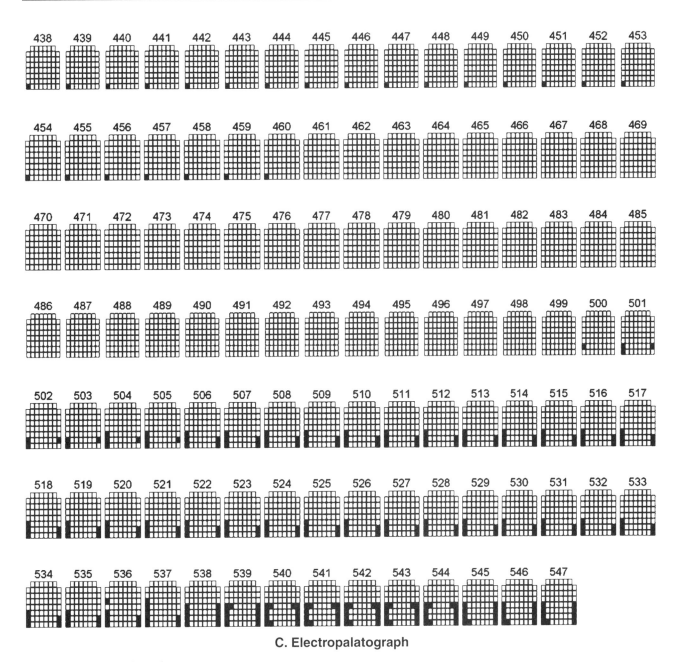

C. Electropalatograph

Figure 30–2. *continued*

spectrogram, waveform and audio data (not shown in Figure 30-2C). The /f/ extends from 438 to 471. The vowel /a/ extends from frames 472 to 505 and has no tongue/palate contact, except for minimal velar contact during coarticulation with the surrounding consonants. The /ð/ extends from 506 to 536 and the final vowel /ə/ from 537 to 547.

Chapter 31

/ɝ/ or /ɜ/

"bird"

The vowel /ɝ/ is described as upper-mid, central, neutral, and rhotic. /ɝ/ is commonly produced within the United States. In comparison, the nonrhotic variety of this vowel is /ɜ/. The vowel /ɜ/ is described as lower-mid, central, neutral and nonrhotic and is commonly produced in the United Kingdom, Australia, and New Zealand.

/ɝ/ (USA)	/ɜ/ (UK, Australia, New Zealand)
Advancement: central	Advancement: central
Height: upper-mid	Height: lower-mid
Tenseness: neutral	Tenseness: neutral
Roundness: neutral	Roundness: neutral
Rhoticity: rhotic	Rhoticity: nonrhotic

STATIC IMAGES OF /ɜ˞/ AND /ʒ/

Figure 31-1 presents static images of the articulatory characteristics of /ɜ˞/.

Photograph

In this photograph (Figure 31-1A), the mouth is open and lips are slightly protruded to produce /ɜ˞/.

A. Photograph

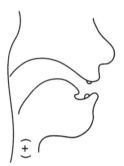

B. Schematic diagram

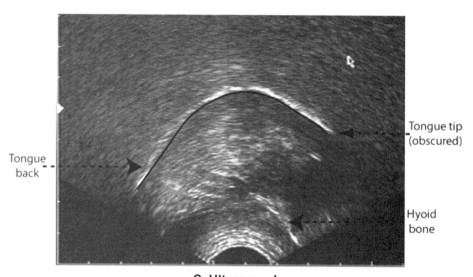

Tongue back

Tongue tip (obscured)

Hyoid bone

C. Ultrasound

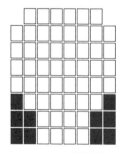

D. Electropalatograph (EPG) (single frame)

Figure 31–1. Static images of the articulatory and acoustic characteristics of /ɜ˞/.

Schematic Diagram

The schematic diagram (Figure 31–1B) shows central-mid position for the vowel /ɝ/. The tongue position for /ɝ/ is more fronted and higher than for the vowel /ʌ/, another central-mid vowel.

Ultrasound

The bright white line on the ultrasound image in Figure 31–1C highlights the tongue surface during production of /ɝ/. The tongue tip is on the right and is directed downward. The body of the tongue is an inverted U shape. Diagonal muscle fibers can be seen below the surface of the tongue and the hyoid bone is seen in the lower right section of the image.

Electropalatograph (EPG)

In the EPG image of /ɜ/ (Figure 31–1D) the tongue contacts the palate along the back lateral margins of the teeth.

DYNAMIC IMAGES OF /ɝ/ AND /ɜ/

To obtain a comprehensive view of the production of this consonant, the dynamic aspects of articulatory and acoustic characteristics of the production of /ɝ/ and /ɜ/ are shown in a filmstrip, spectrogram, and EPG frames (Figure 31–2).

/ɝ/ in the Within-Word Context: "bird"

Filmstrip: /bɝd/ "bird"

The lip configuration for the vowel /ɝ/ shows rounding, protrusion, and opening (Figure 31–2A). These lip

characteristics have also been shown to be important for the vowels /u/ and /ʊ/ in Chapters 32 and 33. The difference among the three vowels may lie in the positioning of the tongue.

Sound Spectrogram: /bɝd/ "bird"

In this sound spectrogram (Figure 31–2B), the vowel /ɝ/ is presented in the medial position in the word "bird." The vowel /ɝ/ has an F1 at approximately 250 Hz and an F2 at approximately 1650 Hz. These formant characteristics indicate that, at least for this speaker, /ɝ/ is a more fronted than centered vowel. The initial consonant is a voiced labial stop. Voicing is indicated by the rising first formant of the vowel /ɝ/, as well as by a -VOT of approximately 175 msec. Labiality is signaled by the rising F2, implying low energy for the labial stop. The final consonant is a voiced fronted stop, denoted by a silence of approximately 100 msec, followed by a plosive burst. The plosive burst is indicated by a thin line, starting at 2000 Hz and terminating at 4200 Hz.

Electropalatograph: /bɜd/ "bird"

The dynamic series of EPG palates for the production of the word /bɜd/[1] "bird" is presented in Figure 31–2C. The /b/ extends from frames 404 to 434. The juncture between the /b/ and /ɜ/ was determined by using simultaneous EPG, sound spectrogram, waveform, and audio data (not shown in Figure 31–2C). The vowel /ɜ/ extends from frames 435 to 483. The sounds, /b/ and /ɜ/, have limited tongue/palate contact, concentrated toward the velar region of the palate. The final /d/ is depicted in frames 484 to 491. The rows of contact are more posterior than in the typical horseshoe shape described in Chapter 5.

---

[1]/bɜd/ is the Australian English pronunciation of "bird."

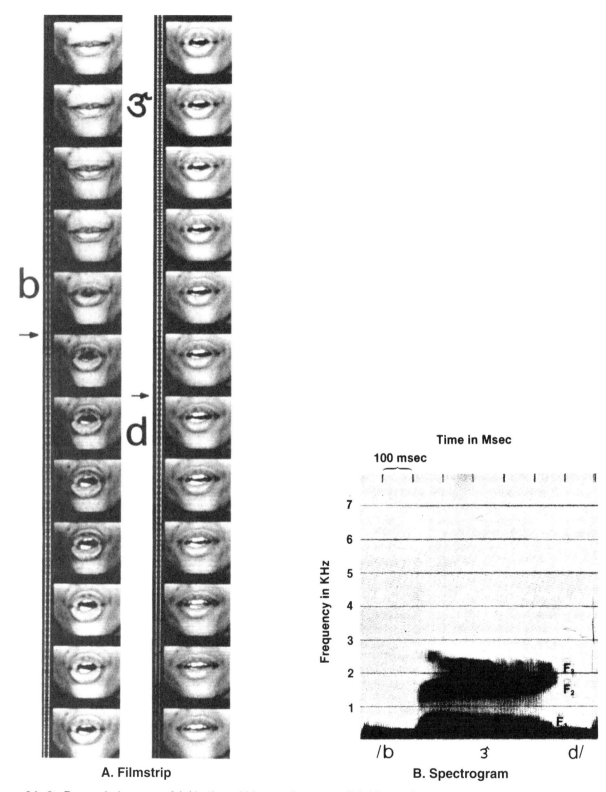

A. Filmstrip

B. Spectrogram

Figure 31–2. Dynamic images of /ɜ/ in the within-word context: "bird." *continues*

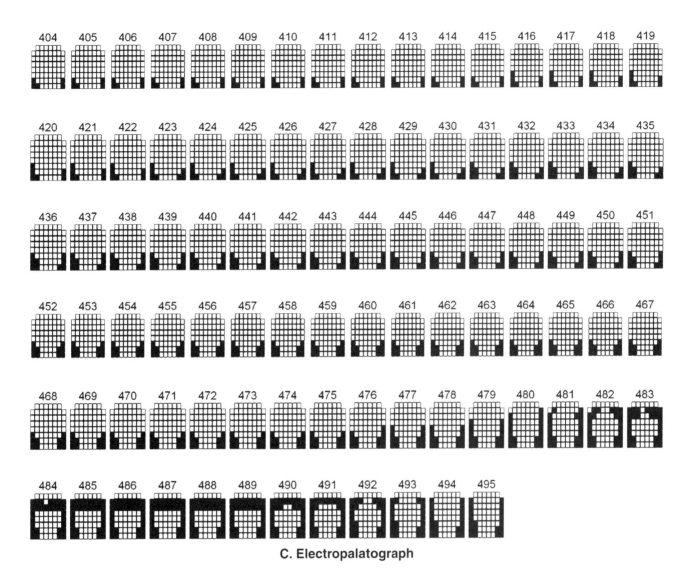

C. Electropalatograph

Figure 31–2. *continued*

Chapter 32

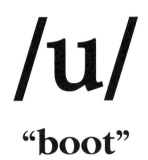

"boot"

The vowel /u/ is described as high, back, tense and rounded.

Advancement: back

Height: high

Tenseness: tense

Roundness: rounded

STATIC IMAGES OF /u/

Figure 32-1 presents static images of the articulatory and acoustic characteristics of /u/.

Photograph

In the photograph (Figure 32-1A), the lips are protruded to produce the rounded vowel /u/. Comparison with the photograph for /ʊ/ in Chapter 33 provides evidence that /u/ is more rounded than /ʊ/.

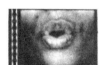

A. Photograph

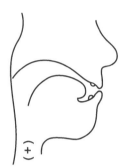

B. Schematic diagram

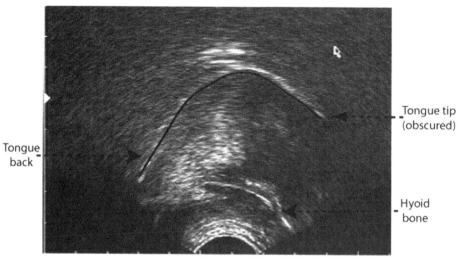

C. Ultrasound

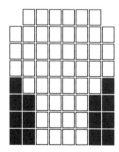

D. Electropalatograph (EPG) (single frame)

Figure 32–1. Static images of the articulatory and acoustic characteristics of /u/.

Schematic Diagram

In the schematic diagram (Figure 32-1B), the tongue is positioned at the back of the oral cavity for the vowel /u/. The height of the tongue is the maximum for a back vowel.

Ultrasound

The bright white line on the ultrasound image in Figure 32-1C shows the tongue surface during production of /u/. The tongue tip is on the right and is directed toward the floor of the mouth. The centre of the tongue is raised in the oral cavity. An air shadow can be seen above the tongue and diagonal muscle fibers can be seen below the surface of the tongue.

Electropalatograph (EPG)

The EPG frame (Figure 32-1D) has tongue contact along the back lateral margins of the palate. There is more tongue/palate contact for /u/ than for /ʊ/ (Chapter 33) due to the increased height of /u/.

DYNAMIC IMAGES OF THE ARTICULATORY AND ACOUSTIC CHARACTERISTICS OF /u/

To obtain a comprehensive view of the production of this consonant, the dynamic aspects of the production of /u/ are shown in a filmstrip, spectrogram, and EPG images (Figure 32-2).

/u/ in Within-Word Context: "boot"

Filmstrip: /but/ "boot"

In the filmstrip (Figure 32-2A) the vowel /u/ is shown at the medial position in the word /but/ "boot." This vowel displays greater lip protrusion, greater lip rounding, and smaller lip opening than the vowel /ʊ/ (Chapter 33). The distances between the upper and lower lips in frames 7 through 14 are 2, 2, 1¾, 1½, 1½, and 1¼ mm, respectively. The primary distinguishing lip characteristics for this vowel are lip protrusion and lip rounding.

Sound Spectrogram: /but/ "boot"

In Figure 32-2B, the vowel /u/ is shown at the medial position in the word /but/, preceded by the voiced labial consonant /b/ and followed by the voiceless front consonant /t/. The F1 of the vowel /u/ is centered at 250 Hz and the F2 at about 1250 Hz. Its long durational character, about 275 msec, may denote the stressed nature of this vowel. The rising F2 and the absence of vocal fold vibration, followed by a long duration plosive burst with energy spread between 2000 and 8000 Hz, indicate the strong release of the final consonant /t/.

Electropalatograph: /but/ "boot"

Figure 32-2C presents the dynamic series of EPG palates for the production of the word "boot" in the phrase "I see a boot again." The /b/ extends from 416 to 441. The vowel /u/ extends from frames 442 to 470 and has tongue/palate contact that is concentrated along the lateral margins of the palate. The juncture between the /b/ and /u/ was determined by using simultaneous EPG, sound spectrogram, waveform, and audio data (not shown in Figure 32-2C). The transition from the /u/ to the /t/ in frames 458 to 470 is marked by broader tongue/palate contact along the lateral margins. The horseshoe shape for the final /t/ is depicted in frames 471 to 483. The friction accompanying the release of the /t/ is shown in frames 484 to 495.

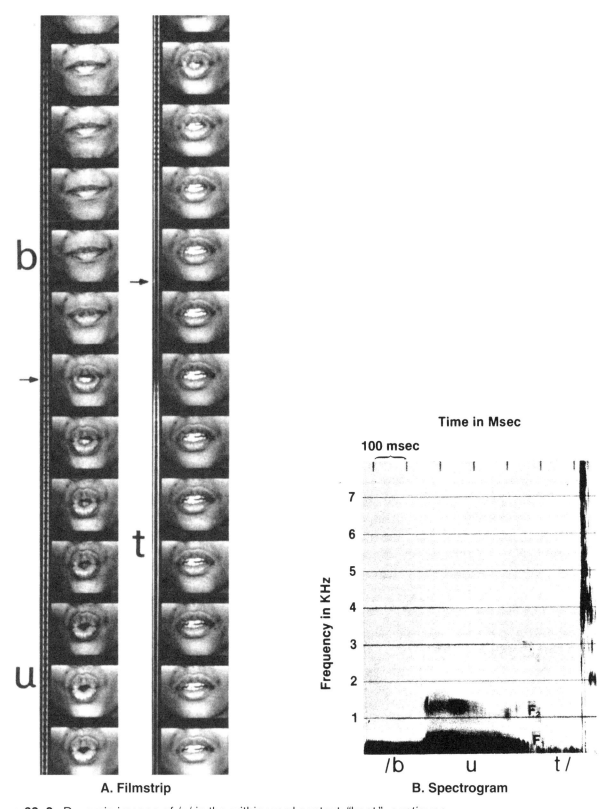

A. Filmstrip

B. Spectrogram

Figure 32–2. Dynamic images of /u/ in the within-word context: "boot." *continues*

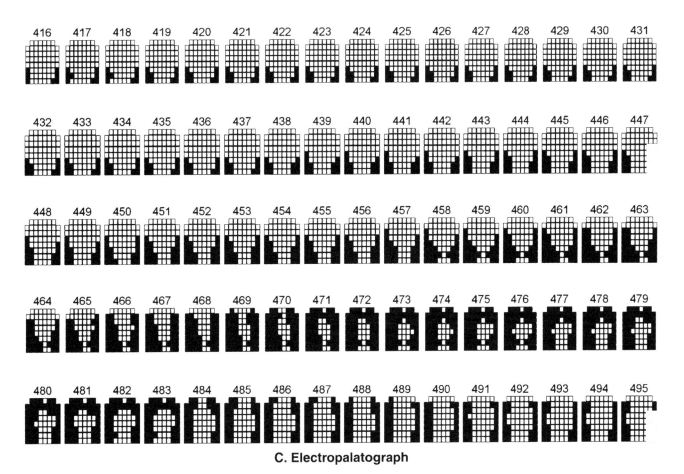

C. Electropalatograph

Figure 32–2. *continued*

Chapter 33

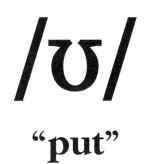

"put"

The vowel /ʊ/ is described as high, back, lax and rounded.

Advancement: back

Height: high

Tenseness: lax

Roundness: rounded

STATIC IMAGES OF /ʊ/

Figure 33-1 presents static images of the articulatory and acoustic characteristics of /ʊ/.

Photograph

In this photograph (Figure 33-1A), the lips are rounded to produce /ʊ/.

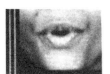

A. Photograph

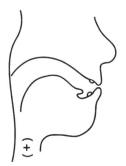

B. Schematic diagram

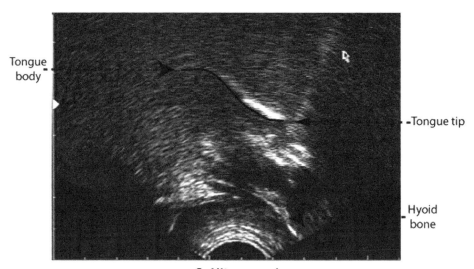

C. Ultrasound

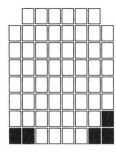

D. Electropalatograph (EPG) (single frame)

Figure 33–1. Static images of the articulatory characteristics of /ʊ/.

Schematic diagram

In Figure 33-1B the tongue is positioned at the back of the oral cavity in the production of the vowel /ʊ/. The height of the tongue is slightly lower than the maximum height for any back vowel. The voicing of this vowel is symbolically represented at the source (the vocal folds) by a plus sign.

Ultrasound

A midsagittal ultrasound image of the tongue surface during production of /ʊ/ is shown in Figure 33-1C. The bright white line is immediately above the tongue surface. The tongue is raised compared to its resting position as described in Chapter 1. The tongue tip is toward the right of the image, but compared with the production of other vowels is retracted more to the center of the image. An air shadow can be seen near the tongue tip and diagonal muscle fibres can be seen below the tongue. The hyoid bone is seen as the bright diagonal line at the bottom right of the image.

Electropalatograph (EPG)

The EPG frame in Figure 33-1D is almost empty, demonstrating limited tongue contact along back margins of the palate. Limited tongue/palate contact is typical for vowel production, particularly vowels that are defined as backed.

DYNAMIC IMAGES OF /ʊ/

To obtain a comprehensive view of the production of this vowel, the dynamic aspects of the articulatory and acoustic characteristics of /ʊ/ are shown in Figure 33-2 via a filmstrip, spectrogram, and EPG frames.

/ʊ/ in the Within-Word Context: "put"

Filmstrip: /pʊt/ "put"

In Figure 33-2A, the vowel /ʊ/ is shown here within the word /pʊt/. The production of this vowel involves lip rounding, lip protrusion, and opening between the upper and lower lips. The distance between the lips is 1 mm in the fifth frame, with increments to 2½, 3½ and 4 mm in frames 6 through 8. The opening remains at a steady 4 mm in frames 7 and 8.

Sound Spectrogram: /pʊt/ "put"

In Figure 33-2B, the vowel /ʊ/ is presented within the word "put." The first formant of this vowel is at approximately 300 Hz, whereas the second formant is at approximately 1200 Hz. This is generally an unstressed vowel in English, exhibiting a duration of only about 150 msec. The falling F2 indicates the labial feature of the preceding consonant. The rising F2 of the vowel /ʊ/ at its termination indicates the high-frequency energy domain of the final consonant /t/.

Electropalatograph: /pʊt/ "put"

The dynamic series of EPG palates for the production of the word "put" is presented in Figure 33-2C. The word "put" was extracted from the sentence "I see a put again." The /p/ extends from 419 to 446. The vowel /ʊ/ extends from frames 447 to 467 and has limited tongue/palate contact, concentrated towards the velar region of the palate. The juncture between the /p/ and /ʊ/ was determined by using simultaneous EPG, sound spectrogram, waveform, and audio data (not shown in Figure 33-2C). The horseshoe shape for the final /t/ is depicted in frames 471 to 486 followed by a series of frames depicting the aspiration frication for the release of the /t/.

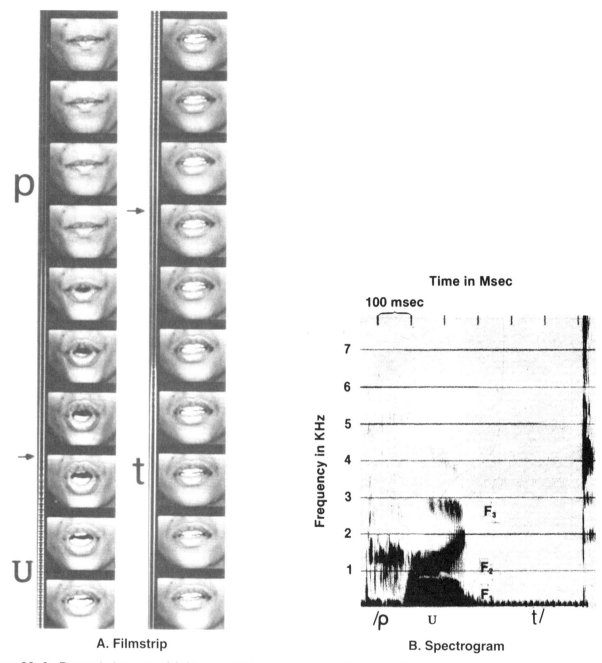

A. Filmstrip

Time in Msec

100 msec

B. Spectrogram

Figure 33–2. Dynamic images of /ʊ/ in the within-word context: "put." *continues*

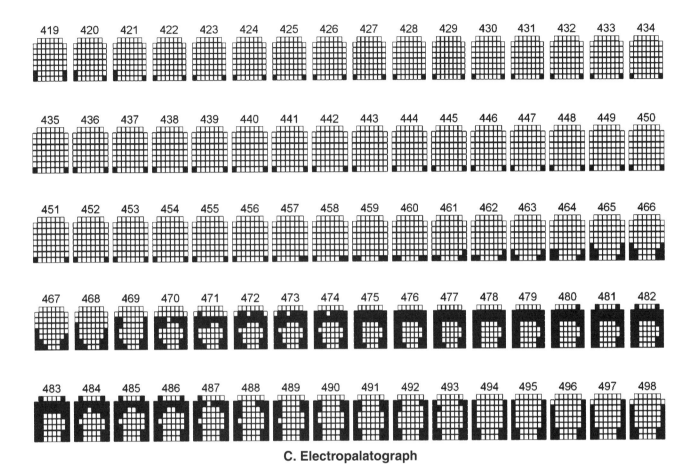

C. Electropalatograph

Figure 33–2. *continued*

Chapter 34

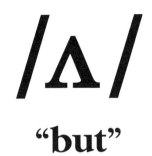

"but"

The vowel /ʌ/ is described as low, central, neutral and unrounded.

Advancement: central

Height: low

Tenseness: neutral

Roundness: unrounded

STATIC IMAGES OF /ʌ/

Photograph

Figure 34-1 presents static images of the articulatory characteristics of /ʌ/.

In the photograph depicted in Figure 34-1A, the mouth is open and the lips are unrounded.

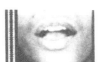

A. Photograph

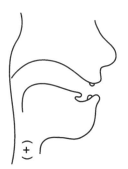

B. Schematic diagram

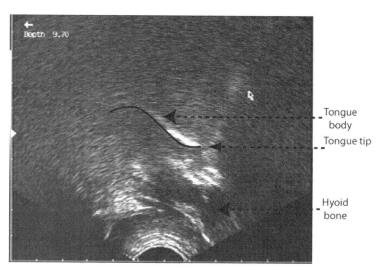

C. Ultrasound

Tongue body
Tongue tip
Hyoid bone

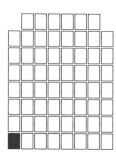

D. Electropalatograph (EPG) (single frame)

Figure 34–1. Static images of the articulatory characteristics of /ʌ/.

Schematic Diagram

In Figure 34-1B, the tongue is shown elevated to approximately the central-mid position for the vowel /ʌ/. A close examination of the lip and tongue position shows that the tongue is further back on the vowel diagram realizing its designation as a low central vowel.

Ultrasound

Figure 34-1C shows the tongue in an ultrasound image during production of the vowel /ʌ/. The surface of the tongue is difficult to see during production of vowels and velars with steeply sloping tongue surfaces (Stone, 2005). In this image the tongue tip is the brighter line pointing towards the floor of the mouth at the center of the image. The lines below the surface of the tongue are the muscle fibers.

Electropalatograph (EPG)

The tongue barely contacts the palate during the production of /ʌ/, as indicated by only one activated electrode on the EPG frame in Figure 34-1D. The vowel /ʌ/ is a low central vowel, thus the lowering of the jaw moves the tongue away from the palate.

DYNAMIC IMAGES OF /ʌ/

To obtain a comprehensive view of the dynamic production of this vowel, the articulatory and acoustic characteristics of /ʌ/ are shown in a filmstrip, spectrogram, and EPG frames in Figure 34-2.

/ʌ/ in Within-Word Context: "but"

Filmstrip: /bʌt/ "but"

In Figure 34-2A the central-mid vowel /ʌ/ is shown within the word /bʌt/. The vowel /ʌ/ is a low central vowel. Frames 8 and 9 show some lip rounding and opening, not unlike that seen for the vowel /ɑ/ in Chapter 30. The 8th frame shows an opening of 5 mm. The opening increases in the 9th frame to 5½ mm and returns to 5 mm in the 10th frame. Although these lip openings and the associated rounding are also characteristic of the vowel /ɑ/, there is a considerable durational difference between these two vowels. The vowel /ɑ/ maintains a distance of 5 mm between the upper and lower lips for six consecutive frames, whereas the vowel /ʌ/ maintains this degree of openness for only three frames.

Sound Spectrogram: /bʌt/ "but"

In Figure 34-2B, the vowel /ʌ/ is presented within the word "but." The first formant of this vowel is centered at about 500 Hz and the second at about 1500 Hz. These center frequencies approximate the theoretical model for a neutral vowel, implying the vocal tract as a linear tube. The duration of this vowel at the medial position is relatively short and, therefore, it is hard to visualize the steady-state portion of the vowel. The initial consonant is a voiced labial stop. Voicing is denoted by a negative voice onset time (−VOT) of approximately 180 msec as well as a rising F1. Labiality is denoted by a rising F2. The consonant following the vowel is a voiceless-front stop. Voicelessness is indicated by the absence of vocal fold vibration at the base of the spectrogram. The stop feature is indicated by the complete silence for 200 msec, followed by a narrow plosive burst of energy, starting at 3300 Hz and terminating at over 7000 Hz. The duration of the plosive burst is also indicative of the devoicing phenomenon. Compare the duration of this consonant /t/ with the duration of the plosive burst (/d/) in the word "bird" in Chapter 31.

Electropalatograph: /bʌt/ "but"

The dynamic series of EPG palates for the production of the word "but" is presented in Figure 34-2C. The word "but" took 0.391 seconds to produce within a sentence context. The /b/ extends from 434 to 461. The vowel /ʌ/ extends from frames 462 to 485 and has limited tongue/palate contact, concentrated toward the velar region of the palate. The juncture between

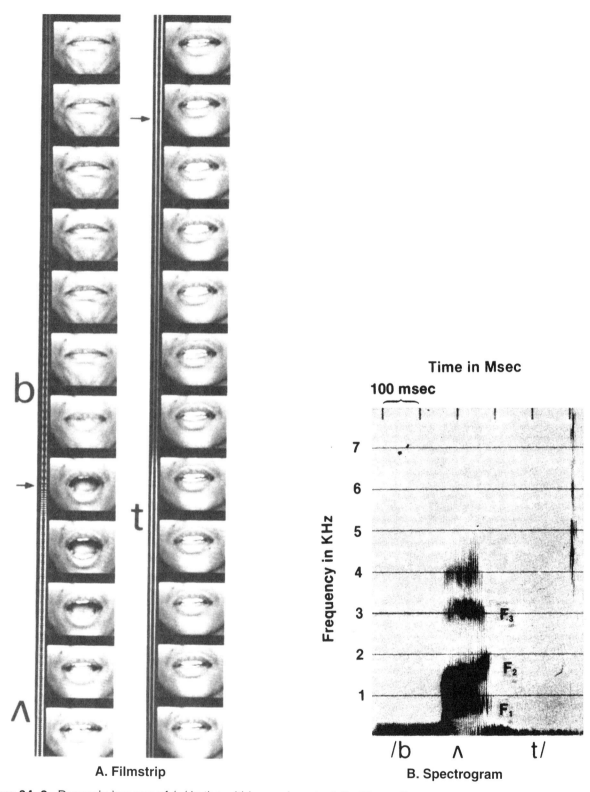

A. Filmstrip

B. Spectrogram

Figure 34–2. Dynamic images of /ʌ/ in the within-word context: "but." *continues*

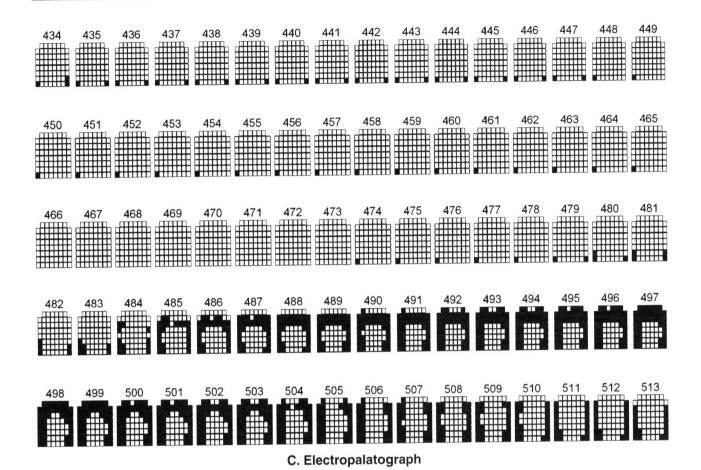

C. Electropalatograph

Figure 34–2. *continued*

the /b/ and /ʌ/ was determined by using simultaneous EPG, sound spectrogram, waveform, and audio data (not shown in Figure 26-2C). The horseshoe shape for the final /t/ is depicted in frames 486 to 503. The aspiration frication following the /t/ is found in frames 504 to 513.

Chapter 35

/ɔ/

"bought"

The vowel /ɔ/ is described as a lower-mid, back, lax, and rounded.

Advancement: back

Height: lower-mid

Tenseness: lax

Roundness: rounded

STATIC IMAGES OF /ɔ/

Figure 35-1 presents static images of the articulatory and acoustic characteristics of /ɔ/.

Photograph

In Figure 35-1A, the photograph exemplifies the lip-rounding that is necessary for the production of /ɔ/.

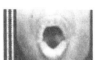

A. Photograph

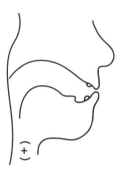

B. Schematic diagram

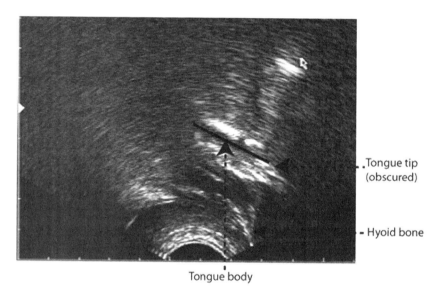

Tongue tip (obscured)

- Hyoid bone

Tongue body

C. Ultrasound

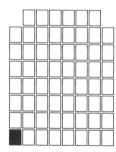

D. Electropalatograph (EPG) (single frame)

Figure 35–1. Static images of the articulatory characteristics of /ɔ/.

Schematic Diagram

In Figure 35-1B, the tongue is positioned at the lower end of the oral cavity with a slight elevation toward the back for the production of the vowel /ɔ/. For this reason, this vowel is labeled as a lower mid-back vowel. A comparison of the tongue involvement of this vowel with that of the vowel /ɑ/ in Chapter 30 shows that /ɔ/ is positioned farther back and slightly higher than the vowel /ɑ/. These two vowels, however, are very similar in tongue position and are sometimes hard to distinguish.

Ultrasound

The ultrasound image in Figure 35-1C is unclear compared with images of vowels such as for /u/ in Figure 32-1C. The brightest and straightest white diagonal line extending upward from right to left represents the air above the tongue surface for the production of /ɔ/.

Electropalatograph (EPG)

Only one electrode is contacted on this EPG frame (Figure 35-1D). This indicates that there is limited tongue/palate contact during the production of /ɔ/. The vowel /ɔ/ is defined a low vowel; thus, the jaw is lowered, moving the tongue away from the palate. The one electrode that is contacted in this EPG frame is at the back of the mouth, supporting the definition of /ɔ/ as a back vowel. Minor asymmetry in tongue/palate contact is common.

DYNAMIC IMAGES OF /ɔ/

To obtain a comprehensive view of the production of this vowel, Figure 35-2 presents dynamic images of the articulatory and acoustic characteristics of /ɔ/ via a filmstrip, spectrogram, and EPG frames.

/ɔ/ in the Within-Word Context: "bought"

Filmstrip: /bɔt/ "bought"

In Figure 35-2A, the vowel /ɔ/ is shown within the word /bɔt/. The lips begin to open and approximate this vowel in the fifth frame. In the subsequent six frames, greater opening and greater rounding can be seen. A comparison of the lip involvement in this vowel with that of the vowel /ɑ/ in Chapter 30 indicates a wider opening and a greater rounding for vowel /ɔ/. The distance between the upper and lower lips is 2 mm in the fifth frame, with a steady increase in the degree of opening in the subsequent six frames: 4, 5, 6, 6½, 7, and 7 mm, respectively, in frames 6 through 11.

Sound Spectrogram: /bɔt/ "bought"

In Figure 35-2B, the vowel /ɔ/ is presented within the word "bought." This is essentially a stressed vowel in English; consequently it shows long duration, approximately 275 msec. The first formant is centered at about 750 Hz and the second formant at about 1250 Hz. The central portion of the vowel exhibits its steady state for approximately 100 msec. The second formant transition can be seen rising toward the high energy of the final consonant /t/.

Electropalatograph: /bɔt/ "bought"

Figure 35-2C contains a sequential series of EPG palates for the production of the word "bought" produced in the sentence "I see a bought again." The 110 frames for the word "bought" took 0.548 seconds. The /b/ extends from 408 to 443. The vowel /ɔ/ extends from frames 444 to 488 and predominantly has no tongue/palate contact. The juncture between the /b/ and /ɔ/ was determined by using simultaneous EPG, sound spectrogram, waveform, and audio data (not shown in Figure 35-2C). The horseshoe shape for the final /t/ is depicted in frames 489 to 504. The coarticulatory influence of the back vowel /ɔ/ can be seen by the closure of the /t/ commencing in the third row of electrodes

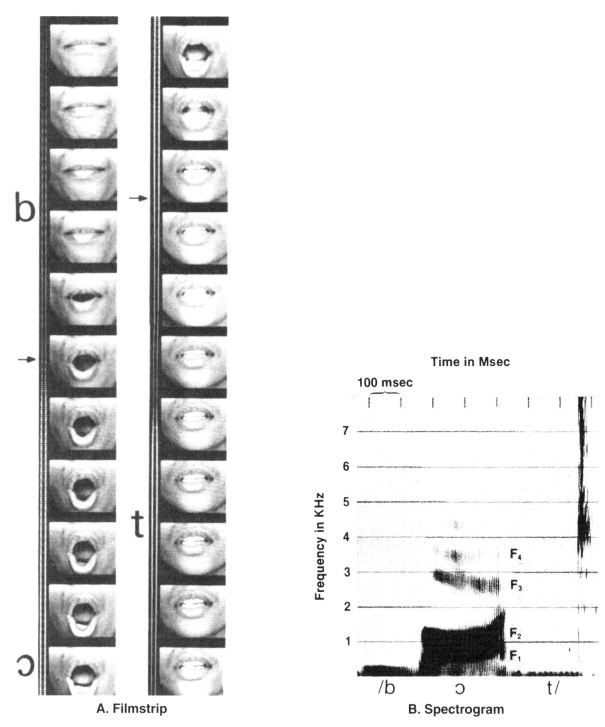

A. Filmstrip

B. Spectrogram

Figure 35–2. Dynamic images of /ɔ/ in the within-word context: "bought." *continues*

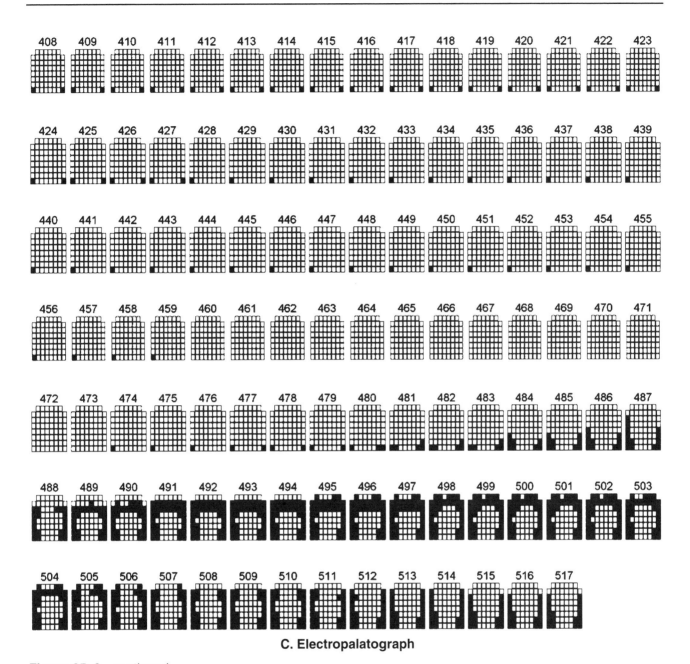

C. Electropalatograph

Figure 35–2. *continued*

in frame 489, the moving forward to the first and second rows of electrodes by frame 498.

Scottish English-Speaking Adults

Gibbon, Smeaton-Ewins, and Crampin (2005) described the speech of five typical Scottish English-speaking adults to provide a comparison with the speech of eighteen children with cleft palate. The participants produced four words containing five different vowels. Figure 35-3 demonstrates the cumulative maximum contact EPG frames for four productions of /ɔ/ spoken by the five adults. A black square indicates that that electrode was contacted at least 67% of the time. Gibbon et al. (2005) indicated that /ɔ/ had the least tongue palate contact, compared with /ʉ/, /o/, /ɪ/ and /i/.

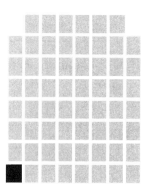

Figure 35–3. Cumulative EPG frame for the production of /ɔ/ by five English-speaking adults (adapted from Gibbon et al., 2005, Figure 3, p. 188).

Chapter 36

Diphthongs

A diphthong is "a vowel-like sound involving a gradual change in articulatory configuration from an onglide to offglide position." (Kent & Read, 2002, p. 302). The five diphthongs commonly produced in General American English are /eɪ/ "bake," /aɪ/ "bike," /ɔɪ/ "boy," /aʊ/ "out," and /oʊ/ "slow." Each of these will be considered in turn. Other English dialects have additional diphthongs, but they are not illustrated in this chapter. For sake of completeness, additional diphthongs produced in countries such as United Kingdom and Australia include: /ɪə/ "near," /ɛə/ "square," and /ʊə/ "cure."

IMAGES OF THE ARTICULATORY AND ACOUSTIC CHARACTERISTICS OF /eɪ/ IN "BAKE"

The diphthong /eɪ/ "bake" has the following features:

> Advancement: from front to front
>
> Height: from mid to high
>
> Tenseness: from tense to lax
>
> Roundness: from unrounded to unrounded

Filmstrip of /beɪk/ "bake"

In Figure 36–1A, the two vowel elements involved in the formation of a diphthong are influenced by each other, like the coarticulatory influence of any two neighboring phonemes. In addition, each of the two vowels involved maintains its independent identity. The diphthong /eɪ/ is at the medial position of the word /beɪk/. It can be seen that, although there is an influence of vowel /e/ on /ɪ/ and vice versa, each vowel maintains its uniqueness for several frames. The vowel /e/, without any influence from the vowel /ɪ/, can be seen in frames 8 through 11. The gliding of the tongue and lip positions continues in frames 12 and 13. The vowel /ɪ/ can be seen in its "pure" state in frames 14 and 15. Two separate frames have been taken, one from the /e/ portion and another from the /ɪ/ portion of the diphthong /eɪ/, when pronounced in isolation. These two portions further support the hypothesis that /e/ and /ɪ/ may have independent phonemic status in the formation of the diphthong /eɪ/.

Schematic Diagram of /eɪ/

In Figure 36–1B, the schematic drawing shows the movement of the tongue from the front-mid position, with the vowel /e/, to the front-high position, with the vowel /ɪ/. The tongue position for the vowel segment /e/ is denoted by a dashed line, whereas the tongue position for the vowel /ɪ/ is denoted by a solid line. These two tongue positions are produced in sequence. First vowel /e/ is produced, then there is a gliding transition to vowel /ɪ/.

Sound Spectrogram of beɪk/ "bake"

In Figure 36–1C, the diphthong /eɪ/ is presented within the word "bake." The diphthong nature of the

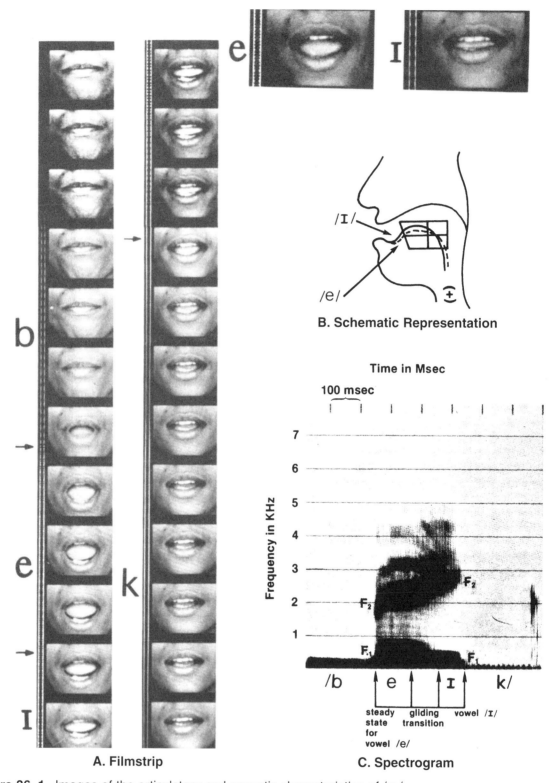

e

I

B. Schematic Representation

/I/

/e/

Time in Msec

100 msec

Frequency in KHz

7

6

5

4

3   F₂

2   F₂

1

F₁   F₁

/b   e   I   k/

steady   gliding   vowel /ɪ/
state   transition
for
vowel /e/

b

e

k

I

A. Filmstrip

C. Spectrogram

Figure 36–1. Images of the articulatory and acoustic characteristics of /eɪ/.

vowel /eɪ/ is such that the individual phoneme boundaries for the vowels /e/ and /ɪ/ are maintained. The formant frequencies for the vowel /e/ are centered at approximately 500 and 2000 Hz, and those of the vowel /ɪ/ at approximately 250 and 2600 Hz. These two steady states are bridged by a gliding transition.

IMAGES OF THE ARTICULATORY AND ACOUSTIC CHARACTERISTICS OF /aɪ/ IN "BIKE"

The diphthong /aɪ/ in "bike" has the following features:

> Advancement: from front to front
>
> Height: from low to high
>
> Tenseness: from neutral to lax
>
> Roundness: from unrounded to unrounded

In the United States, the diphthong /aɪ/ in "bike" is also written as /ɑɪ/ as pronunciation of the onglide /a/ within the Midwest is more similar to the low-back /ɑ/ (Shriberg & Kent, 2003).

Filmstrip of /baɪk/ "bike"

In Figure 36–2A, the filmstrip demonstrates the production of the diphthong /aɪ/ in the word "bike." After the lip closure for the /b/ consonant in the first four frames, the first sign of opening for the vowel /a/ is seen in frame 5. The next four frames (6 through 9) show the production of the vowel /a/. These four frames involved in the production of the /a/ portion of the diphthong may be compared with frames 13 through 18 in Chapter 30, involved in the production of vowel /ɑ/. Their similarities may be noted. Frames 10 and 11 of this module show the glide from the vowel /a/ to the vowel /ɪ/. Frames 12 through 15 show the vowel /ɪ/ independently. Again, these four frames can be compared with frames 11 through 16 of chapter 27, and the similarities in the production of /ɪ/ may be noted. Two separate frames have been taken, one from the /a/ portion and another from the /ɪ/ portion of the diphthong /aɪ/ when produced in isolation. These two portions further support the hypothesis that /a/ and /ɪ/ may have independent phonemic status in the formation of the diphthong /aɪ/.

Schematic Diagram of /aɪ/

In Figure 36–2B, the schematic diagram shows the tongue movement from the central-low vowel /a/ to the front-high vowel /ɪ/. The tongue position for the vowel /a/ is denoted by a dashed line, and the tongue position for vowel /ɪ/, by a solid line. These two tongue positions are produced in sequence.

Sound Spectrogram of /baɪk/ "bike"

In Figure 36–2C, the vowel /aɪ/ is presented within the word "bike." The clear existence of the vowel /a/ is shown in this sound spectrogram by the steady-state vowel formants at approximately 900 and 1400 Hz, which continue for about 150 msec. This steady state is followed by a gliding movement toward the formant frequencies of the vowel /ɪ/. The first formant of the vowel /ɪ/ is centered at 250 Hz and the second formant at 2500 Hz.

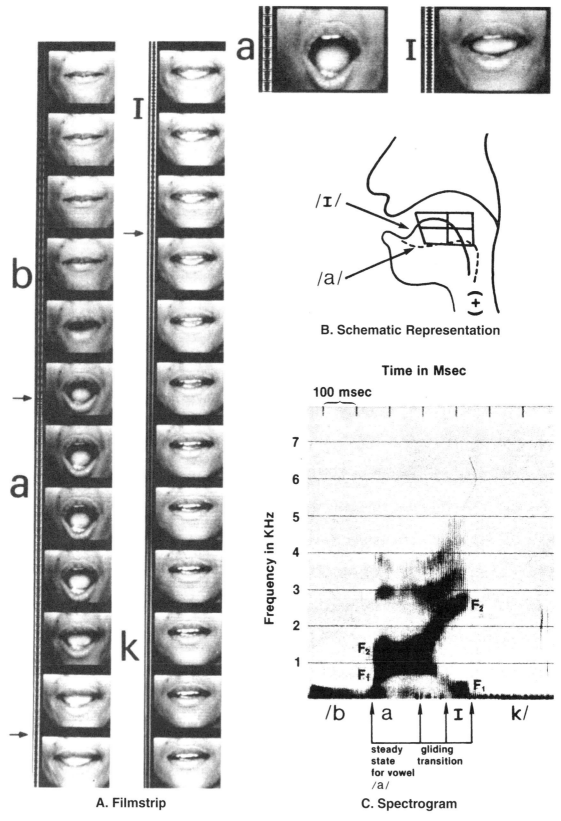

A. Filmstrip

B. Schematic Representation

Time in Msec

100 msec

C. Spectrogram

Figure 36–2. Images of the articulatory and acoustic characteristics of /aɪ/.

IMAGES OF THE ARTICULATORY AND ACOUSTIC CHARACTERISTICS OF /ɔɪ/ IN "BOY"

The diphthong /ɔɪ/ in "boy" has the following features:

Advancement: from back to front

Height: from mid to high

Tenseness: from lax to lax

Roundness: from rounded to unrounded

Filmstrip of /bɔɪ/ "boy"

In Figure 36–3A, the diphthong /ɔɪ/ is shown in the word /bɔɪ/. After three frames of lip closure associated with the consonant /b/, the lips show the first traces of opening in the fourth frame. A rounding of the lips accompanies this opening in frames 5 through 14. Both the rounding of the lips and degree of opening are attributable to the vowel /ɔ/. In the 15th frame, the distance between the lips begins to narrow and is replaced by flattening. In frames 16 through 22, the flattened and less open lip characteristics of the vowel /ɪ/ can be seen.

Schematic Diagram of /ɔɪ/

In this schematic diagram (Figure 36–3B), the tongue position for the vowel segment /ɔ/ is depicted by a dashed line, and the tongue position for vowel segment /ɪ/ by a solid line. These two tongue positions are produced in sequence. To produce the necessary articulatory adjustments for the diphthong /ɔɪ/, the tongue moves from the back-mid to the front-high position.

Sound Spectrogram of /bɔɪ/ "boy"

In Figure 36–3C, the diphthong /ɔɪ/ is presented in the final position in the word "boy." The initial consonant is a voiced labial stop, represented by a long negative voice onset time and rising F1 and F2 formant frequencies. Because of the diphthong nature of /ɔɪ/, it is possible to trisect it into the following segments: the steady state for the first vowel /ɔ/ formants, a gliding transition, and the steady state for the second vowel /ɪ/ formants. The steady state for the first vowel formants can be estimated at 450 and 850 Hz, respectively. Following the long glide, the second formant assumes a steady state at 2400 Hz, approximating the second formant of the vowel /ɪ/.

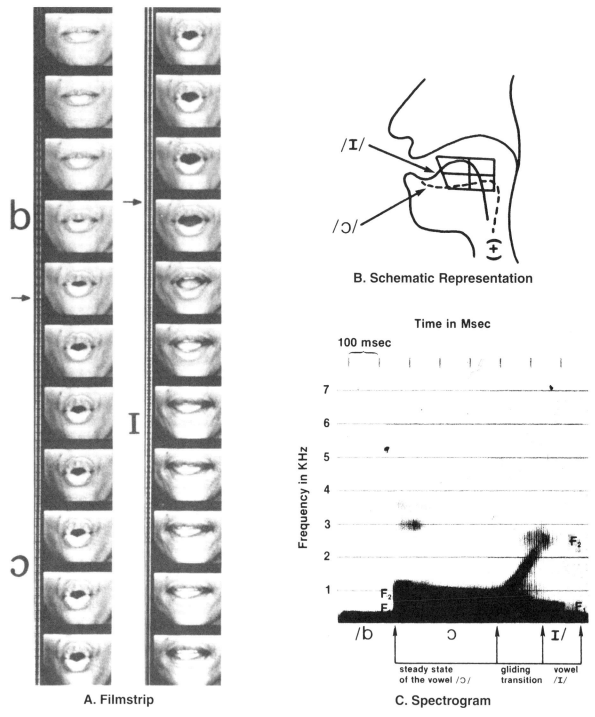

B. Schematic Representation

A. Filmstrip

C. Spectrogram

Figure 36–3. Images of the articulatory and acoustic characteristics of /ɔɪ/.

IMAGES OF THE ARTICULATORY AND ACOUSTIC CHARACTERISTICS OF /aʊ/ IN "OUT"

The diphthong /aʊ/ in "out" has the following features:

> Advancement: from front to back
>
> Height: from low to high
>
> Tenseness: from neutral to lax
>
> Roundness: from unrounded to rounded

Within the United States the diphthong /aʊ/ is also written as /ɑʊ/, as the Midwest pronunciation of the onglide is closer to /ɑ/ than /a/ (Shriberg & Kent, 2003). These two different transcriptions are similar for the diphthong /aɪ/.

Filmstrip of /aʊt/ "out"

In Figure 36–4A, the diphthong /aʊ/ is present in the word "out." Substantial lip opening for the vowel /a/ can be seen in frames 1 through 8. In frames 7 through 9, the lips begin to approximate a more rounded and narrower opening for the vowel /ʊ/.

Schematic Diagram of /aʊ/

In Figure 36–4B, the tongue positions are shown for the diphthong /aʊ/. The displacement of the mandible, associated with the tongue movement for the vowel /a/, is also shown in this diagram. The dashed line shows the back-low tongue position for the vowel /a/. The dashed outline of the mandible indicates a downward excursion in the production of /a/. The solid line shows the back-high tongue position of the vowel /ʊ/. The mandible at this point is shown at the rest position.

Sound Spectrogram of /aʊt/ "out"

In Figure 36–4C, the diphthong /aʊ/ is presented in the initial position in the word "out." The diphthongal nature can be seen in the accommodation of the formant frequencies for the vowel /a/ and the vowel /ʊ/ on a continuum. The vowel segment of this spectrogram can be trisected; the vowel /a/ has an F1 and F2 at 1,200 Hz and 1,500 Hz; the vowel /ʊ/ has an F1 and F2 at 300 Hz and 1,100 Hz; and between these two steady states is a considerable area of glide. Prior to the burst and aspirated energy of the final plosive consonant /t/, there exists an element of silence.

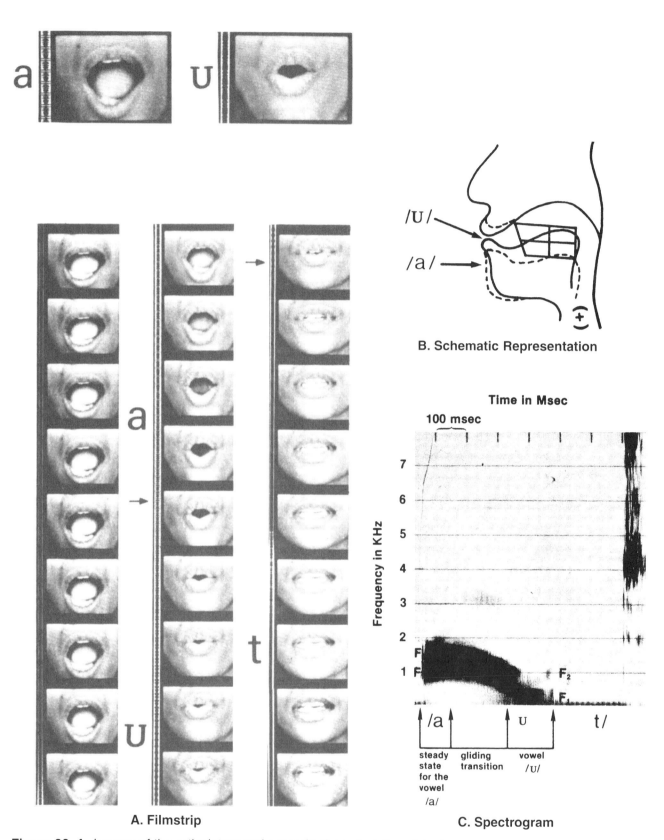

A. Filmstrip

B. Schematic Representation

C. Spectrogram

Figure 36–4. Images of the articulatory and acoustic characteristics of /aʊ/.

IMAGES OF THE ARTICULATORY AND ACOUSTIC CHARACTERISTICS OF /oʊ/ IN "SLOW"

The diphthong /oʊ/ in "slow" has the following features:

Advancement: from back to front

Height: from mid to high

Tenseness: from tense to lax

Roundness: from rounded to rounded

Filmstrip of /sloʊ/ "slow"

The diphthong /oʊ/ in the word "slow" /sloʊ/ can be seen in this filmstrip (Figure 36–5A). The lips open in a rounded position in the 13th frame to approximate the vowel /o/. This opening decreases almost linearly throughout the remaining frames. The change from the vowel /o/ to the vowel /ʊ/ is marked by a lesser degree of lip opening, greater lip rounding, and increasing protrusion.

Schematic Diagram of /oʊ/

In Figure 36–5B, the tongue positions for the vowels /o/ and /ʊ/ are shown separately. The dashed line shows the tongue position for the vowel /o/ at the back-mid position; and the solid line shows the tongue position of the vowel /ʊ/ at the back-high position.

Again, these tongue positions are accomplished sequentially, in a gliding manner, from the /o/ position to the /ʊ/ position.

Sound Spectrogram of /sloʊ/ "slow"

In Figure 36–5C, the vowel /o/ is presented in the final position in the word "slow." The initial consonant /s/ is a voiceless front sibilant. The acoustic representation of voicelessness can be seen by the absence of glottal vibration at the baseline of the sound spectrogram, as well as the lack of a rising first formant transition for the sonorant consonant /l/. The duration of this sibilant /s/ is over 200 msec. The sonorancy of the /l/, can be clearly seen in the formation of its formants, which are patterned after vowels. The F1 of /l/ is about 300 Hz, and the F2 is about 1100 Hz. A comparison of this production of /l/ with /l/ in the word "lily" in Chapter 23 demonstrates the influence of the high F2 for the vowel /ɪ/ in Chapter 23, as compared with the influence of the low F2 for the vowel /o/ on the second formant of the consonant /l/ in this module. Note that the second formant of the consonant /l/ in the word /lili/ (Chapter 23) is centered at 1500 Hz, whereas the second formant for the same consonant /l/ in the word /sloʊ/ is at 1100 Hz. These differences demonstrate the influence of vowel formants on the formants of adjacent sonorant consonants. The distribution of the formants indicates a detectable phoneme boundary for /o/ (F1 at 600 Hz and F2 at 1400 Hz), followed by approximately 100 msec of gliding F2 transition and the steady state of the vowel /ʊ/ (F1 at 250 Hz and F2 at 750 Hz).

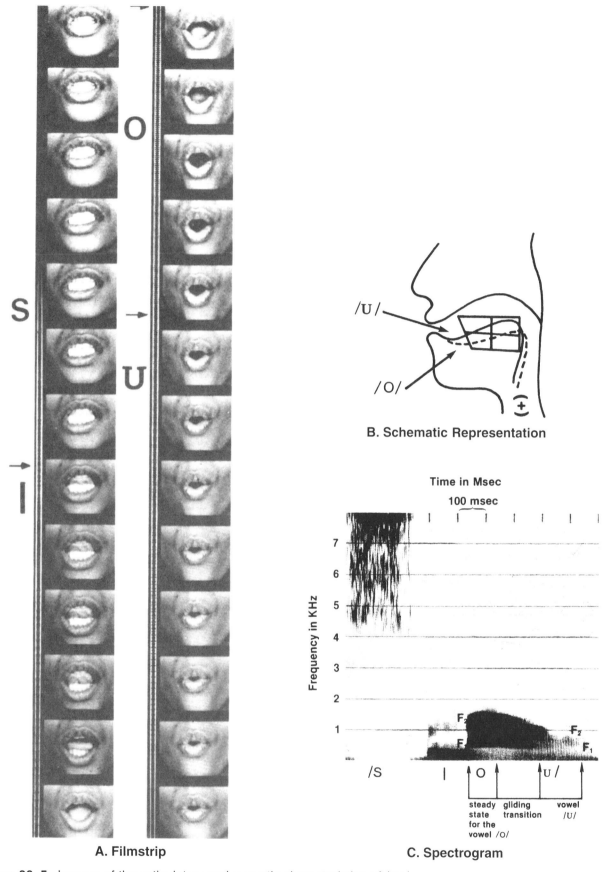

A. Filmstrip

B. Schematic Representation

C. Spectrogram

Figure 36–5. Images of the articulatory and acoustic characteristics of /oʊ/.

Chapter 37

Comparisons Between Speech Sounds

OVERVIEW

This chapter provides comparisons between the static images of English consonants and vowels. Each English consonant and vowel has been described fully in the preceding chapters. In this chapter, similar images are grouped so that visual comparisons can be made. Chapter 1 provides additional information in the interpretation of the images and Chapter 38 provides a description of how the images were created.

COMPARISON BETWEEN CONSONANTS

In the subsequent tables the English consonants are grouped using the format of the International Phonetic Alphabet (IPA) chart (see IPA chart at the front of the book). The columns are organized according to the prominent point of articulation of the consonant within the mouth. Consonants that are made toward the front of the mouth are located in the left-hand columns. Back sounds are located in columns at the right of the table. Consonants that are made in the middle of the mouth are in the central columns. For the voiced and voiceless cognates (such as /f/ and /v/, /t/ and /d/), the voiceless member of the pair is located on the column immediately to the left of the voiced member. The rows of the table are organized according to the manner of production. The first row comprises the stops (also called plosives). The second row comprises the nasal sounds. The third row, contains the majority of the sounds which are the fricatives. The fourth row contains the approximants.

Photographs

Photographs comparing production of English consonants are shown in Figure 37-1. The photographs allow comparison between the way consonants are produced, with particular focus on the shape of the lips and the extent of opening of the mouth. In some images the tongue tip also can be seen. These images will be of particular relevance to people who are interested in lip reading.

Line Drawings

Schematic line drawings comparing production of English consonants are shown in Figure 37-2. These line drawings allow for comparison between use of lips, tongue placement, presence and absence of nasality (shown by the velum being closed or open), and voicing status of the consonant (either a plus or minus symbol at the larynx).

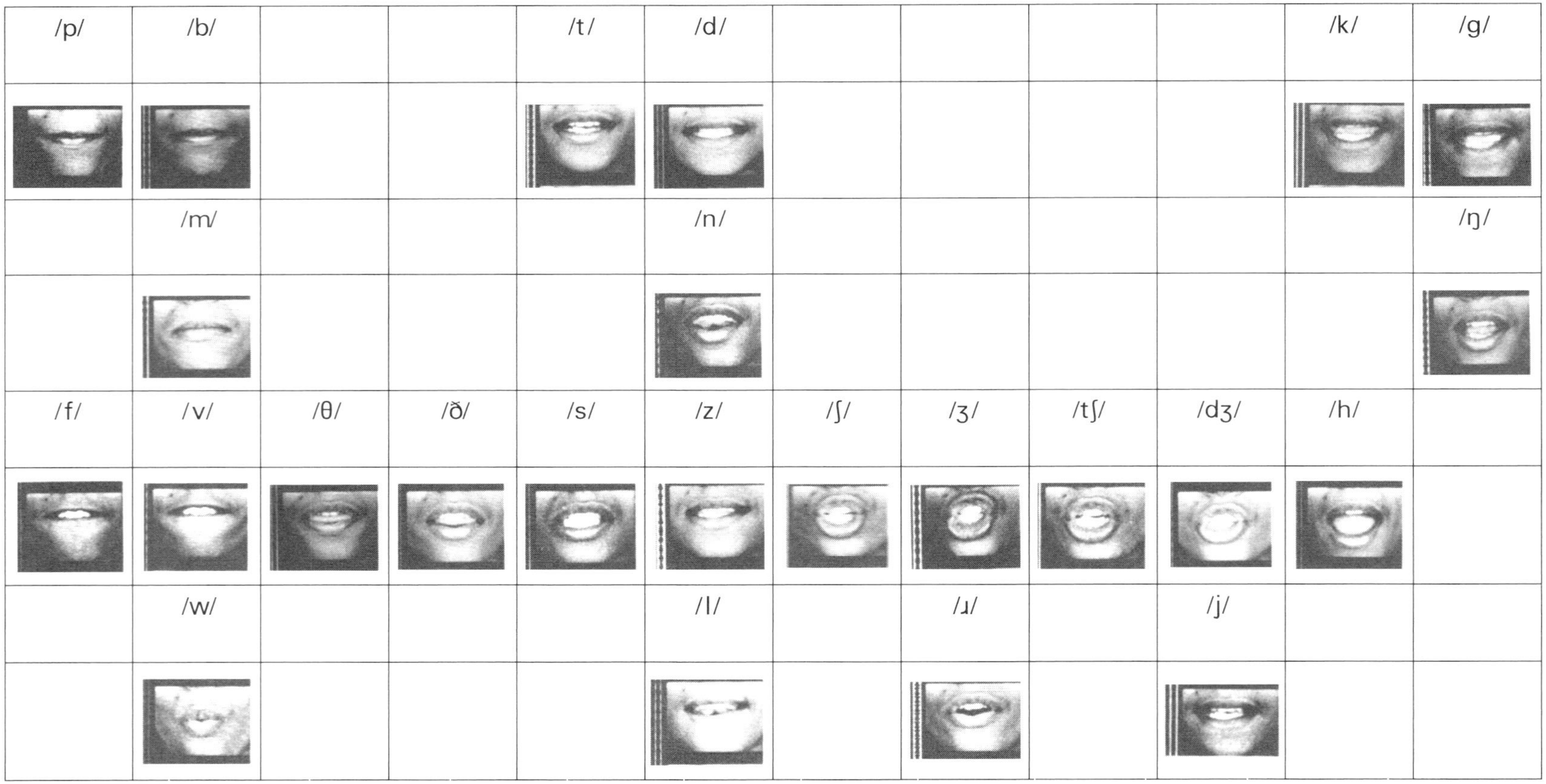

Figure 37–1. Comparison between photographs of the production of English consonants.

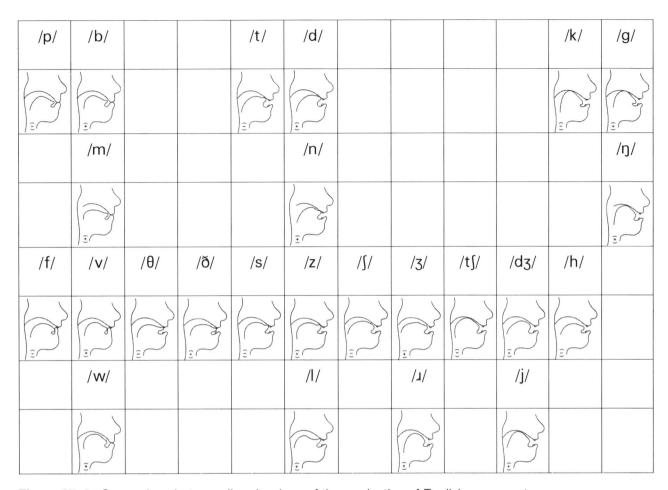

Figure 37–2. Comparison between line drawings of the production of English consonants.

Ultrasound Images

Figure 37-3 provides a comparison of ultrasound images of the production of English consonants. As with the line drawings, the ultrasound images allow comparison between the height and advancement of the tongue in the mouth. It is important to note that the tongue tip is on the right of the ultrasound images. Additionally, approximately 1 cm of the tongue tip is obscured by the acoustic shadow of the jaw (Stone, 2005). The cursor arrow at the top right of each image enables direct comparisons to be made from one image to another as the head was held in a steady state during each of these ultrasound recordings (see Chapter 38).

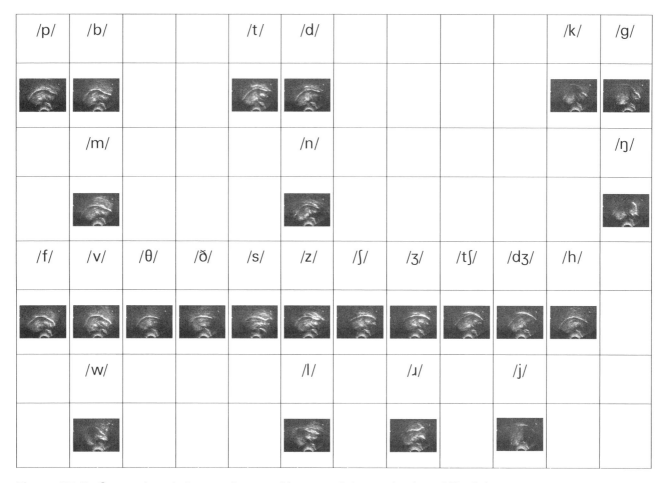

Figure 37–3. Comparison between ultrasound images of the production of English consonants.

Electropalatograph (EPG): Single Frames

Figure 37-4 provides a comparison between the extent and placement of tongue/palate contact during the production of English consonants for one speaker. The top of the image corresponds to the row of the electrodes immediately behind the front teeth on the alveolar ridge. Some frames are asymmetrical because they have been taken from real-time speech (see Chapter 38).

Electropalatograph (EPG): Cumulative Frames

Cumulative EPG images comparing production of English consonants are depicted in Figure 37-5. These images depict the extent of tongue/palate averaged over hundreds of exemplars of eight typical adult speakers' productions. The darker the shading the more contact. The numbers indicate the percentage of contact. The number 100 indicates that that electrode was contacted by each of the eight of the participants 100% of the time.

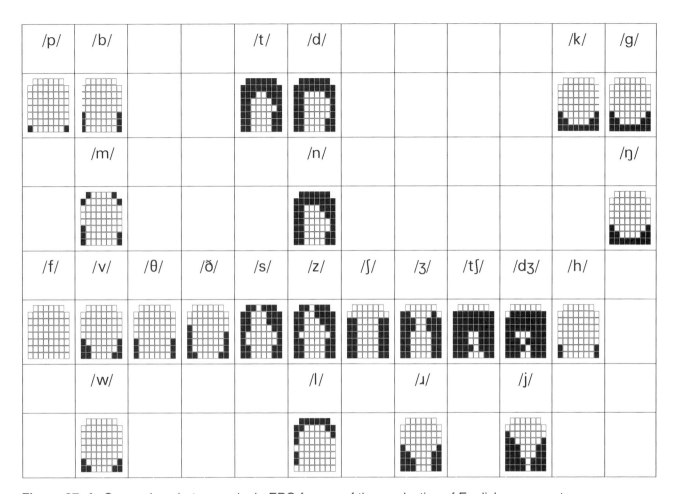

Figure 37–4. Comparison between single EPG frames of the production of English consonants.

Figure 37–5. Comparison between cumulative EPG frames of the production of lingual English consonants.

347

COMPARISON BETWEEN VOWELS

The next series of tables contain comparisons between English vowels. The vowels are grouped using the format of the vowel quadrilateral (Figure 37-6). The columns are organized according to the position within the mouth. Vowels that are made toward the front of the mouth are located in the left-hand columns. Vowels that are made toward the back are located in columns at the right of the table. Vowels that are made in the middle of the mouth are in the central columns. The rows of the table are organized according to the height of the vowel. The first row contains the vowels that are produced with the tongue high in the mouth. The final row contains the vowels that are produced with the jaw open and the tongue lower in the mouth.

Photographs

Photographs comparing production of English vowels are shown in Figure 37-7. The photographs allow comparison between the height of the vowel (depicted by the extent of the opening of the mouth) and the roundness of the vowel (depicted by the extent of lip rounding).

Line Drawings

Line drawings comparing production of English vowels are shown in Figure 37-8. The line drawings allow comparison between the height of the vowel (depicted by the height of the tongue in the mouth) and the advancement of the tongue in the production of the vowel (depicted by how forward the tongue is in the mouth). Lip rounding is also illustrated in these line drawings. All English vowels are voiced, so each image has a plus sign at the vocal cords.

Ultrasound Images

Ultrasound images comparing production of English vowels shown in Figure 37-9. As with the line drawings, the ultrasound images allow comparison between the height of the vowel (depicted by the height of the

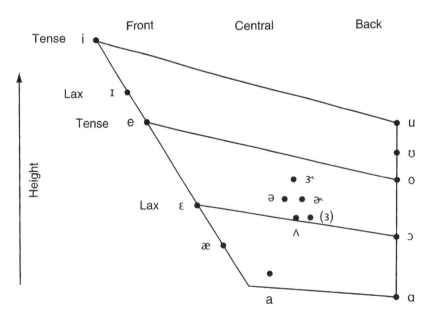

Figure 37–6. The complete set of 15 English vowels representing the advances, height, and tenseness continua shown in the vowel quadrilateral (*Source:* Singh, S. and Singh, K. (2006). *Phonetics: Principles and Practice* (3rd ed.). San Diego, CA: Plural. Figure 4-2, p. 98).

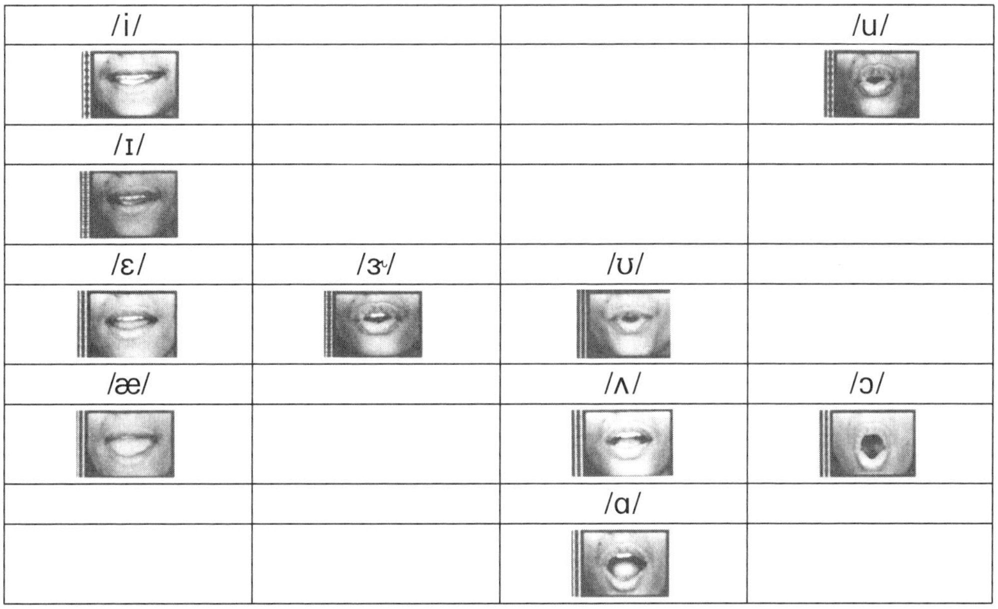

/i/			/u/
/ɪ/			
/ɛ/	/ɝ/	/ʊ/	
/æ/		/ʌ/	/ɔ/
		/ɑ/	

Figure 37–7. Comparison between photographs of the production of English vowels.

/i/			/u/
/ɪ/			
/ɛ/	/ɝ/	/ʊ/	
/æ/		/ʌ/	/ɔ/
		/ɑ/	

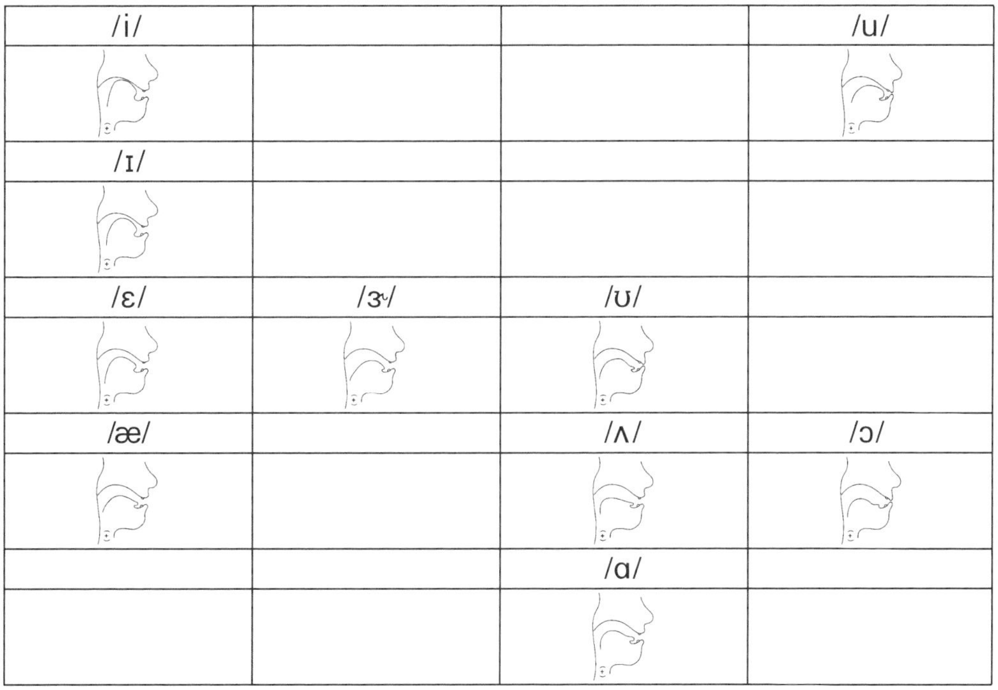

Figure 37–8. Comparison between line drawings of the production of English vowels.

tongue in the mouth) and the advancement of the tongue in the production of the vowel (depicted by how forward the tongue is in the mouth). The tongue tip is on the right of the ultrasound images.

Electropalatography (EPG)

Single EPG images comparing production of English vowels are shown in Figure 37-10. These images depict

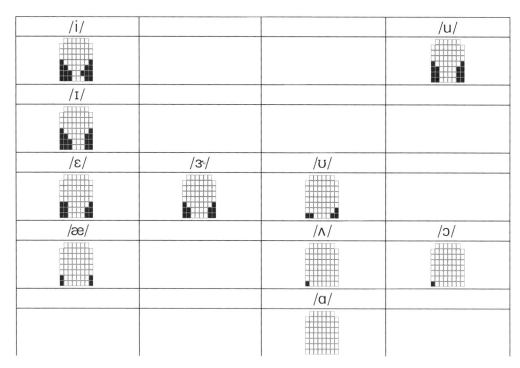

Figure 37–9. Comparison between ultrasound images of the production of English vowels.

Figure 37–10. Comparison between single EPG frames of the production of English vowels.

the extent of tongue/palate contact in the production of English vowels. The EPG is most frequently used to provide information about production of consonants; however, Figure 37-10 demonstrates that differences between the vowel height can be demonstrated using the EPG. When producing high vowels (e.g., /i/, /ɪ/) the tongue contacts the palate at the lateral margins. In contrast, low vowels (e.g., /ɑ/) have limited or no tongue/palate contact.

Chapter 38

Creating Images of Speech Production

CREATION OF STATIC AND DYNAMIC IMAGES OF SPEECH PRODUCTION

The images displayed in the *Speech Sounds: A Pictorial Guide to Typical and Atypical Speech* represent articulatory and acoustic aspects of consonant and vowel production for English. The majority of images have been specifically created for this book.

Creating Photographs and Filmstrips

The picture filmstrips were made from negatives of 35-mm high-speed motion picture film accompanied by a sound tract. It must be noted that these filmstrips are in absolute continuation. The only reason that some are presented in two, or sometimes three, different strips is the limitation of space in this printed book. One uninterrupted strip would have been too long for any reasonable symmetric presentation. The bottom of the first strip continues at the top of the second strip.

Second, it must be noted that these strips have been edited for presentation. The editing was done only at the beginning and at the end of a word. Because of the long duration of prephonatory articulatory gestures, the part of the filmstrip between the neutral stage of the articulators and the first trace of acoustic energy is not included. However, in each filmstrip, certain amounts of prephonatory and postphonatory articulatory gestures are included to show that the articulators are active before and after a sound is emitted. In the left-hand margin, phonemes are indicated using the International Phonetic Alphabet and arrows point to the general area of transition between phonemes.

The individual photographs are a single frame selected from the continuous filmstrip to approximately represent the production of a discrete phoneme.

Creating Schematic Line Drawings

Although the high-speed motion picture presentations provide important information regarding the articulatory gestures involved in the production of speech sounds, these pictures primarily emphasize the outside portion of the mouth. Therefore, a line drawing accompanies each module to emphasize the position of the tongue during the production of a particular consonant or vowel. These schematic diagrams are extremely simplified, showing outlines of the lips, tongue, palate and nasooropharynx. At the position of the larynx a plus (+) sign indicates voicing and a minus (–) sign indicates no voicing. The velum is either closed or open, indicating whether the sound is a nasal or oral sound. The tongue shape for each sound was hand-drawn onto the outline of the nasooropharynx by superimposing ultrasound images of the tongue during connected speech. As described below, the selection of each ultrasound image was verified by simultaneous audio and electropalatographic imaging.

Creating Sound Spectrograms

The sound spectrogram is provided for each consonant, vowel, and diphthong. The words presented in each chapter were spoken by a 25-year-old, multilingual female. The speaker learned English simultaneously with two other Indo-European languages. Her dialect has undergone change over time. She spoke General American English at the time of the recordings. The reader should be aware that spectrograms reflect the dialect and sex differences of speakers. Because the speaker in these modules is female, the overall frequency components are elevated. A comparison of the frequency components of speech sounds presented here with those of male speakers generally found in the literature should be made with this consideration in mind. Xue, Hao, and Mayo (2006) described the effect of race on males' vocal tracts and indicated that volumetric differences in vocal tracts may be responsible for formant frequency differences between speakers from white American, African American, and Chinese descent.

Creating Single Electropalatography (EPG) Images

A female researcher who frequently uses EPG in research and teaching recorded the single EPG images for the *Speech Sounds: A Pictorial Guide to Typical and Atypical Speech*. The speaker spoke Australian English, had no history of hearing difficulties, no speech impairment, and no impairment in oromusculature structure or function.

An individual EPG palate for the speech researcher was made from a dental impression of the upper and lower teeth and palate. In this case, a Reading WIN/EPG palate was used that has 62 electrodes arranged in eight rows (see Chapter 1). The dental impression and Reading WIN/EPG palate worn by the speaker is shown in Figure 38–1. The speaker adapted to the palate by wearing it for 1 hour prior to the recording session. Words and phonemes were embedded within a carrier phrase: "I see a _____ again." At the time of the recording session, the speaker simultaneously recorded the EPG, ultrasound,

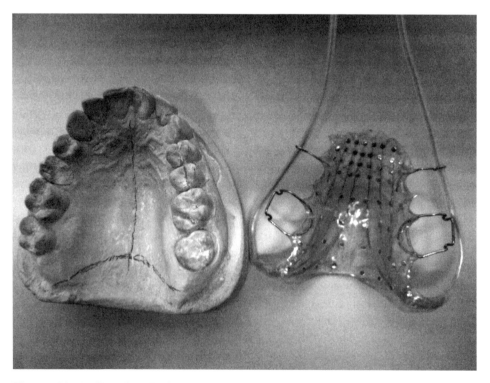

Figure 38–1. Reading EPG palate worn to produce the single EPG images and dental impression used to create the palate.

and acoustic (waveform and spectrographic) data in order to assist with identification of the boundaries and midpoint of the phoneme. Data were collected and analyzed using the Articulate Assistant Advanced (AAA) computer program, version 2.02 (Articulate Instruments, 2006) (Figure 38-2).

Selection of the single EPG frame was based on identifying the midpoint of the phoneme and comparing its similarity with the research data on typical EPG images of maximum contact (e.g., Hardcastle & Edwards, 1992; McLeod & Roberts, 2005; Stone & Lundberg, 1996). In all cases, the selected production was similar (but not necessarily identical) to the typical EPG images published by these researchers. Unlike stylized images of tongue/palate contact, the selected single EPG images within *Speech Sounds: A Pictorial Guide to Typical and Atypical Speech* are at times asymmetric. This is evidence that the images come from real speech. To examine variability in articulation of a specific speech sound, where possible, the single EPG images should be compared with the cumulative EPG productions.

Creating Dynamic Sequences of Electropalatography (EPG) Images

The same speaker who produced the single EPG images also produced the dynamic sequences of EPG images. In each case, the speaker embedded the target words within the phrase "I see a _____ again." Figure 38-3 shows the Articulate Assistant Advanced computer screen for the production of "I see a tat again." The simultaneous display of waveform, spectrogram, electropalatograph, and ultrasound images is apparent. Figure 38-4 shows the complete EPG series of frames for the sentence "I see a tat again" taken from the same recording as shown in Figure 38-3. Due to space considerations, the dynamic EPG sequence of frames shown in Chapters 2 to 27 only include the targeted word selected from the entire sentence. Consequently, Figure 38-5 shows the selected EPG frames to illustrate the word "tat" as presented in Chapter 4. The word boundaries were selected as the frame immediately prior to closure for the initial sounds and immediately following closure for the final sound.

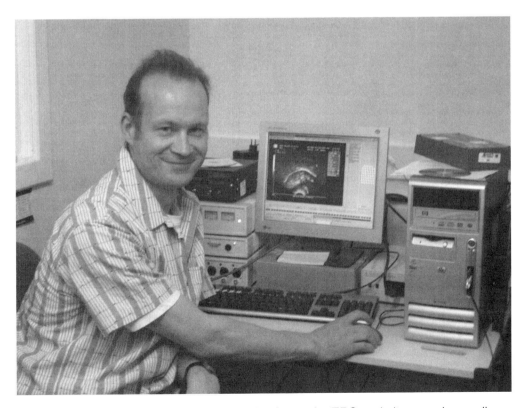

Figure 38–2. Data analysis hardware and software for EPG and ultrasound recordings.

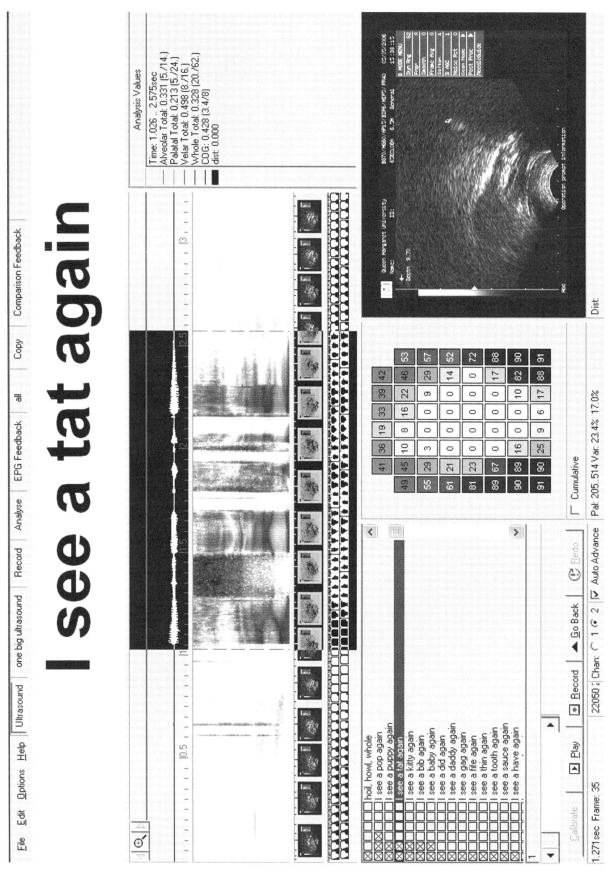

Figure 38–3. Screen image for Articulate Assistant Advanced (AAA) computer program showing simultaneous waveform, spectrogram, EPG, and ultrasound data capture of "I see a tat again."

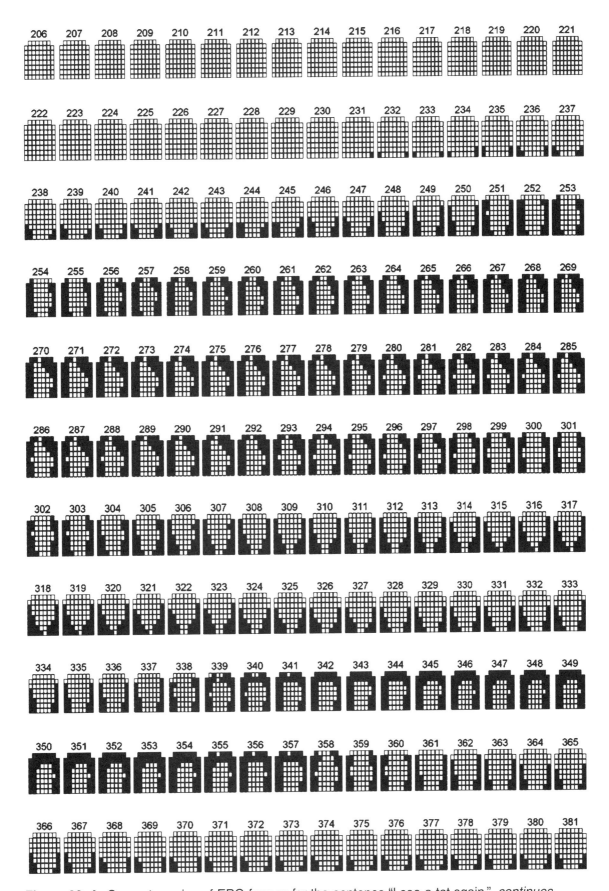

Figure 38–4. Compete series of EPG frames for the sentence "I see a tat again." *continues*

355

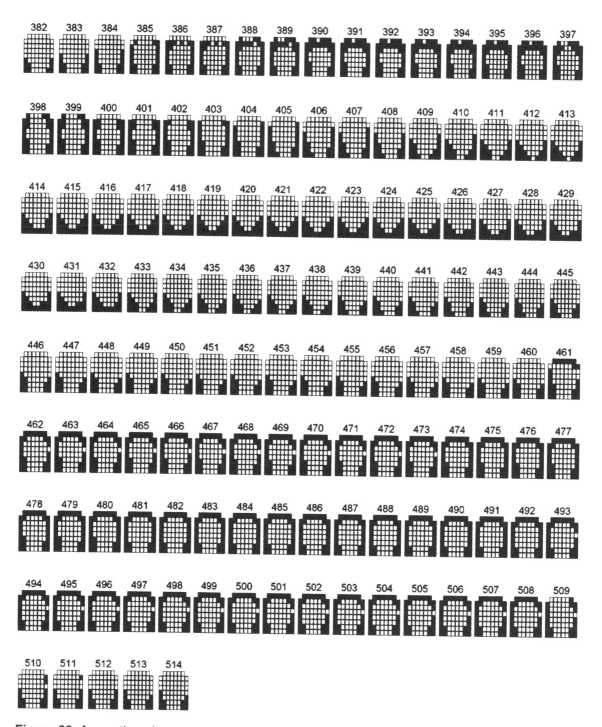

Figure 38–4. *continued*

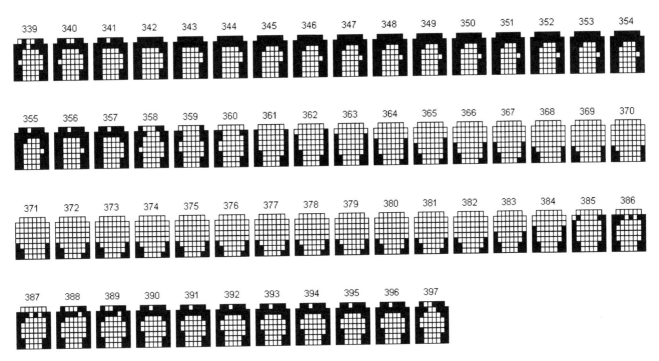

Figure 38–5. Selected EPG frames for the word "tat."

Creating Cumulative Electropalatography (EPG) Images

The cumulative EPG frames were created as part of a large research project (McLeod, 2003); that has been documented in a variety of research papers and presentations (McLeod, 2006; McLeod & Gibbon, 2007; 2008; McLeod & Roberts, 2005; McLeod & Searl, 2006). The participants were four females (F1–F4) and four males (M1–M4) who spoke General Australian English. None had exposure to speech-language pathology or phonetics. None of the participants reported any significant medical history. Prior to data collection, each participant was assessed and found to have normal results on the following measures: hearing, oromusculature, and ability to produce speech tasks that stressed the phonological system (multisyllabic words, tongue twisters and the Grandfather Passage). The participants produced 13 lingual consonants in a variety of syllable shapes (CV, VC, CVC). The consonants (C) studied were: /t, d, k, g, s, z, ʃ, ʒ, n, ŋ, l, r, j/. Each consonant was paired with a phoneme that occurred at the same alveolar place of articulation, then a phoneme at the opposite place of articulation. The syllables contained the following vowels (V) /i, æ, ʌ, ɜ,

u/ representing the extremes of the Australian vowel quadrilateral. The participants produced the stimuli in the same order and the syllables containing the five vowels were recorded within one phrase, for example, "a neat, a gnat, a nut, a nert, a noot."

To acclimatize to wearing the EPG palate the participants wore a pseudo-EPG palate (the same shape, but without electrodes or wires). On day 1, they wore the pseudopalate for 3 hours over a period of 5 hours and on day 2, participants wore the pseudopalate for 0.5 hours, then the EPG palate (see McLeod & Searl, 2006 for full details). Data recording using the EPG palate commenced immediately following the acclimatization phase on day 2. For the next 4 hours, the participants read a word list of approximately 1000 target words three times over. Productions 2 and 3 of each word were analyzed. These were rated "normal/typical" by two experienced speech pathologists. If a production was not considered to be "normal" then production 1 was analyzed (this was rare). The maximum point of contact for each consonant was selected as the reference frame (cf. Hardcastle & Gibbon, 1997).

The EPG files were uploaded using ArticAssist v.1.6 (Wrench, 2002). The waveform and audio recordings were used to identify the point where the consonants were initiated and where they ceased. The frames within these parameters were annotated to represent the series of tongue-palatal contacts for each consonant. The middle 5 frames were then identified and the frame with the greatest amount of contact (maximum point of contact) selected from within these 5 frames.

To exhibit tongue/palate contact patterns for each participant 4 different types of images were created for display in the *Speech Sounds: A Pictorial Guide to Typical and Atypical Speech*:

1. A cumulative display was created by cumulating *all* eight participants' maximum contact frames for their production of all words containing each the consonant.
2. The maximum contact frame from the second production of each word was placed into an extensive table.
3. A cumulative display was created by cumulating all maximum contact frames for *each* participants' production of all words containing each the consonant.

Each of these images was included the *Speech Sounds: A Pictorial Guide to Typical and Atypical Speech* to graphically demonstrate the wide degree of intra- and interparticipant variability for productions of each speech sound.

Creating EPG Images from Others' Research

Throughout the literature, EPG images have been represented in numerous ways. Within each paper, unique varieties of colour (dark to light shading) and shapes (squares, rectangles, and circles) have been used to represent each EPG electrode. To simplify the complexity and individuality of these images and to reduce the need to explain each image separately, all images from others' research have been redrawn using a simple box EPG template. A criterion of at least 67% contact was set for shading of contacted electrodes as black. In almost every instance, it was possible to keep to this criterion and any departure from this criterion is mentioned in the text of the chapter. For example, Guzik and Harrington (2007) reported at least 50% contact in their paper, so it was impossible to use the

67% criterion when reporting their data on three Polish speakers' productions of /s/ in Chapter 15.

There is a substantial body of published literature on electropalatography and its usefulness in understanding typical speech production as well as in the assessment and intervention for people with speech impairment. Due to the size of the corpus of published EPG data, a large amount has not been included in the *Speech Sounds: A Pictorial Guide to Typical and Atypical Speech*. One criterion for the exclusion of data was if researchers had used non-Reading EPG palate designs (such as the Logometrix and Kay designs). These palate designs use a different array and number of electrodes, so it is not appropriate to redraw these images on the 62 electrode Reading EPG palate design. The authors of *Speech Sounds: A Pictorial Guide to Typical and Atypical Speech* would encourage interested readers to read the research from others who have used different EPG palates. Some recommended papers include:

◆ Stone and Lundberg (1996)—typical adults' production of 11 American English vowels + the consonants /l, s, ʃ, θ, n, ŋ/
◆ Stone, Faber, Raphael, and Shawker (1992) – typical adults' production of /s, ʃ, l/
◆ Dagenais (1995) and Dagenais, Critz-Crosby, and Adams (1994)—intervention for children with speech impairment, including lateral lisps

New electropalatography instrumentation is currently being developed. Researchers such as Searl (2003) and Murdoch, Goozee, Veidt, Scott, and Meyers (2004) are developing pressure sensitive EPG palates. Wrench (2007) is developing a new EPG palate enhancing features of the Reading EPG palate used throughout this book. Interested readers can keep in touch with these developments and the new insights that they provide through reading academic journals such as *Clinical Linguistics and Phonetics*.

Creating Ultrasound Images

A female speech researcher who spoke Australian English created the midsagittal ultrasound images of the tongue during speech. In order to stabilize the ultrasound probe so that images could be compared with one another a purpose-built helmet was worn (see Figures 38–3 and 38–4) (for further details, see McLeod & Wrench, 2008). Stone (2005, p. 469) indicates that transducer stabilization is important to ensure "intimate contact with the chin and accurate beam direction." The ultrasound images were created simultaneously with the single and dynamic EPG images described above. In Figure 38–6, the ultrasound probe can be seen under the chin and the cords extending from the EPG palate can be seen leaving the mouth and inserting into the multiplexer (box).

In order to select the ultrasound images for inclusion in the *Speech Sounds: A Pictorial Guide to Typical and Atypical Speech*, the audio file, spectrogram, electropalatograph, and ultrasound image were played simultaneously. Each ultrasound image corresponds exactly to the single EPG image to ensure accurate and compatible identification of tongue shape for each consonant or vowel. This simultaneous identification at the point of maximum tongue/palate contact

using EPG and ultrasound is a unique feature of this text and may explain any differences between ultrasound images found in other texts that have not paired ultrasound and EPG imaging.

Rationale for Selection of Speech Models

As far as possible, the authors purposefully used women as the speech models for *Speech Sounds: A Pictorial Guide to Typical and Atypical Speech*. The majority of texts and research papers on articulatory and acoustic properties of consonants and vowels have used examples from males' speech. Kent and Read (2002, p. 189) indicate the need for exemplars from women and children: "The problem is that the research effort given to the speech of women and children has been on a smaller scale than that given to the speech of men. Consequently, there is a continuing need to gather acoustic data for diverse populations." Kent and Read (2002, Chapter 6) provide an extensive discussion

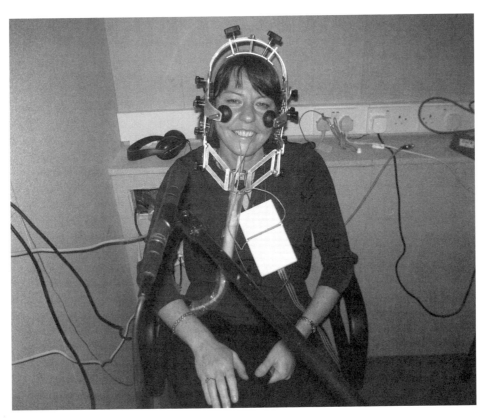

Figure 38–6. Helmet worn to stabilize the ultrasound probe.

of the differences between the acoustic properties of men's, women's, and children's speech. For example, formant frequencies are different for speakers of different gender and ages due to differences in the length of the vocal tract, with an overall trend toward decreasing formant frequencies with age. Females and children tend to have higher formant frequencies than males.

Stone (2005) indicated that the quality of ultrasound images varies according to the speaker. She suggested that images of the tongues of women and children were often clearer than images of men's tongues. She hypothesized that this was possibly due to having smaller and smoother tongue surfaces. She also suggested that people who are thinner have better images than those who are fatter, possibly because fatty tissue in the tongue can refract the sound waves. Furthermore, she suggested that those who are younger have better tongue images than those who are older, possibly because their mouths are moister and they have less fatty tissue.

In comparison, differences between the articulation of sounds are unlikely to be affected by gender. For example, the cumulative electropalatography (EPG) data presented in *Speech Sounds: A Pictorial Guide to Typical and Atypical Speech* have been created by four males and four females. Consideration of these articulatory images indicates that although there are many individual differences, these do not appear to be an artifact of gender. As with texts that primarily use male examples of speech production, the articulatory and acoustic images provided in the *Speech Sounds: A Pictorial Guide to Typical and Atypical Speech* can be used as exemplars for understanding speech production for all people.

Chapter 39

Exercises

FILL IN THE BLANKS

1. In the sound spectrogram of "pop" in Chapter 2, the phoneme /p/ shows lack of aspiration at the _____ position of the word and aspiration at the position of the word.

2. The influence of one phoneme on another in context is called _____.

3. In the schematic diagram of the phoneme /g/ in Chapter 7, the back of the tongue contacts the _____ and stops the airstream.

4. Considerable jaw excursion and unrounded lips are characteristic of the vowel _____.

5. In the filmstrip of "zoom" in Chapter 16, although the first frame is involved in the production of the nonlabial phoneme /z/, it shows a considerable amount of lip rounding because of the influence of _____.

6. In the sound spectrogram of "searching" in Chapter 19, the lowering of energy below 4000 Hz for the sibilant /tʃ/ as compared to the sibilant /s/ is caused by _____ for /tʃ/.

7. In Chapter 22, the frames at the end of the first strip of the film for "wash" are involved in the production of the phoneme _____.

8. In the sound spectrogram of Chapter 34, the (+) voicing characteristic of the phoneme /b/ is denoted by a rising F1, and labiality is denoted by _____.

9. In Chapter 11 for the word "fife," the soundtrack of the filmstrip does not begin until frame _____.

10. In the sound spectrogram of the diphthong /ɔɪ/ in Chapter 36, following the long glide, the second formant of the vowel /ɪ/ assumes a steady state at approximately _____ Hz.

TRUE OR FALSE

1. Frames 1 through 6 in the word "baby" in Chapter 3 and frames 1 through 4 in the word "bathe" in Chapter 14 are similar because they both are involved in the production of /b/.

2. The sound spectrogram and filmstrip in the word "pop" in Chapter 2 exemplify the rule that stops in the final position in a word are always released.

3. The plosive burst for the voiceless stop /t/ shown in the sound spectrogram of the word "tat" in Chapter 4 has energy concentrated in the same frequency area as that for the phoneme /p/ in the word "pop" in Chapter 2.

4. The sound spectrogram in the word "puppy" in Chapter 2 shows that the phoneme /p/ has allophonic variations in the English language.

5. Frames 1 through 9 of the filmstrip in the word "fife" in Chapter 11 are similar to frames 7 through 15 in the word "veal" in Chapter 12, because they represent the same phoneme.

6. The (+) voicing nature of the phoneme /b/ in the sound spectrogram of the word "baby" in Chapter 3 is indicated by the presence of negative voice onset time and a falling F1 for the following vowel.

7. The schematic diagram of the phoneme /d/ in the word "did" in Chapter 5 shows that it is clearly a back consonant.

8. The sound spectrogram in the word "sauce" in Chapter 15 shows that the sibilant /s/ has the same frequency characteristics as the sibilant /z/ in Chapter 16.

9. The weak band of energy below 1000 Hz for the vowel /ɑ/ in the sound spectrogram of the word

"mom" in Chapter 8 is caused by the effect of nasalization.

10. The stop characteristic of the phoneme /ʒ/ can be seen in the schematic diagram in Chapter 18.

11. In the sound spectrogram of the word "bit" in Chapter 27, the second formant of the vowel /ɪ/ is centered at approximately 2800 Hz.

12. A comparison of the filmstrip in the word "bought" in Chapter 35 with that in the word "father" in Chapter 30 shows that the lips are more open and more rounded for vowel /ɔ/ than for vowel /ɑ/.

13. In the diphthong /aɪ/ in Chapter 36, the individual phoneme boundaries for the vowels /a/ and /ɪ/ are both maintained and can be seen in the filmstrip, schematic diagram, and sound spectrogram.

14. The schematic diagrams in Chapters 2 and 22 differ only in the voicing characteristic.

Recommended Background Reading

Ball, M. J., & Lowry, O. (2001). *Methods in clinical phonetics*. London: Whurr.

Ball, M. J., & Rahilly, J. (1999). *Phonetics. The science of speech*. London: Edward Arnold.

International Phonetic Association. (1999). *Handbook of the International Phonetic Association*. Cambridge: Cambridge University Press.

Kent, R. D. (1997). *The speech sciences*. San Diego, CA: Singular.

Kent, R. D., & Read, C. (2002). *Acoustic analysis of speech*. (2nd ed.). Albany, NY: Singular Thomson Learning.

Ladefoged, P. (2000a). *A course in phonetics* (4th ed.). Florence, KY: Heinle.

Ladefoged, P. (2000b). *Vowels and consonants: An introduction to the sounds of languages*. Oxford: Blackwell.

Laver, J. (1994). *Principles of phonetics*. Cambridge: Cambridge University Press.

Shriberg, L. D., & Kent, R. D. (2003). *Clinical phonetics* (3rd ed.). Boston: Allyn & Bacon.

Singh, S., & Singh, K. (2006). *Phonetics: Principles and practice* (3rd ed). San Diego, CA: Plural.

References

Articulate Instruments. (2006). *Articulate Assistant Advanced* (AAA) version 2.02 [computer program]. Edinburgh: Author.

Bacsfalvi, P., Bernhardt, B. M., & Gick, B. (2007). Electropalatography and ultrasound in vowel remediation for adolescents with hearing impairment. *Advances in Speech-Language Pathology, 9*(1), 36–45.

Ball, M. J., Gracco, V., & Stone, M. (2001). A comparison of imaging techniques for the investigation of normal and disordered speech production. *Advances in Speech-Language Pathology, 3*, 13–24.

Bernhardt, B., Gick, B., Bacsfalvi, P., & Adler-Bock, M. (2005). Ultrasound in speech therapy with adolescents and adults. *Clinical Linguistics and Phonetics, 19*, 605–617.

Bernhardt, B., Gick, B., Bacsfalvi, P., & Ashdown, J. (2003). Speech habilitation of hard of hearing adolescents using electropalatography and ultrasound as evaluated by trained listeners. *Clinical Linguistics and Phonetics, 17*, 199–216.

Bressmann, T., Thind, P., Uy, C., Bollig, C., Gilbert, R., & Irish, J. (2005). Quantitative three-dimensional ultrasound analysis of tongue protrusion, grooving and symmetry: Data from 12 normal speakers and a partial glossectomee. *Clinical Linguistics and Phonetics, 19*(6–7), 573–588.

Catford, J. C. (1977). *Fundamental problems in phonetics*. Bloomington: Indiana University Press.

Cheng, Y., Murdoch, B. E., Goozée, J. V., & Scott, D. (2007). Electropalatographic assessment of tongue-to-palate contact patterns and variability in children, adolescents, and adults. *Journal of Speech, Language, and Hearing Research, 50*(2), 375–392.

Chi-Fishman, G. (2005). Quantitative lingual, pharyngeal and laryngeal ultrasonography in swallowing research: A technical review. *Clinical Linguistics and Phonetics, 19*(6–7), 589–604.

Crystal, T. H., & House, A. S. (1982). Segmental durations in connected speech signals: Preliminary results. *Journal of the Acoustical Society of America, 72*, 705–716.

Dagenais, P. A. (1995). Electropalatography in the treatment of articulation/phonological disorders. *Communication Disorders, 28*, 303–329.

Dagenais, P. A., Critz-Crosby, P., & Adams, J. B. (1994). Defining and remediating persistent lateral lisps in children using electropalatography: Preliminary findings. *American Journal of Speech-Language Pathology, 4*, 67–76.

Dagenais, P. A., Lorendo, L. C., & McCutcheon, M. J. (1994). A study of voicing and context effects upon consonant linguapalatal contact patterns. *Journal of Phonetics, 22*, 225–238.

Davidson, L. (2005). Addressing phonological questions with ultrasound. *Clinical Linguistics and Phonetics, 19*(6–7), 619–633.

Dent, H. (2001). Electropalatography: A tool for psycholinguistic therapy. In J. Stackhouse, & B. Wells (Eds.), *Children's speech and language difficulties 2: Identification and intervention* (pp. 205–248). London: Whurr.

Flipsen, P., Shriberg, L., Weismer, G., Karlsson, H., & McSweeny, J. (1999). Acoustic characteristics of /s/ in adolescents. *Journal of Speech, Language, and Hearing Research, 42*, 663–677.

Flipsen, P., Shriberg, L. D., Weismer, G., Karlsson, H. B., & McSweeny, J. L. (2001). Acoustic phenotypes for speech-genetics studies: Reference data for residual /ʒ/ distortions. *Clinical Linguistics and Phonetics, 15*, 603–630.

Fuchs, S., Brunner, J., & Busler, A. (2007). Temporal and spatial aspects concerning the realisations of the voicing contrast in German alveolar and postalveolar fricatives. *Advances in Speech-Language Pathology, 9*(1), 90–100.

Fujiwara, Y. (2007). Electropalatography home training using a portable training unit for Japanese children with cleft palate. *Advances in Speech-Language Pathology, 9*(1), 65–72.

Gibbon, F., & Hardcastle, W. (1987). Articulatory description and treatment of "lateral /s/" using electopalatography:

A case study. *British Journal of Disorders of Communication, 22,* 203–217.

Gibbon, F., & Hardcastle, W. (1989). Deviant articulation in a cleft palate child following late repair of the hard palate: A description and remediation procedure using electropalatography (EPG). *Clinical Linguistics and Phonetics, 3,* 93–110.

Gibbon, F., Hardcastle, W., & Moore, A. (1990). Modifying abnormal tongue patterns in an older child using electropalatography. *Child Language Teaching and Therapy, 6,* 227–245.

Gibbon, F., Smeaton-Ewins, P., & Crampin, L. (2005). Tongue-palate contact during selected vowels in children with cleft palate. *Folia Phoniatrica et Logopaedica, 57,* 181–192.

Gibbon, F., Stewart, F., Hardcastle, W. J., & Crampin, L. (1999). Widening access to electropalatography for children with persistent sound system disorders. *American Journal of Speech-Language Pathology, 8,* 319–333.

Gibbon, F., Whitehill, T. L., Hardcastle, W. J., Stokes, S. F., & Nairn, M. (1998). Cross-language (Cantonese/English) study of articulatory error patterns in cleft palate speech using electropalatography (EPG). In W. Zeligler & K. Deger (Eds.), *Clinical Phonetics and Linguistics* (pp. 165–176). London: Whurr.

Gibbon, F. E. (1999a). Towards a better understanding of abnormal lingual articulation in children with speech disorders. In S. McLeod & L. McAllister (Eds.), *Speech Pathology Australia National Conference* (pp. 12–23). Sydney: Speech Pathology Australia.

Gibbon, F. E. (1999b). Undifferentiated lingual gestures in children with articulation/phonological disorders. *Journal of Speech, Language, and Hearing Research, 42,* 382–397.

Gibbon, F. E. (2004). Abnormal patterns of tongue/palate contact in the speech of individuals with cleft palate. *Clinical Linguistics and Phonetics, 18*(4/5), 285–312.

Gibbon, F. E., & Crampin, L. (2002). Labial-lingual double articulations in speakers with cleft palate. *Cleft Palate-Craniofacial Journal, 39*(1), 40–49.

Gibbon, F. E., Ellis, L., & Crampin, L. (2004). Articulatory placement for /t/, /d/, /k/ and /g/ target in school age children with speech disorders associated with cleft palate. *Clinical Linguistics and Phonetics, 18*(6–8), 391–404.

Gibbon, F. E., Lee, A., & Yuen, I. (2007). Tongue palate contact during bilabials in normal speech. *Cleft Palate-Craniofacial Journal, 44*(1), 87–91.

Gibbon, F. E., McNeill, A. M., Wood, S. E., & Watson, J. M. M. (2003). Changes in linguapalatal contact patterns during therapy for velar fronting in a 10-year-old with Down's syndrome. *International Journal of Language and Communication Disorders, 38*(1), 47–64.

Gibbon, F. E., & Paterson, L. (2006). A survey of speech and language therapists' views on electropalatography therapy outcomes in Scotland. *Child Language Teaching and Therapy, 22*(3), 275–292.

Gibbon, F. E., & Wood, S. E. (2003). Using electropalatography (EPG) to diagnose and treat articulation disorders associated with mild cerebral palsy: A case study. *Clinical Linguistics and Phonetics, 17,* 365–374.

Gibbon, F. E., Yuen, I., Lee, A., & Adams, L. (2007). Normal adult speakers' tongue palate contact patterns for alveolar oral and nasal stops. *Advances in Speech-Language Pathology, 9*(1), 82–89.

Guzik, K. M., & Harrington, J. (2007). The quantification of place of articulation assimilation in electropalatographic data using the similarity index (SI). *Advances in Speech-Language Pathology, 9*(1), 109–119.

Hardcastle, W., & Edwards, S. (1992). EPG-based description of apraxic speech errors. In R. Kent (Ed.), *Intelligibility in speech disorders* (Vol. 1, pp. 287–329). Amsterdam: John Benjamin.

Hardcastle, W. J., & Gibbon, F. (1997). Electropalatography and its clinical applications. In M. J. Ball & C. Code (Eds.), *Instrumental clinical phonetics* (pp. 149–193). London: Croom Helm.

Hardcastle, W. J., Morgan Barry, R. A. & Nunn, M. (1989). Instrumental articulatory phonetics in assessment and remediation: Case studies with the electropalatograph. In J. Stengelhofen (Ed.) *Cleft palate: The nature and remediation of communicative problems* (pp. 136–164). Edinburgh: Churchill Livingstone.

Harrington, J., Cox, F., & Evans, Z. (1997). An acoustic phonetic study of broad, general, and cultivated Australian English vowels. *Australian Journal of Linguistics, 17,* 155–184.

Hewlett, N. (1988). Acoustic properties of /k/ and /t/ in normal and phonologically disordered speech. *Clinical Linguistics and Phonetics, 2,* 29–45.

Hickey, J. (1992). The treatment of lateral fricatives and affricates using electropalatography: A case study of a 10 year old girl. *Clinical Speech and Language Studies, 1,* 80–87.

Hoole, P., Zeigler, W., Hartman, E., & Hardcastle, W. (1989). Parallel electropalatography and acoustic measures of fricatives. *Clinical Linguistics and Phonetics, 3,* 59–69.

Horvath, B. M. (1985). *Variation in Australian English: The sociolects of Sydney.* Cambridge: Cambridge University Press.

Howard, S. (2004). Compensatory articulatory behaviours in adolescents with cleft palate: Comparing the perceptual and instrumental evidence. *Clinical Linguistics and Phonetics, 18*(4/5), 313-340.

Howard, S. (2007). The interplay between articulation and prosody in children with impaired speech: Observations from electropalatographic and perceptual analysis. *Advances in Speech-Language Pathology, 9*(1), 20-35.

Kent, R. D. (1992). The biology of phonological development. In C. A. Ferguson, L.Menn, & C. Stoel-Gammon (Eds.), *Phonological development: Models, research, implications* (pp. 65-90). Timonium, MD: York Press.

Kent, R. D., & Read, C. (2002). *Acoustic analysis of speech* (2nd ed.). Albany, NY: Singular Thomson Learning.

Ladefoged, P. (2005). *Vowels and consonants* (2nd ed.). Oxford, UK: Blackwell.

Lee, A., Gibbon, F. E., Crampin, L., Yuen, I., & McLennan, G. (2007). The national CLEFTNET project for individuals with speech disorders associated with cleft palate. *Advances in Speech-Language Pathology, 9*(1), 57-64.

Liker, M., Gibbon, F., Wrench, A., & Horga, D. (2007). Articulatory characteristics of the occlusion phase of /tʃ/ compared to /t/ in adult speech. *Advances in Speech-Language Pathology, 9*(1), 101-108.

Maclagan, M. & Gillon, G. T. (2007). New Zealand English speech acquisition. In S. McLeod (Ed.), *The international guide to speech acquisition* (pp. 257-268). Clifton Park, NY: Thomson Delmar Learning.

Martin, K. L., Hirson, A., Herman, R., Thomas, J., & Pring, T. (2007). The efficacy of speech intervention using electropalatography with an 18-year-old deaf client: A single case study. *Advances in Speech-Language Pathology, 9*(1), 46-56.

McAuliffe, M. J., Ward, E. C., & Murdoch, B. E. (2003). Variation in articulatory timing of three English consonants: An electropalatographic investigation. *Clinical Linguistics and Phonetics, 17*, 43-62.

McAuliffe, M. J., Ward, E. C., & Murdoch, B. E. (2006a). Speech production in Parkinson's disease I: An electropalatographic investigation of tongue-palate contact patterns. *Clinical Linguistics and Phonetics, 20*(1), 1-18.

McAuliffe, M. J., Ward, E. C., & Murdoch, B. E. (2006b). Speech production in Parkinson's disease II: Acoustic and electropalatographic investigation of sentence, word and segment durations. *Clinical Linguistics and Phonetics, 20*(1), 19-33.

McAuliffe, M. J., Ward, E. C., & Murdoch, B. E. (2007). Intra-participant variability in Parkinson's disease: An electro-palatographic examination of articulation. *Advances in Speech-Language Pathology, 9*(1), 13-19.

McLeod, S. (2003). Mapping tongue/palate contact for intelligible speech production for Australians. *Charles Sturt University Competitive Grant.*

McLeod, S. (2006). Australian adults' production of /n/: An EPG investigation. *Clinical Linguistics and Phonetics, 20*(2/3), 99-107.

McLeod, S. (Ed.). (2007). *The international guide to speech acquisition.* Clifton Park, NY: Thomson Delmar Learning.

McLeod, S. & Gibbon, F. E. (2007, July). *The impact of voicing on the extent of tongue/palate contact.* 5th Asia Pacific Conference on Speech, Language, and Hearing, Brisbane.

McLeod, S. & Gibbon, F. E. (2008). *The impact of place, manner, voicing, syllable and vowel contexts on production of lingual consonants.* Manuscript in preparation.

McLeod, S. & Isaac, K. (1995). Use of spectrographic analyses to evaluate the efficacy of phonological intervention. *Clinical Linguistics and Phonetics, 9*, 229-234.

McLeod, S., & Roberts, A. (2005). Templates of tongue/palate contact for speech sound intervention. In C. Heine & L. Brown (Eds.), *Proceedings of the 2005 Speech Pathology Australia National Conference* (pp. 104-112). Melbourne: Speech Pathology Australia.

McLeod, S., Roberts, A., & Sita, J. (2006). Tongue/palate contact for the production of /s/ and /z/. *Clinical Linguistics and Phonetics, 20*(1), 51-66.

McLeod, S., & Searl, J. (2006). Adaptation to an electropalatograph palate: Acoustic, impressionistic, and perceptual data. *American Journal of Speech-Language Pathology, 15*, 192-206.

McLeod, S. & Wrench, A. (2008). Protocol for restricting head movement when recording ultrasound images of speech, *Asia Pacific Journal of Speech, Language, and Hearing, 11*(1), 23-29.

McNeill, A. M. (2001). *The effect of electropalatography (EPG) therapy on persistent velar fronting in a 10 year old with Down's syndrome.* Unpublished BSc Hons Speech Pathology and Therapy dissertation, Queen Margaret University College, Edinburgh.

Mitchell, A. G. (1946). *The pronunciation of English in Australia.* Sydney, Australia: Angus & Robertson.

Moen, I., & Simonsen, H. G. (2007). The combined use of EPG and EMA in articulatory descriptions. *Advances in Speech-Language Pathology, 9*(1), 120-127.

Murdoch, B. E., Goozee, J. V., Veidt, M., Scott, D. H., & Meyers, I. A. (2004). Introducing the pressure-sensing palatograph—the next frontier in electropalatography. *Clinical Linguistics and Phonetics, 18,* 433–445.

Nicolaidis, K. (2004). Articulatory variability during consonant production by Greek speakers with hearing impairment: An electropalatographic study. *Clinical Linguistics and Phonetics, 18*(6-8), 419–432.

O'Halpin, R. (2001). Intonation issues in the speech of hearing impaired children: Analysis, transcription and remediation. *Clinical Linguistics and Phonetics, 15*(7), 529–550.

Onslow, M., Stocker, S., Packman, A., McLeod, S. (2002). Speech segment timing in children after the Lidcombe Program of early stuttering intervention. *Clinical Linguistics and Phonetics, 16,* 21–33.

Oxley, J., Buckingham, H., Roussel, N., & Daniloff, R. (2006). Metrical/syllabic factors in English allophony: Dark /l/. *Clinical Linguistics and Phonetics, 20*(2-3), 109–117.

Pantelemidou, V., Herman, R., & Thomas, J. (2003). Efficacy of speech intervention using electropalatography with cochlear implant. *Clinical Linguistics and Phonetics, 17*(4-5), 383–392.

Penner, H., Miller, N., Hertich, I., Ackermann, H., & Schumm, F. (2001). Dysprosody in Parkinson's disease: An investigation of intonation patterns. *Clinical Linguistics and Phonetics, 15*(7), 551–566.

Rahilly, J. (2007). Irish English speech acquisition. In S. McLeod (Ed.), *The international guide to speech acquisition* (pp. 204–220). Clifton Park, NY: Thomson Delmar Learning.

Recasens, D. (2004). Darkness in [l] as a scalar phonetic property: Implications for phonology and articulatory control. *Clinical Linguistics and Phonetics, 18*(6-8), 593–603.

Robb, M. P., Maclagan, M. A., & Chen, Y. (2004). Speaking rates of American and New Zealand varieties of English. *Clinical Linguistics and Phonetics, 18,* 1–15.

Roberts, A., McLeod, S., & Sita, J. (2002). Describing normal and impaired /s/ and /z/ using the EPG. *ACQuiring Knowledge in Speech, Language and Hearing, 4*(3), 158–163.

Ryalls, J., Cliche, A., Fortier-Blanc, J., Coulombe, I., & Prud'Hommeaux, A. (1997). Voice onset time in younger and older French-speaking Canadians. *Clinical Linguistics and Phonetics, 11,* 205–212.

Samuelsson, C., & Lofqvist, A. (2006). The role of Swedish tonal word accents in children with language impairment. *Clinical Linguistics and Phonetics, 20*(4), 231–248.

Schmidt, A. M. (2007). Evaluating a new clinical palatometry system. *Advances in Speech-Language Pathology, 9*(1), 73–81.

Scobbie, J. M. Mennen, O. & Matthews, B. (2007). Scottish English speech acquisition. In S. McLeod, (Ed.), *The international guide to speech acquisition* (pp. 221–240). Clifton Park, NY: Thomson Delmar Learning.

Scobbie, J. M., Wood, S. E., & Wrench, A. A. (2004). Advances in EPG for treatment and research: An illustrative case study. *Clinical Linguistics and Phonetics, 18,* 373–389.

Searl, J. (2003). Comparison of transducers and intraoral placement options for measuring lingua-palatal contact pressure during speech. *Journal of Speech, Language, and Hearing Research, 46,* 1444–1456.

Shannon, J. (2001). *Stability of articulatory patterns for /t/, /s/ and /b/ targets in cleft palate speech.* Unpublished Honours Project, Queen Margaret University College, Edinburgh.

Shriberg, L. D., & Kent, R. D. (2003). *Clinical phonetics* (3rd ed.). Boston: Allyn & Bacon.

Simonsen, H. G., & Moen, I. (2004). On the distinction between Norwegian /ʃ/ and /ç/ from a phonetic perspective. *Clinical Linguistics and Phonetics, 18*(6), 605–620.

Smit, A. B. (2004). *Articulation and phonology: Resource guide for school-age children and adults.* Clifton Park, NY: Thomson Delmar Learning.

Snow, D. (2001). Imitation of intonation contours by children with normal and disordered language development. *Clinical Linguistics and Phonetics, 15*(7), 567–584.

Stokes, S. F., & Zhen, F. (1998). An electropalatographic description of Putonghua fricatives and affricatives. *Asia Pacific Journal of Language and Hearing, 3,* 69–78.

Stone, M. (2005). A guide to analyzing tongue motion from ultrasound images. *Clinical Linguistics and Phonetics, 19,* 455–501.

Stone, M., Faber, A., Raphael, L., & Shawker, T. (1992). Cross-sectional tongue shape and linguopalatal contact patterns in [s], [ʃ], and [l]. *Journal of Phonetics, 20,* 253–270.

Stone, M., & Lundberg, A. (1996). Three-dimensional tongue surface shapes of English consonants and vowels. *Journal of the Acoustical Society of America, 99,* 3728–3737.

Tabain, M. (2001). Variability in fricative production and spectra: Implications for the hyper- and hypo- and quantal theories of speech production. *Language and Speech, 44,* 57–94.

Umeda, N. (1977). Consonant duration in American English. *Journal of the Acoustical Society of America, 61,* 846–858.

van Doorn, J., & Sheard, C. (2001). Fundamental frequency patterns in cerebral palsied speech. *Clinical Linguistics and Phonetics, 15*(7), 585–601.

Vazquez Alvarez, Y., Hewlett, N. & Zharkova, N. (2004, March). *An ultrasound study of the "trough effect."* Poster at the British Association of Academic Phoneticians Colloquium 2004 (BAAP), University of Cambridge, UK.

Wang, Y., Kent, R. D., Duffy, J. R., Thomas, J. E., & Weismer, G. (2004). Alternating motion rate as an index of speech motor disorder in traumatic brain injury. *Clinical Linguistics and Phonetics, 18*(1), 57–84.

Weismer, G. (1980). Control of the voicing distinction for intervocalic stops and fricatives: Some data and theoretical considerations. *Journal of Phonetics, 8,* 427–438.

Wells, J. C. (1982). *Accents of English.* Cambridge: Cambridge University Press.

Wrench, A. A. (2002). Articulate Assistant, Version 1.6 [Computer Software]. Edinburgh: Articulate Instruments.

Wrench, A. A. (2007). Advances in EPG palate design. *Advances in Speech-Language Pathology, 9*(1), 3–12.

Xue, S. A., Hao, G. J. P., & Mayo, R. (2006). Volumetric measurements of vocal tracts for male speakers from different races. *Clinical Linguistics and Phonetics, 20*(9), 691–702.

Index